Advance Praise for *Living a Healthy Life with HIV*

"This is an essential guide that will allow long and healthy survival despite HIV— something we only imagined when this epidemic began. Highly recommended!"

> —Paul Volberding, MD
> University of California, San Francisco Department of Medicine,
> Director of the UCSF AIDS Research Institute

"An excellent resource for patients as they navigate living with HIV."

> —Jason E. Farley, PhD, MPH, NP, FAAN
> Johns Hopkins University School of Nursing

"The perspective of self-empowerment provided by this book will be helpful for people living with HIV."

> —Kenneth Mayer MD,
> Infectious Disease Attending and Director of HIV
> Prevention Research, Beth Israel Deaconess Medical Center,
> Professor of Medicine, Harvard Medical School

"Everyone working in the HIV community—advocates, counselors, community-based organizations, and church outreach ministries—we all need this book as a reference for our work with men, women, and children living with this virus. We need to make it available to our HIV people—not just for saving lives, but for improving the quality of life with dignity for all those impacted by the HIV virus."

> —Father Joseph I. O'Brien, O.P.
> Executive Director, Saint Therese Center HIV Outreach,
> Las Vegas, Nevada

"A cross between a self-help motivational discourse and an easy-to-follow health manual, this book offers invaluable advice . . ."

> —Publishers Weekly

"The focus is not on what is wrong, but on how to keep things as right as possible . . ."

—Library Journal

"When I was first diagnosed with AIDS, I thought all that was left for me to do was go home and die. In discovering the book Living a Healthy Life with HIV *through a class offered by Stanford University, I discovered there is LIFE to be enjoyed and shared, and that taking care of myself is key . . . I plan to share the book with my mother and other members of my family as well!"*

—David, HIV positive since 2005

"This book gives information on how to succeed with the changes you may want to make in your life by using an action plan. It also helps you problem-solve. Living a Healthy Life With HIV *is helping me be a better self."*

—Robert, AIDS for over twenty years

"This book has taught me that, these days, having HIV is similar to having any other chronic condition, and with the right combination of medications and self-management tools, one can lead a healthy and fulfilling life. For me personally, this book 'normalizes' living with HIV, and it has helped me stop worrying about the stigma associated with living with HIV and to get on with my life.

By following the advice in the book, I have increased energy levels, I am getting a better night's sleep, and feel in control living with HIV. Living a Healthy Life with HIV *has improved my confidence and self-esteem and I now have a better relationship with my doctor, putting me in greater control of my health."*

—Richard, recently diagnosed as HIV positive

FOURTH EDITION

Living a Healthy Life with HIV

Allison R. Webel, RN, PhD • **Kate Lorig**, DrPH
Diana Laurent, MPH • **Virginia González**, MPH
Allen L. Gifford, MD • **David Sobel**, MD, MPH
Marian Minor, PT, PhD

Bull Publishing Company
Boulder, Colorado
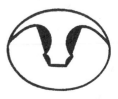

Published by Bull Publishing Company
P.O. Box 1377
Boulder, CO, USA 80306
www.bullpub.com

Library of Congress Cataloging-in-Publication Data

Names: Webel, Allison R., author.
Title: Living a healthy life with HIV / Allison R. Webel, RN, PhD [and six others].
Other titles: Living well with HIV and AIDS
Description: Fourth edition. | Boulder, Colorado : Bull Publishing Company, [2016] | Revison of:
    Living well with HIV and AIDS / Allen L. Gifford . . . [et al.]. c2005. 3rd ed.
Identifiers: LCCN 2015039959 | ISBN 9781936693726 (paperback)
Subjects: LCSH: AIDS (Disease)—Popular works. | HIV (Viruses)—Popular works. | BISAC: HEALTH
    & FITNESS / Diseases / AIDS & HIV.
Classification: LCC RC606.64 .L58 2016 | DDC 616.97/92—dc23
LC record available at http://lccn.loc.gov/2015039959

Summary: "This book combines the latest medical advice, ideas from people living with HIV, and
proven practices for self-management based on research conducted at Stanford University School of
Medicine. It includes current care guidelines from the Centers for Disease Control and Prevention.
The easy content will help patients, friends, family, and others who support anyone with HIV. Includes
tips, ideas, and resources about how to become an HIV self-manager.—Provided by publisher.

Printed in U.S.A.

21 20 19 18 17 16   10 9 8 7 6 5 4 3 2 1

Interior design and project management: Dovetail Publishing Services
Cover design and production: Shannon Bodie, BookWise Design
Manuscript editors: Erin Mulligan and Jon Ford

To Chris Adams and Vivian Vestal

Acknowledgments

This book was produced with the help of many people. None, however, deserve greater appreciation or more acknowledgment than the many people with HIV, and their friends, families, and loved ones, who have brought their own life experiences to bear, and have made suggestions about things to include in this book, and ways to improve it. Doctors, nurses, health educators, and other health professionals who have devoted themselves to improving the lives of people with HIV have all contributed many of the ideas included here.

Other important individuals deserve special mention. Chris Adams helped conceive and plan our original project, and his intelligence, wit, irreverence, and bravery in facing his own illness inspired us all. Vivian Vestal was for many years our very dear friend and the very best and most dedicated of our peer leaders in the Positive Self-Management Program for HIV.

We'd like to thank the professionals who have assisted us with this edition of the book: John Brion, Bonnie Bruce, Joe DiMilia, Sahera Dirajlal-Fargo, James Miller, Yvonne Mullan, and

Blair Voyvodic. We'd like also to thank Rayden Marcum, who broadened our knowledge and understanding of sexual identity issues.

Finally, many thanks to Jim Bull, Claire Cameron, and the team at Bull Publishing. Bull Publishing has been a strong supporter of health-related books for more than 40 years. Jim's support and encouragement have been essential to the development of this book. We couldn't have done it without you!

If you would like to learn more about our continuing research, online programs, trainings, and materials, please visit our website:

http://patienteducation.stanford.edu

We are continually revising and improving this book. If you have any suggestions or comments, please send them to

self-management@stanford.edu.

Contents

Disclaimer

This book is not intended to replace common sense, professional medical or psychological advice. You should seek and get appropriate professional evaluation and treatment for problems—especially unusual, unexplained, severe, or persistent symptoms. Many symptoms and diseases require and benefit from specific medical or psychological evaluation and treatment. Don't deny yourself proper professional care.

- If your symptoms or problems persist beyond a reasonable period despite using self-care recommendations, you should consult a health professional. What is a reasonable period will vary; if you're not sure and you're feeling anxious, consult a health care professional.

- If you receive professional advice in conflict with this book, you should rely upon the guidance provided by your health care professional. He or she is likely to be able to take your specific situation, history and needs into consideration.

- If you are having thoughts of harming yourself in any way, please seek professional care immediately.

This book is as accurate as its publisher and authors can make it, but we cannot guarantee that it will work for you in every case. The authors and publisher disclaim any and all liability for any claims or injuries that you may believe arose from following the recommendations set forth in this book. This book is only a guide; your common sense, good judgment, and partnership with health professionals are also needed.

CHAPTER 1

Overview of HIV and Self-Management

NOBODY WANTS TO HAVE HIV, but just because you have HIV doesn't mean life is over. Far from it! We wrote this book to help people with HIV explore healthy ways to live the life they want.

This may seem like a strange concept. How can you have an illness like HIV and still live a healthy life? To answer this, we need to look at what happens with most chronic (long-term) health problems. These diseases—whether HIV, heart disease, diabetes, depression, bipolar disorder, emphysema, or any one of a host of others— cause most people to experience symptoms such as fatigue and often to lose physical strength and endurance. They may cause emotional distress, such as frustration, anger, fear, or a sense of helplessness. Health is soundness of body and mind, and a healthy life is one that seeks that soundness. Therefore, a healthy way to live with a chronic health problem is to overcome the physical, mental, and emotional problems caused by the condition.

Can people with HIV live healthy lives? Of course. HIV is a chronic disease like many others. For people with HIV, there are more treatments available now than ever before. The challenge is to learn how to function at your best regardless of the

1

difficulties life presents. The goal is to achieve the things you want to do and to get pleasure from life. That is what this book is all about.

Remember, times have changed. When we wrote the first edition of this book in the early 1990s, the dream of HIV being considered another chronic illness was just that—a dream. Today it is a reality. Most people in treatment for HIV can and do live full, active lives for many, many years. With proper diagnosis and treatment, HIV has become a chronic condition similar to diabetes or heart disease. This is a big step forward.

Although we all celebrate this advance, it has brought with it many new questions. How do I balance my medication and my quality of life? I look and feel healthy—so who should I tell that I have HIV? This book will help you answer these and many other questions.

Before we go any further, let's talk about how to use this book. Throughout this book, you will find information to help you learn and practice self-management skills—that is, being proactive about living with your condition. This is not a textbook; rather, you might think of it as a reference book. You do not need to read every word in every chapter. Instead, read the first two chapters and then use the table of contents to find the specific information you need. You may want to start with some background information

about HIV and its symptoms and treatments. Or you may want to start by learning about exercise, healthy eating, and stress reduction. Anyone with HIV may find it useful to know how to figure out whether a new symptom is a common "bug" or an urgent condition that needs to be checked out by the medical team. Feel free to skip around and to take notes right in the book. This will help you learn the skills you need to live a healthy life with HIV.

You will not find any miracles or cures in these pages. Rather, you will find tips, ideas, and resources about how to become an HIV self-manager and live your life better. This advice comes from physicians, nurses, psychologists, other health professionals—and, most importantly, from people like you who have learned to positively manage living with their HIV.

In this chapter, we discuss HIV as a chronic illness, as well as pointing out some of the most common problems caused by this disease. You will soon see that the problems and self-management skills of those with HIV have a lot in common with other chronic illnesses—more than you might think. Therefore, learning skills for managing chronic illness allows you to successfully manage not only HIV but other health conditions—and even life—as well. We hope the book gives you the tools you need to become a great manager of your HIV and all other aspects of your life.

What Exactly Is a Chronic Health Condition?

Health problems can be characterized as either "acute" or "chronic." Acute health problems usually begin suddenly, have a single cause, are

often quickly diagnosed, last a short time, and get better with medication, medical treatment, rest, and time. Sometimes, as in the early days of

Table 1.1 **Differences Between Acute and Chronic Disease**

	Acute Disease	**Chronic Disease**
Example	*Pneumocystis* Pneumonia	HIV
Beginning	Usually rapid	Slow
Cause	Usually one, identifiable	Often uncertain, especially early on. HIV, however, does have a specific cause
Duration	Short	Usually for life
Diagnosis	Commonly accurate	Sometimes difficult
Tests	Give good answers	Often of limited value
Role of professional	Select and conduct treatment	Teacher and partner
Role of patient	Follow the treatment plan	Partner of health professionals, responsible for daily management

HIV, acute conditions can end in death. But most people with acute illnesses are cured and return to normal health. There is usually relatively little uncertainty for the patient or the doctor; both usually know what to expect. The illness typically follows a cycle of getting worse for a while, responding to careful treatment after observing the symptoms, and then getting better. Finally, the care of acute illness depends on the body's ability to heal itself and sometimes on a health professional's knowledge and experience in finding and administering the correct treatment.

Appendicitis is an example of an acute illness. It typically begins rapidly, signaled by nausea and pain in the abdomen. The diagnosis of appendicitis, once established by examination, leads to surgery for removal of the inflamed appendix. There follows a period of recovery and then a return to normal health.

Chronic illnesses are different (see Table 1.1). They usually begin slowly and proceed slowly. For example, a person may slowly develop blockage of the arteries over decades and then might have a heart attack or a stroke. Arthritis generally starts with brief annoying twinges that gradually increase. Unlike acute disease, most chronic illnesses usually have multiple causes that vary over time. These causes may include heredity, lifestyle (smoking, lack of exercise or sleep, poor diet, stress, and so on), and exposure to environmental factors such as secondhand smoke or air pollution and to physiological factors such as low levels of thyroid hormone or changes in brain chemistry that may cause depression.

Although HIV is a chronic condition, it has characteristics of both acute and chronic illness. Its beginning is slow and it usually lasts for life. We do know the specific cause, the HIV virus, which can be identified by specific blood tests. Therefore, diagnosis of HIV is usually relatively clear, and tests, especially for HIV viral load, can be very helpful in selecting and maintaining medications. (We will talk more about viral load tests in Chapter 7, "Making Treatment Decisions.") The roles of the patient and the health care provider are similar to the roles for any other chronic condition.

HIV in many ways is quite similar to other chronic diseases, such as heart disease, stroke, and diabetes. Like them, HIV is sometimes interrupted by acute flares or episodes of worsening symptoms. For example, a person with HIV may experience such daily symptoms as fatigue, and then have a brief, acute episode of pneumonia that needs to be diagnosed and treated. Knowing the difference between the acute and chronic conditions associated with HIV is quite important, because the acute conditions can sometimes be infections (referred to as "opportunistic" infections) that need special treatment. Today, with increased use of medications to treat HIV, it is also important to know the difference between drug side effects and HIV symptoms.

The many causes and unknown factors of chronic conditions can be frustrating for those of us who want quick answers. It is difficult for both the doctor and the patient when clear answers aren't available. In some cases, even when diagnosis is rapid, as in the case of a stroke, heart attack, or HIV, the long-term effects may be hard to predict. The lack of a regular or predictable pattern is a major characteristic of HIV and most other chronic illnesses.

Unlike acute disease, where full recovery is expected, chronic illness often leads to more symptoms and loss of physical or mental functioning. With chronic illness, many people assume that the symptoms they are experiencing are due to the disease itself. Although the disease can certainly cause pain, shortness of breath, fatigue, and the like, it is often not the only cause. What's more, each of these symptoms can contribute to the other symptoms, and they can feed on each other. For example, depression causes fatigue, fatigue and pain can cause physical limitations, and physical limitations can lead to poor sleep, more fatigue, more pain, and more depression. The interactions of these symptoms make the condition worse. It becomes a vicious cycle that only gets worse unless we find a way to break the cycle (see Figure 1.1 on the next page). One of the challenges of living with HIV is dealing with this cycle.

Throughout this book, we examine ways of breaking the cycle and getting away from the problems of physical and emotional helplessness.

Another way in which chronic illness differs from acute illness is that chronic illnesses such as heart disease, diabetes, and HIV often have to be treated with medications that need to be taken every day, for life. Using medications properly is a big part of living with HIV. We discuss medications at length in Chapter 8, "Managing Medications for HIV," and Chapter 9, "Side Effects of Medications."

Managing medications is just one part of self-management. Before discussing HIV in more detail, it is important to briefly discuss self-management.

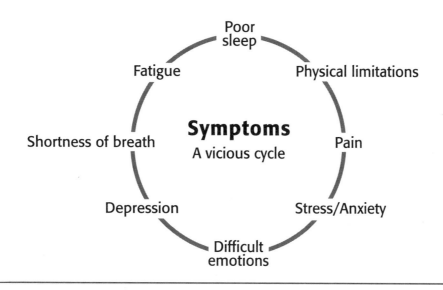

Figure 1.1 **The Vicious Cycle of Symptoms**

Same Disease, Different Response

James has HIV. He experiences fatigue most of the time and can't sleep. He took early retirement because of his HIV and now, at age 55, he spends his days sitting at home bored. He avoids most physical activity because of fatigue, weakness, and depression. He has become very irritable. Most people, including his family, don't enjoy his company. It even seems too much trouble when the grandchildren he adores come to visit.

Isabel, age 66, also has HIV. Every day she manages to walk several blocks to the local library or the park. When she feels fatigue or depression, she practices relaxation techniques and tries to distract herself. She works several hours a week as a volunteer at a local hospital. She also loves going to see her young grandchildren and even manages to take care of them for a while when her daughter has to run errands.

James and Isabel both live with the same condition and with similar physical problems. Yet their abilities to function and enjoy life are very different. Why? The difference lies largely in their attitudes toward HIV and their lives. James has allowed his physical capacities and enjoyment of life to wither. Isabel has learned to take an active role in managing her chronic illness. Even though she has limitations, *she* controls her life instead of letting the illness control it.

Attitude alone cannot cure chronic illness, but a positive attitude and certain self-management skills can make it much easier to live with. Much research now shows that the experience of fatigue, depression, and disability can be modified by circumstances, beliefs, mood, and the attention we pay to symptoms.

Two people with similar chronic conditions can sometimes be affected very differently. One may be able to minimize the effect of symptoms, while the other is extremely disabled. One may focus on healthy living, while the other is completely concentrated on the disease. In other words, one of the keys in shaping the impact of any disease is how effective and engaged the person is in self-management.

HIV and Self-Management

For a person with HIV, it may seem overwhelming to think about being responsible for its management. Unfortunately, there is no other way to self-manage a chronic condition.

So if you have HIV, what are your options? You can go home and do nothing. You can decide to not take medications recommended by your physician and instead use alternative treatments. You can decide to take a "vacation" from all HIV drugs and stop using them temporarily. Or you can choose to follow your doctor's treatment plan to the letter. These are all management decisions that only you can make.

In this book, we cannot tell you how to manage your HIV. This is up to you. What we *can* do is give you all the information we have, including all the tools that others have found helpful in managing their HIV. Using this knowledge, as well as the tools and advice you get from health professionals, family, and friends, you will make your own management decisions. There is no one best way—only the way that works best for you. Experience shows that active self-managers do better. The bottom line is that *you* want to run your disease, not let your disease run you.

We will talk more about self-management later in this chapter and at length in Chapter 2, "Becoming an HIV Self-Manager." Now let us examine exactly what HIV is and some of the conditions that can accompany it.

Understanding HIV

HIV is a disease of the immune system caused by the human immunodeficiency virus. People infected with HIV slowly develop damage to their immune system. This usually takes months or years. When the immune damage is minimal, a person with HIV doesn't notice anything and may be perfectly healthy. If the immune damage gets worse, the person may notice swollen lymph nodes or experience certain mild infections of the skin or mouth. If the immune damage becomes severe, people with HIV lose the ability to fight off serious infections and even cancers.

In the next pages, we discuss how HIV is (and isn't) caught from other people and what HIV does to the immune system. Some readers may find this information frightening, but it's essential to know the basics to be an effective self-manager. As you learn the medical details about HIV, it is important to not lose track of three vital facts:

- HIV is treatable. People in treatment who self-manage well can feel better now and live long, healthy lives, more so than they ever could in the past.

- Treatments for HIV are improving all the time. They're increasingly effective and easy to take. People on treatment today have many more therapy options than ever before.

- Each person with HIV has a unique experience. People can give you probabilities, but no one can say what will happen to you. For example, it's a mistake to assume you will experience side effects from anti-HIV medications just because you may know or have read about someone who did.

How Do People Catch HIV?

HIV is a virus that infects only humans. The only way HIV is transmitted is when the virus travels from inside an infected person to the bloodstream of another person. Many other viruses are different. Influenza virus (flu) concentrates in the lungs, so coughing spreads flu. Chicken pox concentrates in the skin, so touching an infected person can spread the disease. HIV is different. HIV concentrates in the blood, vaginal fluid, breast milk, and semen, and there aren't many ways to transfer these substances from one person to another.

Essentially, all the known cases of HIV infection have been transmitted in one of four ways:

- Having sex
- Injection with intravenous (IV) needles

- Transmission from a mother to her unborn child

- Transfusions of blood or blood products

Remember, you can pass on HIV to someone else in these ways even if you are infected but don't know it, even if you are taking HIV medication, and even if your HIV viral load is very low or even undetectable. (Again, you can read more about viral load tests in Chapter 7, "Making Treatment Decisions.")

Sexual Contact

There is always risk when an HIV-positive person has unprotected sex (sex without a condom) with someone who is HIV negative. The exact risk depends on what you do during sex. Unprotected anal sex is the most effective way to sexually transmit HIV. When a man with HIV puts his bare penis into another person's anus, the receiving person, whether a man or woman, is at very high risk of catching HIV. Unprotected vaginal sex is also risky. Because the virus is present in blood, vaginal fluids, and semen, it can get into the other person's blood through tiny cracks in the skin and soft tissues. Oral sex involves some risk of transmitting HIV, especially if sexual fluids enter the mouth and if there are sores in the mouth or bleeding gums. Pieces of latex or plastic wrap over the vagina, or condoms over the penis, can be used as barriers during oral sex.

There are three reasons why it is vital to practice safer sex:

- *To protect other people.* You would not want to expose someone else to a serious illness.

- *To protect yourself.* Even if you are already HIV positive, you could be infected with a new, possibly more dangerous strain of HIV, such as one that is resistant to anti-HIV drugs. You will stay healthier longer if you can avoid any new HIV infection. If you have HIV, because your immune system is compromised, you are also at increased risk of getting other diseases such as syphilis, gonorrhea, and hepatitis through unsafe sex. If you get one of these diseases, your body will be less able to resist the infection and heal itself.

■ *Because it is doable!* With the right knowledge and partner, sex can be safe, healthy, and enjoyable.

There are ways to limit the risks to yourself and others during sex. Be aware of your body and your partner's body. Cuts, sores, or bleeding gums increase the risk of spreading HIV. Even small injuries to the skin give HIV a way to enter the body. Use a barrier such as a condom to prevent contact with blood or sexual fluid. The most common artificial barrier is the latex condom for the penis. You can also use a female condom to protect the vagina or rectum during intercourse. Lubricants can reduce the chance that condoms or other barriers will break. Do not use oil-based lubricants such as Vaseline, oils, or creams, which can damage condoms and other latex barriers. Only use water-based lubricants.

Needles and Syringes

People who use a needle and syringe (the plastic plunger attached to the needle) to inject drugs always leave a small amount of blood inside the needle or syringe. If the needle or syringe of an HIV-positive person is reused by someone else without being properly sterilized, the first person's blood will then be injected into the next person, causing HIV infection to pass between them.

The best way to avoid HIV infection or transmission is never to use IV drugs to get high. But if you do inject drugs, *always* be sure to use a new syringe and needle, or clean the one you have with the following procedure:

1. Fill the syringe to the top with clean water, shake it, and squirt it out. Do this three times.

2. Repeat the procedure with 100 percent bleach, leaving the bleach in the syringe for at least 30 seconds each time you fill the syringe. Do this three times as well.

3. Finally, fill the syringe with clean water, shake, and squirt the water out. Again, do this three times.

Mother to Child

The placenta is the organ inside a pregnant woman that allows food and oxygen from the mother to go to the unborn baby. If an HIV-positive woman is pregnant, the HIV in her blood can sometimes cross from the placenta and enter her baby's blood while the fetus is still in the womb or during birth. If the mother and baby don't receive treatment, this kind of HIV transmission will happen in about one-third of babies born to HIV-positive women, and the baby will be born infected with HIV. *But*—and this is important—if women with HIV take medications while they are pregnant and the baby also gets medication at birth and afterward, this will block passage of HIV to the baby. So if you are pregnant and have HIV, it is vital to go to your doctor and get care as early as possible. Be sure to tell your doctor about your HIV status. If you are pregnant and not sure about your HIV status, get tested as soon as possible. Your baby's future health depends on you.

HIV can also pass from mother to baby in breast milk, although this kind of transmission is much less common. If safe alternatives to breast milk are available, most doctors recommend that women with HIV not breast-feed their babies. If baby formula and clean bottles are not available, breast milk may be the healthiest option for feeding your baby, even if you have HIV. We discuss this in more detail in Chapter 4, "HIV Through a Lifespan."

Blood Transfusion

Blood transfusions used to be one of the ways that people caught HIV. Before blood tests for HIV were developed in 1985, blood banks couldn't tell whether the blood they received contained the HIV virus. Now all blood is thoroughly screened for HIV (and other diseases), so the risk of getting HIV from a blood transfusion is extremely low, essentially zero.

Are There Other Possible Ways to Catch HIV?

Everyone agrees how unsafe it is to have unprotected sex or to share dirty injection needles, but we are not certain about some other activities, such as kissing deeply with exchange of saliva. Saliva contains extremely low amounts of HIV, so infection from saliva is unlikely. Also, saliva has natural properties that limit the power of HIV to infect. On the other hand, mouth sores, bleeding gums, and small injuries from bites are common and not always easy to detect. So deep kissing with your mouth open could in rare cases transmit HIV. Oral sex (using the mouth on someone else's penis, vagina, or anus) can also transmit HIV, though that too is rare. The U.S. Centers for Disease Control and Prevention website (www.cdc.gov/hiv/basics/transmission.html) has good information about what is and is not risky.

Catching HIV from an HIV-Positive Person

Definitely Risky	Less Risky	Not Risky
Unprotected anal sex	Mouth-to-genitals sex*	Shaking hands
Unprotected vaginal sex	Kissing with saliva exchange	Sharing bathroom/toilets
Sharing needles	Sharing razor or toothbrush	Touching doorknobs
	Mouth-to-anus sex	Casual social contact
		Contact with sweat
		Insect bites

*Although unprotected oral sex is not as risky as anal or vaginal sex, research shows that it can transmit HIV.

What Does HIV Infection Do?

Without treatment, the immune system of a person with HIV deteriorates slowly. The various components of the immune system are vital to staying healthy. White blood cells fight infection and defend us against certain types of cancer. Messenger chemicals signal parts of the system to turn on and off, depending on what invader is causing problems. Natural human toxins ("killer" chemicals) destroy invading organisms. Finally, special proteins "tag" invaders, making it easier for other immune cells to do their work.

All these parts of the immune system are important, but HIV attacks only one part—a type of white blood cell known as the T cell (also called the T helper, T4, or CD4 cell). People with HIV have problems with specific types of infections and cancers that are controlled by normal T cell function. You can read more about monitoring T cells in Chapter 7, "Making Treatment Decisions."

HIV can also infect brain and nerve cells, cells inside the bones (the bone marrow), and cells in the lining of the intestines. Because of the effect on brain cells, some people with untreated HIV may develop confusion and memory problems. Because blood cells are made in the bone marrow, the presence of HIV in the marrow can lead to decreased blood count (anemia). HIV in the intestines can cause chronic problems with diarrhea.

Even without treatment, it usually takes years for HIV to start causing symptoms. Now that we have stronger and better HIV medications, people who are tested early and take the prescribed medications can do well for longer periods than in the past—even for decades.

HIV infection can be divided into four stages:

1. Primary HIV infection, also called acute HIV
2. Healthy HIV carrier state
3. Early symptomatic HIV infection
4. AIDS (acquired immunodeficiency syndrome)

Primary HIV infection occurs within two to four weeks after a person first becomes infected. Not everyone develops symptoms from primary HIV infection, but some people may experience fever, rash, sore throat, aching muscles, cough, swollen lymph nodes, diarrhea, nausea, and vomiting. In other words, it can be like a bad flu infection. Primary HIV infection usually lasts only a few weeks, but it still is a good time to see a doctor and start early anti-HIV therapy if HIV is detected. Unfortunately, most people don't display symptoms, or they don't realize that their symptoms are from primary HIV.

After primary infection, a person with HIV goes into what's called a carrier state, when they do not display symptoms. During this phase, which may last for years, many people do not know that they have HIV, and they feel fine. Unfortunately, they can still transmit HIV to others.

People who develop symptomatic HIV infection start to experience fatigue, fevers, skin and mouth infections, and abnormal blood tests. These early symptoms of HIV infection are signs that the immune system is weakened.

If HIV infection remains untreated, the immune system becomes so weak that the person can develop very serious infections and cancers. This stage is AIDS (acquired immunodeficiency syndrome), the most advanced of the four stages. When HIV infection becomes AIDS, the disease is serious and can cause many symptoms. The line between symptomatic HIV and "full-blown" AIDS is not sharp; it is really a matter of degree of damage to the immune system. Doctors use certain blood test measurements and refer to the presence of other infections in an HIV-positive person to define what they mean by "AIDS." Once a person has AIDS, there has been a lot of damage to their T cells and immune system. If they get a serious infection such as *Pneumocystis* pneumonia, they are really sick.

But people who have AIDS can still rebuild their immune system, return to health, and often become asymptomatic again. That is the goal of HIV medications. But it depends on getting the right treatment and practicing good self-management.

Health Problems and HIV

Infections and cancers are the most common HIV-related severe health problems. These occur when the immune system is weak. Because of better medications, rates of HIV-related infections and cancers are dropping. We can usually prevent nearly all of these illnesses by using anti-HIV medications to boost the immune system. The most common HIV-related illnesses are discussed in Chapter 3, "Health Problems of People with HIV."

The medications prescribed for HIV are multidrug combinations, known as highly active antiretroviral therapy (HAART), or just

antiretrovirals (ART). ART always combines at least three or more anti-HIV drugs that are taken together. The good news is that these medications are usually combined, so there are fewer pills to take.

Even though the medications can be lifesavers, they can cause side effects. Therefore, treatment for HIV also includes managing drug side effects. Such side effects may include high cholesterol levels, muscle pains, high blood sugar, and increases in body fat. Because of drug side effects, and because people are living longer with HIV, they also may suffer from chronic heart disease, kidney disease, high blood pressure, and liver problems, just as other people do as they get older. These problems are usually not caused directly by HIV or the use of HIV medications. They are more often the result of aging, genetics, and lifestyle choices such as smoking, excessive drinking, and drug use. However, they do occur more frequently in people living with HIV. So when we talk about health problems with HIV, we really need to think about a lot of different things. Living a full, long life with HIV is great, but as we explained above, living a long life means that you may have to manage HIV-related conditions and other chronic diseases.

HIV as a Chronic Disease

Uncontrolled, HIV can be similar to other chronic diseases. Damage to the immune system may cause problems with the lungs, for example, so the body does not get enough oxygen. HIV can lead to loss of function in other ways. Nerve cell damage caused by HIV can result in numbness or discomfort in the feet and hands. Problems in the intestines may decrease the absorption of fluids and important nutrients. Bones can become thinner and break more easily. Furthermore, the work that the body has to do to fight HIV can lead to energy loss and fatigue. These things do not always happen—far from it. However, if any one of them does happen, it can lead to pain and disability.

We do not always know that a chronic disease is present until the symptoms start (shortness of breath, fatigue, pain, and so on). Illness is more than cellular malfunction; it also includes problems with everyday life, such as not being able to do the things you want to do, or needing to change your social activities, or needing to adapt life around medications or tests.

Although the biological causes of chronic diseases differ, the problems they create are similar. For example, most people with chronic disease suffer fatigue and loss of energy. Sleeping problems are common. Some people may have pain, whereas others may have trouble breathing. Disability, to some extent, is usually part of chronic disease.

Another common problem with HIV and other chronic illnesses is depression, or just "feeling blue." It is hard to be cheerful when your condition causes serious health problems and limitations. Along with the depression come anger, fear, and concern for the future. Will I be able to remain independent? If I can't care for myself, who will care for me? What will happen to my family? Will I get worse? What will happen as I age? Will I be alone? Disability and depression bring loss of self-esteem.

This all may seem overwhelming, but we are here to help. In this book, we talk about learning to manage HIV by applying the principles that have been used to successfully manage other chronic illnesses. Before we discuss specific management techniques, however, it is necessary to explain what we mean by self-management.

Understanding Your Chronic Illness Path

The first task of any manager is to understand what is being managed. Initially, this may seem like an impossible job. After all, HIV is a complicated and challenging disease that sometimes stumps the best of specialists. But understanding HIV is not as difficult as it might seem. Many people find that as a result of daily living with HIV, they and their families become familiar with the way HIV affects them and what their treatment does for them. You will know better than anyone what problems you encounter with medications and side effects. With experience, you may become better able than health professionals to judge the course of your disease and the effects of your treatments.

In other words, *you* can become the expert in the day-to-day changes in your health. Most chronic illnesses go up and down in intensity; they do not have a steady course. Therefore, being able to identify the ups and downs is essential for good management. Recognizing these patterns can be important in making decisions about medications for pain, breathing problems, nausea, or other symptoms.

Your experience and understanding of the natural rhythms of your chronic illness is often a more useful indicator to your doctor than laboratory tests or other measures. If the doctor encourages you to observe and to learn, and you respond by participating in decisions, a partnership is born. To be most effective, self-management of HIV requires such a partnership. In general, symptoms should be checked out with your doctor if they are unusual, severe, or persistent or if they occur after starting a new medication or treatment plan. Some other important guidelines about when to be concerned about symptoms are provided in Chapter 10, "Evaluating Common Symptoms of HIV."

Throughout this book, we give specific examples of what actions to take if you experience certain symptoms. But this is where your partnership with your health care team becomes critical. Self-management does not mean going it alone. Get help or advice when you are concerned or uncertain.

Both at home and in the business world, managers direct the show. But they don't do everything themselves; they work with others, including consultants, to get the job done. What makes them managers is that they are responsible for making decisions and making sure that their decisions are carried out.

As the manager of your illness, your job is much the same. You gather information and hire a consultant or team of consultants consisting of your physician and other health professionals. Once they have given you their best advice, it is up to you to follow through. All chronic illnesses need day-to-day management. We have all noticed that some people with severe physical problems get on well while others with lesser problems seem to give up on life. The difference often lies in their management style.

Managing a chronic illness, like managing a family or a business, is a complex undertaking. There are many twists, turns, and midcourse corrections. By learning self-management skills, you can ease the problems of living with your condition.

The key to success in any undertaking is, first, deciding what you want to do; second, deciding how you are going to do it; and, finally, learning a set of skills and practicing them until they have been mastered. Success in chronic disease self-management is the same. In fact, mastering such skills is one of the most important tasks of life.

Self-Management Skills

Besides overcoming the physical and emotional problems associated with a chronic condition such as HIV, it is important to learn problem-solving skills and ways to respond to the trends in your disease. These tasks and skills include using medications appropriately and minimizing their side effects, developing and maintaining health with appropriate exercise and nutrition, managing symptoms, making decisions about when to seek medical help, working effectively with your doctor, finding and using community resources, talking about your illness with family and friends, and changing social interactions, if necessary. The most important skill of all is learning to respond to your illness on an ongoing basis to solve day-to-day problems as they arise.

Self-Management Skills

- Problem solving and responding as your disease gets better and worse
- Maintaining a healthy lifestyle with regular exercise, healthy eating, sound sleep habits, and stress management
- Managing common symptoms
- Making decisions about when to seek medical help and what treatments to try

- Working effectively with your health care team
- Using medications safely and effectively while minimizing side effects
- Finding and using community resources
- Talking about your illness with family and friends
- Adapting social activities

What you do about something is largely determined by how you think about it. For example, if you think that having HIV is like running in the dark toward a cliff, not knowing when you will fall over the edge, you might feel no control over what happens and therefore do nothing at all to help yourself. The thoughts you have can greatly determine what happens to you and how you handle your health problems.

Some of the most successful self-managers are people who think of their illness as a path. This path, like any path, changes as you travel along it. Sometimes it is flat and smooth. At other times the way is rough. To negotiate this path one has to use many strategies. Sometimes you can go fast; other times you must slow down. There are obstacles to negotiate.

Good self-managers are people who have learned three types of skills to negotiate this path:

- **Skills needed to deal with the illness.** Any illness requires that you do new things. These may include sticking to complicated medications schedules or dealing with side effects. You may need frequent interactions

with your doctor and the health care system. Sometimes there are new exercises or a new diet. All of these constitute the work you must do just to manage your illness.

- **Skills needed to continue your normal life.** Just because you have HIV does not mean that life stops. There are still chores to do, friendships to maintain, jobs to perform, and family relationships to continue. Things that you once took for granted can become much more complicated in the face of HIV. You may need to learn new skills or adapt the way you do things in order to maintain the things you need and want to do.

- **Skills needed to deal with emotions.** When you are diagnosed with HIV, your future changes, and with this come changes in plans and emotions. Many of the new emotions are negative. They may include anger ("Why me? It's not fair"), fear ("I am afraid of becoming dependent on others"), depression ("I can't be normal anymore, so what's the use?"), frustration ("No matter what I do, it doesn't make any difference. I can't do what I want to do"), or isolation ("No one understands; no one wants to be around someone who is infected"). Negotiating the path of HIV, then, also means learning skills to work with these difficult emotions. We will teach you some of these skills.

With this as background, you can think of self-management as the use of skills to manage the work of living with your illness, continuing your daily activities, and dealing with emotions brought about by chronic illness.

Final Points to Ponder

- **You do not deserve to be sick.** All chronic diseases, including HIV, involve a combination of genetic, biological, environmental, and psychological factors. For example, stress alone does not cause most chronic illnesses. And if you fail to recover, it is not because of lack of the right mental attitude. Mind matters, but mind cannot always triumph over matter. On the other hand, there are many things you *can* control that will help you cope with chronic illness. Remember, you do not deserve to have HIV, but you are responsible for taking action to manage your illness.

- **Don't do it alone.** One of the side effects of chronic illness is a feeling of isolation. This is often a big issue with HIV. As supportive as friends and family members may be, they often cannot understand what you are experiencing. However, there are thousands of others who know firsthand what it is like to live with HIV. Connecting with these people can reduce your sense of isolation, help you understand what to expect, offer practical tips on how to manage symptoms and feelings on a day-to-day basis, give you the opportunity to help others cope with their illness, help you appreciate your strengths, and inspire you to take a more active role in managing your illness. Support can come from reading a book or newsletter about the experiences of others. Or it can come from talking with others on the telephone, in local community support groups, or even online through Internet support groups.

- **You're more than your disease.** When you have HIV, it can consume you. But you are more than your disease. And life is more than trips to the doctor and managing symptoms. It is essential to cultivate areas of your life that you enjoy. Small daily pleasures can help balance the times when you have to manage uncomfortable symptoms or emotions. Find ways to enjoy nature

Chris has HIV. Since his diagnosis, he lives more fully than ever: "I was lost and aimless—using drugs and being self-destructive. It seems strange, but honestly I feel as if HIV has improved my life. I got a wake-up call, and now I'm exercising and eating well. I'm clean and sober, and I take my medications and feel really healthy. I do things that feel important to me. Surprisingly, I feel less afraid of living."

by growing a plant or watching a sunset, indulge in the pleasure of human touch or a tasty meal, or celebrate companionship with family or friends. Finding ways to introduce moments of pleasure into your life is vital to chronic disease self-management. Focus on your abilities and strengths rather than disabilities and problems. Helping others is one way to increase your own sense of what you can do instead of focusing on what you can't. Celebrate small improvements. If chronic illness teaches anything, it is to live each moment more fully. Within the true limits of whatever disease you have, there are ways to enhance your function, sense of control, and enjoyment of life.

- **Illness can be an opportunity.** Illness, even with its pain and disability, can enrich our lives. It can make us reevaluate which things are really important, shift priorities, and move us in exciting new directions. It can give us an opportunity to explore.

In this book, we will describe many skills and tools to help relieve the problems caused by HIV. We do not expect you to use all of them. Pick and choose. Experiment. Set your own goals. *What you do is important, and so is the sense of confidence and control that comes from successfully doing something you want to do.*

Just knowing the skills, however, is not enough. We all need ways of incorporating these skills into our daily lives. Whenever we try a new skill, the first attempts may be clumsy, slow, and show few results. It is easier to return to old ways than to continue trying to master new and sometimes difficult tasks. The best way to master new skills is through taking small steps, practicing, and evaluating the results.

Additional Resources

AIDS.gov: www.AIDS.gov

The Body: The Complete HIV/AIDS Resource: www.thebody.com

Catie: Canada's Source for HIV and Hepatitis C Information: www.catie.ca/en/basics/hiv-and-aids

Centers for Disease Control and Prevention. www.cdc.gov/hiv

HIV Medicine Association Provider Directory: https://www.hivma.org/cvweb/cgi-bin/memberdll.dll/OpenPage?WRP=hivma_member_search.htm&wmt=none

HIV-Age: www.hiv-age.org

HIVPlus Magazine: www.hivplusmag.com

New York State Department of Health AIDS Institute: www.hivguidelines.org

NHS (National Health Service): www.nhs.uk/Conditions/HIV/Pages/Introduction.aspx

U.S. Department of Veterans Affairs: www.hiv.va.gov

Suggested Further Reading

To learn more about the topics discussed in this chapter, we suggest that you explore the following resources:

Cousins, Norman. *Anatomy of an Illness as Perceived by the Patient.* New York: Norton, 2005.

Gruman, Jessie. *AfterShock. What to Do When the Doctor Gives You—or Someone You Love—a Devastating Diagnosis.* New York: Walker, 2010. (See also Gruman's website, which offers a selection of further resources: www.aftershockbook.com.)

Selak, Joy H., and Steven M. Overman. *You Don't Look Sick: Living Well with Invisible Chronic Illness.* Binghamton, N.Y.: Haworth Medical Press, 2005.

Sobel, David, and Robert Ornstein. *The Healthy Mind, Healthy Body Handbook.* Los Altos, Calif.: DRx, 1996.

Sobel, David, and Robert Ornstein. *Healthy Pleasures,* 2nd ed. Reading, Mass.: Addison-Wesley, 1997.

Sobel, David, and Robert Ornstein. *Mind and Body Health Handbook: How to Use Your Mind and Body to Relieve Stress, Overcome Illness, and Enjoy Healthy Pleasures,* 2nd ed. Los Altos, Calif.: DRx, 1998.

Weil, Andrew. *Healthy Aging: A Lifelong Guide to Your Physical and Spiritual Well-Being.* New York: Knopf, 2005.

CHAPTER 2

Becoming an HIV Self-Manager

IT IS IMPOSSIBLE TO HAVE A CHRONIC CONDITION like HIV without being a self-manager. Some people manage by withdrawing from life. They stay in bed or socialize less. The disease becomes the center of their existence. Other people with the same condition and symptoms somehow manage to get on with life. They may have to change some of the things they do or the way that things get done. Nevertheless, life continues to be full and active.

The difference between these two extremes is not the illness but rather how the person with a chronic condition decides to manage the illness. Please note the word *decides*. Self-management is always a decision: a decision to be active or a decision to do nothing, a decision to seek help or a decision to suffer in silence. This book will help you with these decisions.

Like any skill, active self-management must be learned and practiced. This chapter will start you on your way by presenting the three most important self-management tools: problem solving, decision making, and action planning. Remember: you are the manager. Like the manager of an organization or a household, you must do all of the following things:

1. Decide what you want to accomplish.

2. Look for various ways to accomplish this goal.

3. Draft a short-term action plan or agreement with yourself.

4. Carry out your action plan.

5. Check the results.

6. Make changes as needed.

7. Reward yourself for your success.

Problem Solving

Problems sometimes start with a general uneasiness. Let's say you are unhappy but not sure why. Upon closer examination, you find that you miss contact with some relatives who live far away. With the problem identified, you decide to take a trip to visit these relatives. You know what you want to accomplish, but now you need to make a list of ways to solve the problem.

In the past you have always driven, but you now find driving tiring, so you consider various ways to make it less burdensome. You consider leaving at noon instead of early in the morning and making the trip in two days instead of one. You consider asking a friend along to share the driving. There is also a train that stops within 20 miles of your destination, or you could fly. You decide to take the train.

The trip still seems overwhelming, as there is so much to do to prepare. You decide to write down all the steps necessary to make the trip a reality. These include finding a good time to go, buying a ticket, figuring out how to handle luggage, seeing if you can make it back and forth to the train station, researching if you can get food and have access to the bathroom aboard the train, and figuring out how you will take your medications while en route. Each of these steps can be an action plan (more about action plans to follow).

To start making your action plan, you promise yourself that this week you will call and find out just how much the railroad can help. You also decide to plan out how exactly you will carry your different medications, and how you will make them easily accessible when you're traveling. You then carry out your action plan by calling the railroad and looking for appropriate "travel" pill containers.

A week later you check the results. Looking back at all the steps to be accomplished, you see that a single call answered many questions. The railroad can help people who have mobility problems and has ways of dealing with many of your concerns. However, you are still worried about the medications. You know that when you're out of your routine, you sometimes are late with a dose. Even though you generally do well, you want to keep on a perfect schedule, even away from home. You make a change in your plan by asking your pharmacist about this, and they suggest programming a reminder into your mobile phone. Although you don't always like the sound, you realize that the reminder will give you the extra security you need with the change in routine.

You have just engaged in problem solving to achieve your goal to take a trip. Now let's review the specific steps in problem solving.

Steps in Problem Solving

1. **Identify the problem**. This is the first and most important step in problem solving—and usually the most difficult step as well. You may know, for example, that stairs are a problem, but it will take a little more effort to determine that the real problem is fear of falling.

2. **List ideas to solve the problem.** You may be able to come up with a good list yourself, but you may sometimes want to call on your "consultants." These can be friends, family, members of your health care team, or community resources. One note about using consultants: these folks cannot help you if you do not describe the problem well. For example, there is a big difference between saying that you can't walk because your feet hurt and saying that your feet hurt because you cannot find walking shoes that fit properly. The first is a vague complaint; the second is an identifiable problem that can be addressed.

3. **Select one method to try.** Start with the idea that you feel has the most promise to solve your problem. As you try it, remember that new activities are difficult sometimes. Be sure to give your potential solution a fair chance before deciding it won't work. For most things, two weeks is a good trial.

4. **Check the results** after you've given your idea a fair chance. If all goes well, your problem will be solved.

5. **Pick another idea.** If you still have the problem, pick another idea from your list and try again.

6. **Use other resources** (your consultants) for more ideas if you still do not have a solution.

7. **Accept that the problem might not be solvable right now.** Finally, if you have gone through all of the steps until all ideas have been exhausted and the problem is still unsolved, you may have to accept that your problem may not be solvable right now. This is sometimes hard to do. The fact that

Problem-Solving Steps

1. Identify the problem.
2. List ideas to solve the problem.
3. Select one method to try.
4. Check the results.
5. Pick another idea if the first didn't work.
6. Use other resources.
7. Accept that the problem may not be solvable right now.

a problem can't be solved right now doesn't mean that it won't be solvable later or that other problems cannot be solved. Even if your path is blocked, there are probably alternative paths. If you are going through difficult times, don't give up. Keep going.

Living with Uncertainty

Living with uncertainty is one of the hardest self-management tasks. It is something that most of us cannot avoid and can be the cause of emotional ups and downs. The diagnosis of HIV or any chronic condition takes away some of our sense of security and control. It can be frightening. We are following our life path, and suddenly we are forced to detour to a different, unwanted path. And even as we work with health professionals and start new treatments, this uncertainty continues. Of course, we all have an uncertain future, but most people do not think about this. When we have a chronic condition, however, this becomes an important part of our lives. We are uncertain about our future health, and perhaps about our ability to continue to do the things we want, need, and like to do. Many people find it very challenging to make decisions while accepting uncertainty. If you feel uncertain about your life with HIV, know that this is a normal reaction and it is something you can learn to address.

Making Decisions: Weighing the Pros and Cons

Decisions making is an important tool in our self-management toolbox. The following steps to help us make decisions are a little like problem solving:

1. **Identify the options.** Sometimes the options are to change something or to not change at all. For example, you may have to decide whether to get help in the house or continue to do all the work yourself.

2. **Identify what you want.** It may be important for you to continue your life as normally as possible, to have more time with your friends or family, or to not have to shovel the walkways, cut the grass, or clean the house. Sometimes identifying your deepest, most important values (like spending time with family or friends) helps set priorities and increases your motivation to change.

3. **Write down pros and cons for each option.** List as many items as you can for each side. Don't forget the emotional and social effects.

4. **Rate each item on the list** on a 5-point scale, with 0 indicating "not at all important" and 5 indicating "extremely important."

5. **Add up the ratings for each column** and compare them. The column with the higher total should give you your decision. If the totals are close or you are still not sure, go to the next step.

Figure 2.1 **Decision-Making Example**

Should I get help in the house?

Pro	Rating	Con	Rating
I'll have more time	4	It's expensive	3
I'll be less tired	4	It's hard to find good help	1
I'll have a clean house	3	They won't do things my way	2
		I don't want a stranger in the house	1
Total	11		7

6. **Apply the "gut test."** For example, your total may be slightly higher for going back to work part-time, but does it feel right? If so, you have probably reached a decision. If not, the way you feel should probably win out over the math.

Look at the total points for the each list. The decision in this example would be to get help because the pro score (11) is significantly higher than the con score (7). If this feels right in your gut, you have the answer.

Now it's your turn! Try making a decision using the following chart. It's okay to write in your book.

The key to successful problem solving and decision making is taking action. We will talk about this next.

Figure 2.2 **Decision to be Made**

Decision to be made:

Pro	Rating	Con	Rating
Total			

Taking Action

You have looked at a problem or made a decision, but simply knowing what to do is not enough. It is time to do something, to take action. We suggest that you start by doing one thing at a time.

Goal Setting

Before you can take action, you must first decide what you want to do. You must be realistic and specific when stating your goal. Think of all the things you would like to do. One self-manager, Patty, wanted to climb 20 steps to her parents' home so that she could join her family for a holiday meal. Another, Fernando, wanted to overcome anxiety about disclosing his HIV status and start to date again. And Ian wanted to continue to ride a motorcycle but could no longer handle his 1,000-pound bike like he used to.

One of the problems with goals is that they often seem like dreams. They are so far off, big, or difficult that we are overwhelmed and don't even try to accomplish them. We'll tackle this problem next. For now, take a few minutes and write your goals below (add more lines if you need to).

Goals

_____

_____

_____

_____

Put a star (★) next to the goal you would like to work on first.

There are many ways to reach any specific goal. For example, our self-manager who wanted to climb 20 steps to a family gathering could start off with a slow walking program, start to climb a few steps each day, or look into having the family gathering at a different place. The person who wanted to date could start by asking others about HIV disclosure and when and how it was best to do this. Our motorcycle rider could buy a lighter motorcycle, use a sidecar, put "training wheels" on the bike, buy a three-wheeled motorcycle, ride the motorcycle with a friend, or focus on a different goal.

As you can see, there are many options for reaching each goal. The job here is to list the options and then choose one or two to try out.

Sometimes it is hard to think of all the options yourself. If you are having problems, it is time to use a consultant. Share your goal with family, friends, and health professionals. Use the Internet to research options, or call community organizations such as the AIDS Foundation. (For tips on finding other resources, see Chapter 18 "Finding Resources.") Just don't ask the consultant what you *should* do; rather, ask for *suggestions* about what to do. It is a subtle but important distinction. It is always good to have a list of options, but in the end *you* must prioritize them and pursue the ones that you feel are the most promising.

A note of caution: many options are never seriously considered because you assume they don't exist or are unworkable. Never make this assumption until you have thoroughly investigated the option. One person we know, Virginia, had lived in the same town all her life and felt she knew all about the community resources. When she was having problems with her health insurance, a friend from another city suggested contacting an insurance counselor. However, Virginia dismissed this suggestion because she was certain that this service did not exist in her town. It was only when, months later, the friend came to visit and called the Area Agency on Aging (which exists in most counties in the United States) that Virginia learned that there were three insurance counseling services nearby. Then there's our motorcycle rider, Ian, who thought that putting training wheels on a Harley was a crazy idea, but he overcame his skepticism and investigated the possibility. They added 15 years to his riding life. In short,

never assume anything. Assumptions are major self-management enemies.

Write the list of options for your main goal here. Then put a star (★) next to the two or three options on which you would like to work.

Options

_____

_____

_____

_____

_____

Making Short-Term Plans: Action Planning

Once you have made a decision about a goal, you have a pretty good idea of where you are going. However, this goal may be overwhelming. *How will I ever move? How will I ever be able to paint again? How will I ever be able to _____?* (You fill in the blank.) The secret is to not try to do everything at once. Instead, look at what you can realistically expect to accomplish within *the next week*. We call this an action plan: something that is short-term, is doable, and sets you on the road toward your goal.

Action plans are probably your most important self-management tool. Let's go through all the steps for making a realistic one.

First, decide what you will do *this week*. For a step climber, this might be climbing three steps on four consecutive days. The person who wants to continue riding a motorcycle might spend half an hour on two days researching lighter motorcycles and motorcycle training wheels.

Make sure your plans are "action-specific"; that is, rather than just deciding "to lose weight" (which is not an action but the result of an action), you will "replace soda with tea."

Also make sure your action plan has a realistic chance for success. An action plan can help you do the things you know you should do, but it is best to start with what you *want* to do.

Next, make a specific plan. Deciding what you want to do is worthless without a plan to do it. The plan should answer all of the following questions:

- Exactly **what** are you going to do? Are you going to walk? How will you eat less? What distraction techniques will you practice?

- **How much** will you do? This question is answered with something like time, distance, portions, or repetitions. Will you practice relaxation exercises for 15 minutes, walk one block, eat half portions at lunch and dinner, or take two flights of stairs every afternoon?

■ *When* will you do this? Again, this must be specific: before lunch, in the shower, upon coming home from work. Connecting a new activity with an old habit is a good way to make sure it gets done. For example, brushing your teeth can serve as a reminder to take your medication. Another trick is to do your new activity before an old favorite activity, such as reading the paper or watching a favorite TV program.

■ **How often** will you do the activity? This is a bit tricky. We would all like to do things every day, but that is not always possible. It is usually best to decide to do an activity three or four times a week to give yourself "wiggle room" if something comes up. If you are able to do more, so much the better. However, if you are like most people, you will feel less pressure if you can do your activity three or four times a week and still feel successful. (Note that taking medications is an exception. This must be done exactly as directed by your doctor.)

Here are some tips to help you write a successful action plan:

1. **Choose wisely.** An action plan is a tool to help you do what *you* want to do or accomplish. Do not make action plans to please your friends, family, or doctor.

2. **Start slowly.** Begin where you are and very gradually improve. If you can walk for only one minute, start your walking program by walking one minute once every hour or two, not by trying to walk a block. If you have never done any exercise, start with a few minutes of warm-up. A total of five or ten minutes is enough. If you want to lose weight, set a goal based on your existing eating behaviors, such as switching to half portions, rather than trying a radical new diet.

3. **Be specific.** This is important, so it bears repeating. For example, "losing a pound this week" is not an action plan because it does not involve a specific action. "Not eating after dinner for four days this week," by contrast, would be a fine action plan.

4. **Give yourself some time off**. All people have days when they don't feel like doing anything. That is a good reason for saying that you will do something three times a week instead of every day. If you plan to do something every day, then the first time you miss a day, you are more likely to become frustrated and abandon the whole plan.

5. **Use the confidence test**. Once you've made your action plan, ask yourself the following question: "On a scale of 0 to 10, with 0 being totally unsure and 10 being totally certain, how sure am I that I can complete this entire plan?"

   If your answer is 7 or above, it is probably a realistic action plan. If your answer is below 7, you should look again at your action plan. Ask yourself why you are unsure. What problems do you foresee? Then see if you can either solve the problems or change your plan to make it easier and make yourself more confident of success.

6. **Write down your action plan.** Once you have made a plan you are happy with, write it down and post it where you will see it every

Basics of a Successful Action Plan

- It is something *you* want to do.

- It is achievable (something you can expect to be able to accomplish in a given week).

- It is action-specific.

- It answers the questions *What? How much? When?* and *How often?*

- On a scale from 0 (not at all sure) to 10 (absolutely sure), you are confident you will complete your entire plan at a level of 7 or higher.

day. Thinking through an action plan is one thing. Writing it down makes it more likely you will take action. Keep track of how you are doing and the problems you encounter. A blank action plan form is provided at the end of this chapter. (You may wish to make photocopies of it to use weekly.) See also the Resources section for an action-planning app for your smartphone or tablet.

As we age or develop a chronic illness, physical abilities and self-image may decline. For many people, it is discouraging to find that they can't do what they used to do or want to do. By changing and improving one area of your life, whether it is boosting your physical fitness or learning a new skill, you regain a sense of optimism and vitality. By focusing on what you can do rather than what you can't do, you're more likely to lead a more positive and happier life.

Carrying Out Your Action Plan

If the action plan is well written and realistically achievable, completing it is generally pretty easy. Ask family or friends to check with you on how you are doing. Having to report your progress is good motivation. Keep track of your daily activities while carrying out your plan. Many

Success Improves Health

The benefits of successful change go beyond the payoffs of adopting healthier habits. Obviously, you will feel better when you exercise, eat well, keep regular sleeping hours, stop smoking, and take time to relax. But regardless of the behavior that's altered, there's evidence that your health will improve just from the feelings of self-confidence and control over your life that come from making *any* successful change in your life. This is one important reason why you need an action plan that sets yourself up for success—no matter how small.

good managers have lists of what they want to accomplish. Check things off as they are completed. This will give you guidance on how realistic your planning was and will also be useful in making future plans. Make daily notes, even of the things you don't understand at the time. Later these notes may be useful in establishing a pattern to use for problem solving.

For example, Patty, our stair-climbing friend, never did the climbing. Each day there was a different problem: not enough time, being tired, the weather being too cold, and so on. When looking back at her notes, she began to realize that the real problem was fear of falling with no one around to help. She then decided to use a cane while climbing stairs and to do it when a friend or neighbor was around.

Checking the Results

At the end of each week, check on how well you have fulfilled your action plan and if you are any nearer to accomplishing your goal. Are you able to walk farther? Have you lost weight? Are you less anxious? Taking stock is important. You may not see progress day by day, but you should see a little progress each week. If you find you are still having problems after each week, this is the time to use your problem-solving skills.

Making Midcourse Corrections (Back to Problem Solving)

When you are trying to overcome obstacles, the first plan is not always the most workable plan. If something doesn't work, don't give up. Try something else: modify your short-term plans so that your steps are easier, give yourself more time to accomplish difficult tasks, choose new steps toward your goal, or check with your consultants for advice and assistance. If you are not sure how to go about this, go back and read page 18.

Rewarding Yourself

The best part of being a good self-manager is the reward that comes from accomplishing your goals and living a fuller and more comfortable life. However, don't wait until your goal is reached; rather, reward yourself frequently for your short-term successes. For example, decide that you won't read the news on the Internet until after you exercise. Thus reading the news becomes your reward. One self-manager buys only one or two pieces of fruit at a time and walks the half-mile to the supermarket every day or two to get more fruit—the walk is the short-term goal, the fruit the reward. Another self-manager who stopped smoking used the money that would have been spent on cigarettes to have the house professionally cleaned, and there was

How People Change

Thousands of studies have been done to learn how people change—or why they don't change. Here's what we have learned:

- Most people change by themselves, when they are ready. Although physicians, counselors, partners or spouses, and self-help groups may coax, persuade, nag, and otherwise try to assist people to change their lifestyle and habits, most people do so without much help from others.

- Change is not an all-or-nothing process. It happens in stages. Most of us think of change as occurring one step at a time, each step an improvement over the one before it. Although a few people do make changes this way, it is rare. More than 95 percent of people who successfully quit smoking, for example, do so only after a series of setbacks and relapses.

- In most cases, change resembles a spiral more than a straight line, with people reverting to previous stages before proceeding further ("two steps forward, one step back"). So relapses are not failures but setbacks, which are an integral part of change. And dealing with relapse is frequently a helpful way for people to learn how to maintain change. Relapsing provides feedback about what doesn't work.

- Efficient self-change depends on doing the right things at the right time. There's evidence that people who are given strategies inappropriate to their particular stage are less successful in changing than people who receive no assistance at all. For example, making an elaborate written plan of action when you really haven't decided you want to change is a prescription for failure. You're likely to get bored, discouraged, or frustrated before you even start.

- Confidence in your ability to change is the key ingredient for success. Your belief in your own ability to succeed predicts whether you will attempt change in the first place, whether you will persist if you relapse, and whether you will ultimately be successful in making the change.

even enough left over to go to a baseball game with a friend. Rewards don't have to be fancy, expensive, or fattening. Sometimes just congratulating yourself on being successful is enough. Celebrate yourself. There are many healthy pleasures that can add enjoyment to your life.

One last note: not all goals are achievable. Chronic illness may mean having to give up some options. If this is true for you, don't dwell too much on what you can't do. Rather, start working on another goal you would like to accomplish. One self-manager we know who uses a wheelchair talks about the 90 percent of things they *can* do. This person devotes life to developing this 90 percent to the fullest.

Tools for Becoming a Self-Manager

Now that you understand the meaning of self-management, you are ready to begin learning to use the tools that will make you a successful self-manager of your HIV. Most self-management skills are similar for all diseases. Chapters 1, 3, 4, 5, 9, and 10 in this book all contain useful information about HIV. The rest of the book is devoted to general but important tools of the trade. These include exercise, nutrition, symptom management, communication, making decisions about the future, finding resources and information about advance directives for health care, and sex and intimacy.

Additional Resources

Stanford Patient Education Research Center (app for keeping track of your action plans on your mobile device): http://patienteducation.stanford.edu/myactionplanner

Suggested Further Reading

To learn more about the topics discussed in this chapter, we suggest that you explore the following resources:

Dean, Jeremy. *Making Habits, Breaking Habits: Why We Do Things, Why We Don't, and How to Make Any Change Stick.* Boston: Da Capo Press, 2013.

Duhigg, Charles. *The Power of Habit: Why We Do What We Do in Life and Business.* New York: Random House, 2014.

Halvorson, Heidi Grant. *Succeed: How We Can Reach Our Goals.* New York: Plume, 2012.

Scott, S. J. *Habit Stacking: 97 Small Life Changes That Take Five Minutes or Less.* Ridgewood State, N.J.: Oldtown Publishing, 2014.

My Action Plan

In writing your action plan, be sure it includes all of the following:

1.　What you are going to do (a specific action)

2.　How much you are going to do (time, distance, portions, repetitions, etc.)

3.　When you are going to do it (time of the day, day of the week)

4.　How often or how many days a week you are going to do it

Example: This week, I will walk (what) around the block (how much) before lunch (when) three times (how often).

This week I will _____ (what)

_____ (how much)

_____ (when)

_____ (how often)

How sure are you? (0 = not at all sure; 10 = absolutely sure) _____

Comments

Monday _____

Tuesday _____

Wednesday _____

Thursday _____

Friday _____

Saturday _____

Sunday _____

CHAPTER 3

Health Problems of People with HIV

To be a good HIV self-manager, you need to know about HIV and what to expect. Most people with HIV feel fine. This is the goal of HIV medications. However, people with HIV are at increased risk of illness caused by HIV or other non-HIV illnesses. Unhealthy behaviors such as smoking, taking drugs, drinking, or having unprotected sex can also cause health problems. Finally, aging often brings its own set of health issues. In this chapter we look at some of the health issues that may affect you and how good self-management will help you successfully address these issues.

Effective HIV medications are now available. This means that the rates of HIV-related opportunistic infections, cancers, and nerve problems have dropped sharply. People who are tested for HIV before they get sick and who start on medications and stay on them usually do not develop serious HIV-related problems. These people have controlled HIV. When HIV is not controlled, the immune system weakens. The brain and nerves can also be harmed. This can lead to serious problems, including memory loss and pain.

HIV-Related Opportunistic Infections

Opportunistic infections are caused by other, non-HIV infectious agents (viruses, bacteria, fungi, and parasites) that typically do not cause problems in people who do not have HIV and have healthy immune systems. When HIV weakens the immune system, these infectious agents can cause a range of complications. People with HIV can avoid most of these infections by regularly taking medications as directed. These medications lower HIV in your body and boost your immune system. If you stop taking your medication, take a "drug holiday," or do not take your medications as directed, the medications won't work and you become vulnerable to opportunistic infections. In the following section, we discuss the most common HIV opportunistic infections.

Pneumocystis Pneumonia (PCP)

Pneumocystis jiroveci is a common fungus that causes *Pneumocystis* pneumonia (PCP). PCP is an HIV-related pneumonia (lung infection) that was once the most common AIDS-related illness. As an opportunistic infection, it causes pneumonia (see below) only in those who have a weakened immune system. PCP causes cough, fever, and labored breathing. Over the years, the medical community has learned a lot about PCP and is now better at preventing it. People who regularly take HIV medications seldom get PCP. Even people with weakened immunity who are at higher risk for PCP can still avoid getting it by taking daily low doses of antibiotics such as trimethoprim/sulfamethoxazole (Septra® or Bactrim®).

Pneumonia

Pneumonias caused by common bacteria or viruses can also be a problem for people with HIV. You can often prevent these illnesses by getting a yearly flu vaccine and a vaccine for pneumonia every five years. As a good self-manager, your job is to remind your health care provider to give you these vaccinations. The medicines to prevent *Pneumoncystis* pneumonia (such as Septra® or Bactrim®, discussed above) may also help to prevent some bacterial or viral pneumonias.

Candida (Thrush)

Candida, also called thrush, is a fungus that appears in the mouth, digestive tract, skin, and vagina. If you have candida inside your mouth, you may see white spots or patches clinging to your cheeks. Sometimes these spots can be red and sore. The white spots can be scraped off easily. Candida of the esophagus (the tube between the mouth and stomach) causes painful swallowing and interferes with eating. Candida of the vagina can be a mild irritation but is sometimes painful.

Candida, no matter where it is found, is often the first sign of immune system problems. Fortunately, it is easy to treat. Antifungal medicines such as fluconazole are usually very effective and quickly decrease the discomfort associated with candida.

Kaposi's Sarcoma (KS)

Kaposi's sarcoma (KS) is a slow-growing cancer. It starts on the skin as a purple, brown, or pink bump. It may be small and not cause much trouble, but sometimes it spreads widely and travels to the liver, lungs, and other internal organs. Kaposi's sarcoma is caused by infection with herpes virus 8 (HHV8). Fortunately, KS is not common in people who regularly take the new HIV medications.

Toxoplasmosis (Toxo)

Toxoplasmosis, also called toxo, is caused by a parasite (*Toxoplasma gondii*). It is a common infection in humans and many animals, but it usually does not cause serious problems in people with healthy immune systems. Toxo is found in undercooked meat as well as in cat litter boxes, soil, and other places where animals leave their waste. Because of this, people with HIV should wear gloves when handling meat, changing cat litter, or working in the garden to prevent getting the parasite on their hands and accidentally ingesting it. If someone with weakened immune function contracts toxo, the infection can move from the digestive system to other internal organs. In the brain, toxo infection causes weakness, seizures, or problems with speech or walking. For people at risk for toxo (those with a low T cell count of less than 50), taking trimethoprim/sulfamethoxazole (Septra® or Bactrim®) can prevent the disease. (We'll talk more about T cell count in Chapter 7, "Making Treatment Decisions.") In its early stages, toxo can be controlled with a combination of medicines such as pyrimethamine, sulfadiazine, and leucovorin.

Mycobacterium avium Complex (MAC)

Mycobacterium avium complex (MAC) is a bacteria that can spread widely through the blood and internal organs. People with advanced HIV are especially at risk from MAC infection. MAC can occur when the T cell count has dropped below 100, so people with a low T cell count should take an antibiotic such as azithromycin to prevent MAC. Once a MAC infection starts and is in the blood, however, treatment is difficult. Treatment may involve taking two or three types of antibiotics for long periods, sometimes forever. As with all opportunistic infections, the best way to prevent and treat MAC is to take your regular HIV medication as prescribed to keep your T cell count high and your immune system strong.

Cytomegalovirus (CMV)

Cytomegalovirus (CMV) is a common virus. Most people have been exposed to it, and CMV only causes problems when the immune system is weak. The virus can damage the back of the eye (CMV retinitis), causing loss of vision or even blindness. In the gut (CMV colitis or enteritis), CMV causes pain, ulcers, bleeding, and diarrhea. Like MAC, CMV usually causes disease only when the T cell count has dropped below 100. Medication can slow and sometimes even stop CMV problems. Boosting T cells with HIV medications will help slow or stop CMV effects.

Tuberculosis (TB)

Tuberculosis (TB) is caused by a bacterium, *Mycobacterium tuberculosis*. TB is a common and serious infection. Anyone can get TB, but those with a weak immune system are most at risk. This bacterium usually infects the lungs, although it can spread throughout the body. If a person is sick with a TB lung infection, they can easily spread the disease by coughing. TB symptoms include cough, fever, and weight loss.

Fortunately, there are tests that help identify people who have been exposed to TB. The infection can be treated with six months or more of oral medications.

If you contract TB, it is very important that, once treatment is started, you continue taking all of your medications. If you stop, the TB may change into a form that is resistant to treatment. If you stay on treatment, you also cannot pass the disease to others by coughing.

Herpes Virus Infections

People with or without HIV can contract herpes, but for a person with HIV, herpes can be one of the first symptoms of a weak immune system. There are two main types of herpes viruses: herpes simplex and herpes zoster. There are two types of herpes simplex. Herpes simplex type I causes sores (commonly known as cold sores) mostly on the mouth and lips. Herpes simplex type II usually causes sores on the genitals (the penis and vagina) and anus. Sometimes herpes simplex can spread to other parts of the body. Medication is available to treat herpes simplex infections.

The second virus, herpes zoster, is the same virus that causes chicken pox and shingles later in life. Shingles occurs when the virus left in the body from an earlier chicken pox infection is reactivated. The first sign of shingles may be an area of painful, hypersensitive skin. Then a painful rash appears as a patch or strip of small blisters, usually on one side of the body or face. In rare cases, shingles can spread to other parts of the body. If you think you might have shingles, see a doctor right away. The doctor might be able to give you medication that will reduce the intensity and duration of the outbreak. A

shingles vaccination is recommended for HIV-negative adults after age 50, but this vaccine is not typically recommended for adults with HIV.

Cryptosporidiosis

Cryptosporidium parvum is a parasite that infects the intestines, causing a disease called cryptosporidiosis. Symptoms include diarrhea and stomach cramps. Many animals carry this parasite and pass it to people in food or water. People with normal immune systems get rid of the parasite quite easily. People with weakened immune systems have more trouble. Cryptosporidiosis is very difficult to treat but can improve when the immune system is strengthened. If you have cryptosporidiosis, it is important to drink lots of fluids to prevent dehydration. The best thing you can do if you have the disease is to strengthen your immune system by taking HIV medications.

Lymphoma

Lymphoma is a cancer of the lymph node system caused by uncontrolled growth of abnormal white blood cells. It can occur in people with or without HIV. People with HIV are at higher risk for developing lymphoma as well as experiencing a more severe form of the disease. For people with HIV, non-Hodgkin's lymphoma is the most common form. Symptoms include fever or night sweats, as well as painless swelling of a lymph node (gland) in only one part of the body. If lymphoma starts in the brain, it may cause headaches, localized weakness, speech problems, or seizures. Non-Hodgkin's lymphoma is a serious cancer, but it can often be treated with chemotherapy and other cancer treatments.

Human Papillomavirus (HPV)

Human papillomavirus (HPV) is an infection transmitted by sexual contact. If a person gets HPV, years later it can cause cancer of the cervix (the opening of the womb in the vagina), anus, or rectum. Women or men who have both HIV and HPV are at higher cancer risk. HPV can be prevented with a vaccine, usually given when a person is in their teens or early twenties. The medical community recommends the vaccine for people between 13 and 26 with or without HIV.

For women with HIV, it is important to have regular pap smears. Cellular changes in the cervix can be detected long before a cervical cancer appears. If caught early by a pap smear, these changes can be prevented from developing into cancer of the cervix. Women with HIV should be sure to have regular pelvic examinations so that if a problem develops, it is detected and treated early. Smoking may increase the risk of cervical cancer (as well as lots of other bad things!). (For additional information on how to quit smoking, see page 58–61.)

Other Health Problems of People Living with HIV

People living with HIV experience other health problems not caused by the virus or their weakened immune systems. In fact, HIV medications are now so effective that we need to think about the *other* health problems of people with HIV—problems that come with aging, or with habits like smoking, or from exercising too little. These problems are called comorbidities. In the following section, we discuss the most common comorbidities.

HIV Wasting Syndrome

When you lose weight that you do not intend to lose, it is called wasting. For people with HIV, this is called HIV wasting syndrome. People with HIV can lose weight for two reasons: the virus itself may cause the weight loss, or they may have problems eating or absorbing food. The condition is often associated with fevers and lack of energy. If you unintentionally lose weight, it can be very difficult to regain it. Los-

ing more than 10 percent of body weight (for example, 15 pounds in a 150-pound person) is a sign of HIV wasting syndrome, but even losing as little as 5 percent of body weight is significant.

It is important to treat wasting syndrome quickly, because advanced wasting can be dangerous. If you experience wasting, your doctor will first check for another cause for your digestive problems. The best way to prevent and treat wasting is to take your HIV medications every day. High-calorie food supplements and nutritional drinks can help. There are also medications to increase your appetite and to boost your body's hormones. These allow your body to better store calories and nutrients.

Depression

Many people with HIV can experience serious depression. Sometimes just coping with having HIV can seem overwhelming. You might feel alone and unable to talk to others. You may feel like hurting yourself or others. You may have trouble eating or sleeping, or feel tired all the time, or feel worthless and guilty. All of these are signs of depression. One person described this as having the "blahs"—but for some people the blahs can become severe, even dangerous. Be very careful about drugs and alcohol—they may seem like ways to help you cope, but for people with depression they just make matters worse.

Depression can be treated. However, your doctors cannot treat you if you do not tell them how you feel. Unfortunately, many people don't talk to their doctors about depression, and the doctors may not ask. If you think you are depressed, you must let your doctor know. If you start on an antidepressant medication, expect it to take two to four weeks before you notice any improvement. For more about depression, see Chapter 11, "Understanding the Symptom Cycle."

Fat and Metabolism

Some people using HIV medications may notice changes in the way fat is distributed on their bodies. Lipodystrophy, or change in body shape, is a complication of HIV. It can be a side effect of taking protease inhibitors (one of the main types of anti-HIV medications) or related to the HIV virus itself. Fortunately, the medications currently being prescribed usually don't cause lipodystrophy. Additional factors associated with lipodystrophy are age (it's more common in older people), race (more common in Caucasians), how long you have been living with HIV, and your T-cell count. Poor habits such as too little exercise or eating too much fat and sugar can also cause these changes.

Lipodystrophy can be annoying and sometimes frightening. Fat moves from the legs and buttocks to the abdomen, breasts, and neck. You might find yourself with a fat back or fat belly. Your cholesterol levels and blood sugar may also rise. High blood sugar may be a sign of diabetes, which in turn can cause heart disease or stroke. These are drug side effects that can be treated by changing medication and sometimes by surgery.

Not too long ago, doctors usually did not talk to their HIV patients about weight, smoking, diet, or exercise. In those days, people with HIV were not expected to reach old age, so it was thought changes in lifestyle would not make much of a difference. Thankfully, things have changed. People living with HIV can expect to live well into old age. Healthy eating, not smoking, and exercise are essential to living long and well. Several chapters in this book address these topics: Chapter 13, "Physical Activity for Fun and Fitness," is about exercise, and Chapter 14, "Healthy Eating," is about making good food choices. For information on stopping smoking, see page xxxx.

Hepatitis

Hepatitis refers to damage to the liver caused by infection or toxins. The most common toxin that causes hepatitis is alcohol. Unfortunately, liver damage is common in people with HIV. This is because many people with HIV drink too much alcohol (beer, wine, or hard liquor). Also, people who use needles to inject drugs to get high often get hepatitis virus infections from the needles, and these can harm the liver.

Hepatitis C virus (HCV) is transmitted when the virus travels from one infected person to the bloodstream of another person, usually by sharing needles and sometimes through sex. HCV works slowly; some people don't feel sick from it for many years. Eventually the virus damages the liver and can cause liver failure. It is *very* important that people with HCV avoid things that cause more liver damage, including drinking alcohol and sharing needles. People with HCV should have regular liver tests. Treatments for HCV have improved greatly, and today hepatitis C can often be cured. If you have HCV, taking the drugs to treat it may be worth the time and effort. Discuss the options with your doctor.

Hepatitis B virus (HBV) is another blood-borne disease that can be contracted by sharing needles. Similar to HCV, it may act very slowly and not cause symptoms for many years. Some people with HBV can benefit from medications. Discuss your options with your medical team. There is also a vaccination to prevent HBV. If you have not been exposed to HBV and haven't yet had this vaccination, get it.

Neuropathy

Peripheral neuropathy causes pain or tingling in the feet or hands. It is caused by HIV and other conditions such as diabetes or spine problems. Neuropathy can be very uncomfortable and can make it hard to function. Treatment depends on the exact cause of the problem. Some people will improve if they adjust their HIV medications. Many people with neuropathy benefit from taking medications that act directly on the nerves.

Osteoporosis

Osteoporosis is thinning of the bones. Although often associated with older people (it is most common in older women), people with HIV often have osteoporosis. We are unsure why this

happens, but it may be related to the HIV infection or some types of HIV medications. The problem with thin bones is that you are more likely to have a fracture.

Osteoporosis can be prevented or delayed. There is a good screening test to measure bone density to determine your risk for osteoporosis. Ask your doctor about this. If you have osteoporosis or are at risk, your doctor may wish to adjust your HIV medications or add a specific medication for strengthening bones. Weight-bearing exercises such as walking and lifting light weights can also help strengthen bones. Because cigarette smoking is a major cause of bone thinning, quitting smoking is very important. Talk with your doctor about taking calcium and vitamin D supplements. Vitamin D comes from the sun, so if you get outdoors every day for a half hour or so, you probably get enough vitamin D already. You can get calcium in your diet from dairy products as well as some dark green vegetables (See Chapter 14, "Healthy Eating.")

Neurocognitive Disorders

Up to 50 percent of adults living with HIV may experience HIV-associated neurocognitive disorder (HAND). HAND is a group of disorders that occur when HIV enters the nervous system and harms the nerve cells. This then leads to impairments in various cognitive abilities such as attention, memory, language, problem-solving, and decision-making.

There are different types of neurocognitive disorders. The first type is referred to as asymptomatic impairment; it shows that a person has some loss of cognitive function, but it does not affect everyday functioning. Then there is mild neurocognitive impairment, which is the most common form. This type indicates that the person experiences some interference with everyday functioning. The most severe form of neurocognitive impairment is dementia, which greatly affects the person's ability to learn new information, process information, maintain attention, and concentrate. The person is significantly limited and not able to function well on a daily basis at home, work, and during social activities.

Although symptoms can vary widely, the first problem many people notice is forgetfulness severe enough to affect their ability to function at home or work or to enjoy lifelong hobbies. HIV-related cognitive impairment may also cause a person to lose attention, become confused, have trouble making decisions, misplace things, have trouble with language, and experience headaches or pain. They may also have difficulty with movement. The disease gets worse over time, especially if not treated.

If you suspect that you or someone you know with HIV is experiencing symptoms of cognitive impairment, it is important to seek a diagnosis as soon as possible. There is currently no cure for these HIV-related cognitive disorders, but if you have impairment, taking your HIV medications every day and early detection allow you to get the maximum benefit from available treatments—treatments that may relieve some symptoms and help you maintain your independence longer. Early detection also allows you to take part in decisions about care, transportation, living options, and financial and legal matters. You can also start building a social network sooner and increase your chances of participating in clinical drug trials that help advance research.

If you are concerned about HIV-associated neurocognitive disorder or a similar condition, contact your doctor. Don't hesitate to reach out to some of the organizations listed under Additional Resources at the end of this chapter as well. Help is available 24 hours a day, 7 days a week.

Given the potential health problems that people with HIV may face, it is vitally important to understand your symptoms and carefully manage your medical treatments. Nearly all of the opportunistic infections and complications of HIV can be prevented or managed by being tested early and catching the problem before it causes much damage, and by starting HIV medications early and continuing treatment. The chapters that follow provide information on how to assess and manage symptoms, the roles and uses of medications, how to work with your doctor, and how to make treatment decisions.

Additional Resources

AIDS Info (guidelines for prevention and treatment of opportunistic infections):
   https://aidsinfo.nih.gov/guidelines/html/4/adult-and-adolescent-oi-prevention-and-treatment-guidelines/318/introduction

AIDS Info (information on HIV/AIDS-related conditions):
   http://aidsinfo.nih.gov/hiv-aids-health-topics/topic/53/hiv-aids-related-conditions

AIDS InfoNet: www.aidsinfonet.org

AIDS.gov: www.aids.gov/hiv-aids-basics

AIDS.org—Information, Education, Action: www.aids.org/topics/hiv-and-related-diseases

American College of Rheumatology: www.rheumatology.org/Practice/Clinical/Patients/
   Diseases_And_Conditions/HIV_and_Rheumatic_Disease

American Diabetes Association: www.diabetes.org

American Lung Association: www.lung.org/assets/documents/ALA_LDD08_HIV_FINAL.PDF

Centers for Disease Control and Prevention (CDC): www.cdc.gov/hiv

Depression and Bipolar Support Alliance: www.dbsalliance.org

Freedom from Fear: www.freedomfromfear.org

Hepatitis Foundation International: www.hepatitisfoundation.org

HIV and Hepatitis.com: www.hivandhepatitis.com

NAM aidsmap: www.aidsmap.com/topics

National Alliance on Mental Illness (NAMI): www.nami.org

National Institute of Mental Health (NIMH): www.nimh.nih.gov

National Institute of Neurological Disorders and Stroke:
   www.ninds.nih.gov/disorders/aids/detail_aids.htm

National Suicide Prevention Lifeline: www.suicidepreventionlifeline.org or 1-800-273-8255

Substance Abuse and Mental Health Services Administration (SAMSHA): www.samhsa.gov

U.S. Department of Veterans Affairs:
   www.hiv.va.gov/patient/diagnosis/related-conditions-single-page.asp

U.S. National Library of Medicine: www.nlm.nih.gov/medlineplus

The Well Project: www.thewellproject.org/hiv-information/health-and-medical-issues

CHAPTER 4

Living with HIV through a Lifespan

WITH THE AVAILABILITY OF MORE EFFECTIVE TREATMENTS, HIV is now considered a manageable chronic disease. People with HIV can and do live long and full lives. Unfortunately, HIV still affects people of all ages. Babies are still being born with HIV infection, and other groups (youth, young adults, middle-age adults, and older adults) continue to be infected. In addition, people living with HIV are now living to become senior citizens. As people age with HIV, their needs, priorities, and circumstances change. The types of care, services, and self-management skills they need also change with time. In this chapter, we discuss some of these special concerns and issues that people with HIV face at different life stages.

Youths, Young Adults, and HIV

Worldwide, fewer infants are being born with HIV infection than in the past. However, youths between the ages of 12 and 18 and young adults between the ages of 19 and 25 continue to be infected with HIV. No matter what age a person is, there are some self-management tasks required of everyone living with HIV. Some of these include taking HIV medications every day, working and talking with doctors and other members of the health care team, monitoring and reporting changes in symptoms, eating a healthy diet, being physically active, getting enough rest, and getting help and social support.

Infants, children, and teenagers must work with their parents or guardians to complete these different self-management tasks. Accepting help and working with a parent or guardian can be challenging, especially for preteens and teens. At this stage of life, young people are becoming independent. There is a push and pull between making their own decisions and yet still sometimes wanting and needing help. It is a confusing time for everyone. Often, this is when young people challenge authority; they may argue, ignore, defy, and even rebel against their parents' or guardians' wishes. If this is happening, good communication skills are important, as is working closely with the whole health care team, or maybe even a family therapist who can help the young person and parent or guardian negotiate these important issues. Tips for improving communication skills can be found in Chapter 16, "Communicating with Family, Friends, and Everyone Else."

Taking Your Medications

If you are a youth living with HIV, you are usually in the early stages of the disease. This makes you a perfect candidate for taking HIV medication. We now know that the earlier you start medication after infection, the better your overall health. Unlike adults, the type and dose of medication will depend on where you are in your puberty development. If you have not yet completed puberty, your medications may be a bit more complex.

It is important to work closely with your doctor and parent or guardian to find what works best for you. If you hear information that makes you nervous from friends or see something interesting on the Internet or television about medications, write that information down and take it to your doctor. No question is stupid or unimportant. Discussing all of your concerns before you start a medication will help you to get the best treatment and to stick to it. The reward is a long and healthy life.

Once you, your parent or guardian (if appropriate), and your doctor have decided which medications and what dosages you will take, you can work together to figure out the schedule for taking them. It is important for you to develop a plan to help you remember to take your medications every day. When you are growing up, there are many changes in how you think, how your body behaves, and in your emotions. These can make remembering to take medications very challenging. Some teens ask their doctors or a trusted family member to text them each day at the same time to remind them to take the medication. Other teens set an alarm. Some even take pictures of themselves taking the medication to text to their social worker. It often helps to pair taking your medication with something you normally do every day, such as brushing your teeth. Other ideas for remembering to take medications are provided in Chapter 8, "Managing Medications for HIV." Whatever strategy you decide on, make sure it is something that works for you.

Communicating with Your Doctor

Generally, your doctor will want to see you at least twice a year, sometimes more depending on your needs. They will talk with you about your medications, check and discuss blood or other lab test results, conduct a physical exam, and discuss your concerns or questions. In addition to these checkups, you should always schedule an appointment any time you notice any changes in how you feel.

Your doctor works with a team of people—nurses, case managers, social workers, registered dietitians, health educators, and others—to provide you with the best possible health care. The members of this team will help you understand HIV and how to improve your health. They can help with insurance, provide counseling and referrals for other services, and coordinate your medical appointments. Ask team members who you should call first if things change and how they communicate with each other. Also, talk with them about what information you want them to share or not share with your parents or guardians. Be sure to take advantage of the referrals your health care team will have for you for social support, online resources, community-based organizations, and other services

that can help you live well with HIV. For more information on working with your health care providers, see Chapter 6, "Working with Your Health Care Team."

As you get older, you will eventually transition from your pediatric HIV health care team to an adult HIV health care team if you have not already. As an adult, you will have different health needs. An adult team will better understand how to take care of you. This transition can sometimes be difficult, especially since your pediatric health care team may have become like good friends or family to you. You do not want to lose them. It is always difficult to go from the known to the unknown.

To help make this transition successfully, when you start to go through puberty, ask your doctor about when and how the transition to an adult team will occur. Ask your doctor to work with you to develop a plan to ensure that all of your health needs are met as you transition to the adult clinic. This plan will detail what you are hoping to find in a new provider (for example, experience, attitude, or specific types of services); what information you and your family need about the new doctor; how to transfer your clinic records; how and when to schedule appointments; and how to get the appropriate support services you need at the new clinic. The actual transition process takes place over several visits as you determine which doctor is best for you. Often, the adult doctor will meet you at your pediatric clinic. You will slowly transition to seeing your adult health care team at the adult clinic.

You are in charge of this transition so if you are uncomfortable or want to see a different doctor, just say so. It is important that you find the right doctor for you—one who will best help you manage your HIV. If this transition is going to happen more abruptly because you are moving or going away to school, talk to your health care team members and ask if they know a good source of care in your new location. If you are heading to school, remember that you are not the first person with HIV to show up at a student health center. Be honest. The people who work in student centers are experienced professionals and should be very helpful in finding you the right care team.

Finding Social Support

Living with HIV can be lonely. People sometimes feel guilty or ashamed of having HIV, or they may fear stigma (see the box "HIV Stigma"). When this happens, people often withdraw from family and friends. Whereas an adult might understand that there is no reason to feel guilty or ashamed about living with HIV, young people often think and feel differently. They like to feel and believe they are similar to their peers. Having HIV or anything that makes you seem different may make you feel separate from others. You may feel or actually be rejected. This can lead to depression and isolation.

To help overcome this tendency to withdraw, try to develop a positive social support network. This can help you manage your HIV and help you help others and be helped by others. Finding social support may not be easy. It means telling others about your HIV status. Who you choose to tell is one of the hardest decisions. (There is more information about disclosure in Chapter 16, "Communicating with Family, Friends, and Everyone Else.") Remember, you don't have to tell anyone about your HIV, except

your sexual partners. However, many young people who do disclose their HIV status to their family, friends, and teachers experience social and emotional benefits. In addition to finding support from your family and friends, you can also participate in support groups.

Sometimes disclosure does not work out the way we hoped. You may find former friends and even family becoming distant. The sections that follow will help you find other people like you who have made it through this difficult time.

Peer-Based Support Groups

Your HIV clinic probably has at least one support group for young people. If they do not run one directly, a member of your health care team should be able to refer you to a local group. These support groups are exclusively for youth living with HIV and are usually facilitated by a social worker or nurse. The groups are designed to be safe places and offer continual support for people. Some groups may also offer additional activities, such as education about HIV and related health issues (medication, feeling sad, sex, etc.); social activities such as games, going out to dinner, watching movies, makeovers, etc.; and discussion groups. There are also camps specifically for youth with HIV or young people whose lives are affected by HIV. All of these support activities are offered at low or no cost to the participants. The resources at the end of this chapter list contact information for some groups like these.

Online Support Groups

In addition to in-person social support groups, there are online support networks available for young people with HIV. For example, your

HIV Stigma

HIV-related stigma and discrimination refers to prejudice, negative attitudes, and behaviors directed at people living with HIV and AIDS. HIV stigma reinforces existing social inequalities based on gender, race, social class, health and illness, and sexual orientation. The effects of HIV stigma are widespread and directly impact people living with HIV. It can lead to depression, isolation, and withdrawing from care. Many organizations are fighting to change policies and social norms that allow stigma to perpetuate, including the Stigma Project, the Center for HIV Law and Policy, and the National AIDS Trust (in the UK).

Although these organizations are working on long-term solutions to HIV stigma, sometimes what they are doing may not seem to help those who are currently dealing with stigma. If you are dealing with HIV stigma, connect yourself with a supportive social network that can help you face stigma with other people who are also dealing with its effects. You are not alone. There are a number of resources provided at the end of chapter that can connect you with people in your area.

HIV clinic may have a private online discussion group. This is one way to find information about other groups or resources in your community. Additionally, national and international adolescent HIV Facebook pages also provide support and important information. One such page is Teen Club International (www.facebook.com/teenclubinternational). The organization healthMpowerment (www.healthmpowerment.org) is another online support resource currently being tested by researchers. Often your health care team can tell you about these resources as they become available.

HIV, Youth, and Sex

As we grow, at some point, almost everyone starts to think about sex. As a young person living with HIV, you may be facing some questions that other young people do not have. How do I have sex? Should I have sex and should I ever think about having children? The following information is intended to help you answer those questions.

Should I have sex?

HIV is a sexually transmitted disease; therefore, it is natural to wonder whether it is safe for you to have sex. For all people with HIV, not just young people, there are times when sex is not safe. (See Chapter 1, "Overview of HIV and Self-Management," and Chapter 5, "Barriers to HIV Self-Management.") However, in general, if you feel you are emotionally and physically ready to have sex and can do so safely, then yes, you can have sex. For more details on safe sex, taking your HIV medications and sex, and partner notification, please see Chapter 5, "Barriers to HIV Self-Management."

Should I have children?

If you want to be a parent, having HIV should not stop you. An HIV-positive person can take medications during pregnancy, labor, and delivery to prevent the child from being infected with HIV (see below). There are a few other strategies you can use to prevent your child from becoming HIV infected. You can undergo a process called sperm washing in which sperm are washed free of HIV before being inseminated. You can also use sperm from a donor or adopt a child. For more information about any of these methods, talk with your health care provider who can refer you to the appropriate resource. The important thing to remember is that there are many options and there will probably be more in the future.

Women and HIV

In the United States, about 25 percent of the people with HIV are women; it is estimated that approximately 28 percent of transgender women are infected with HIV, with black/African American transgender women being at highest risk. Worldwide, about 50 percent of those who are HIV positive are women. Women with HIV have many of the same health concerns as men with HIV, but often face additional challenges due to family responsibilities (e.g., child care or caring for a parent), current and past trauma, social and structural factors (e.g., poverty), gynecological issues, and childbearing

Family Responsibilities

There are still too few resources available to assist people caring for children or parents. This is true for all people but especially those with HIV. If you find that these responsibilities make it difficult for you to attend your medical appointments, take your medications, or manage other health tasks, talk with your health care provider. Often it is possible to schedule your appointments around your daily tasks. Also, some clinics and HIV service organizations offer child care. Similarly, if caring for others interferes with taking your medications, exercising, or eating healthy, discuss this with your health care team. They can help you develop a plan to stay healthy. You might also seek help from employee assistance where you work. The important thing is to tell people you need help so they can work with you to develop the best plan to meet your obligations while staying healthy.

Women and girls living with HIV are disproportionally affected physical and emotional trauma which can negatively impact their ability to self-manage their HIV. Many HIV clinics provide "trauma-informed care" in which all members of the health care team recognize how common trauma is and are committed to addressing it and the impact trauma has on one's current symptoms and health. To read more about this subject, see Chapter 5, page 64.

Gynecological Care

HIV can make women with HIV more likely to have an abnormal Pap smear, and more susceptible to invasive cervical cancer and recurrent yeast infections. Therefore, it is important to get regular gynecological care that includes an annual pelvic exam and Pap test. HIV clinics may have a gynecologist on site, or they may be able to refer you to a gynecologist. If you are seeing a gynecologist who does not specialize in HIV, it is important to tell them that you have HIV. Also, tell the gynecologist what medications you are taking, and provide them with your HIV doctor's contact information in case they need to confer.

Having Children

As a woman living with HIV, you may be facing some questions about having children that relate to your health. The following information is intended to help you answer those questions.

Should I get pregnant?

If you want to have a child, HIV should not stop you from becoming a parent. Each year thousands of people with HIV give birth to children who are not HIV infected.

Be sure to inform your doctor and health care team when you are thinking about pregnancy or become pregnant. They can quickly help you get and stay as healthy as possible. You may need to change your HIV medications so that they do not harm your unborn child. Also, to help prepare your body for pregnancy, it is important for all pregnant women to take vitamins with folic acid and to eat healthy foods. Remember to take your HIV medications as prescribed to help keep your HIV viral load as low as possible (undetectable). If you smoke and are pregnant, stop smoking. Stop using any drugs or alcohol. All women who get prenatal care early, regardless of HIV status, have healthier babies.

Will pregnancy affect my health?

Pregnancy affects each person differently; therefore, it is important to take good care of your-self. Taking prenatal vitamins, eating healthy foods, staying physically active, getting enough rest, taking your HIV medications, and seeing your doctors on a regular basis will help you to maintain your health.

Will HIV infect my baby?

No, not necessarily. The best way to prevent transmission to your child is to take the following steps:

- Take your HIV medications during pregnancy
- Take intravenous (IV) HIV medications along with your oral HIV medications during labor and delivery
- Give your newborn baby liquid HIV medications for approximately six weeks after birth

Your HIV doctor, your obstetrician, and your pediatrician will need to work together to have a healthy outcome for you and your baby. Line up your prenatal, pregnancy, and childbirth team as soon as possible, even before you become pregnant, if possible.

Is HIV in my breast milk?

Yes. However, the recommendations about whether or not to breastfeed differ and depend on whether you have access to high-quality formula. If you do have access to high-quality formula, then you should not breastfeed but instead feed formula to your baby. If safe formula is not available, your safest choice may be to breastfeed. Whether or not you choose to breastfeed, you should continue taking your HIV medications to reduce the amount of HIV in your breast milk.

Transgender People and HIV

According to the organization GLAAD, transgender "is an umbrella term for people whose gender identity and/or gender expression differs from what is typically associated with the sex they were assigned at birth." Among transgender people, there are some special considerations when it comes to HIV. This is especially true for transgender women, who have a much higher rate of HIV infection than any other group.

Transgender People, HIV, and Sex

Transgender people contract HIV exactly like everyone else. However, studies have shown that there are some special factors that can make them more at risk. Because of self-esteem issues, substance abuse, or depression in some transgender people, they may be less likely to demand the use of condoms or other barriers. In addition, because of stigma, discrimination, and bad experiences with or lack of access to safe health care, some members of this group may be much less likely to seek HIV testing and treatment. Finally, there is an additional risk for transgender people who inject hormones and do not have access to clean needles.

It is easy to understand the risk but much harder to find a solution. If you are an HIV-positive transgender person, follow all the advice in this book. In addition, seek out transgender-friendly health facilities and support groups specifically for transgender people.

It is healthy and normal for transgender women to use their penises for sex. If you are a transgender woman taking hormones, it's important to recognize that you will need some of the hormone testosterone to keep your erection. Keep in mind that, even if you are taking hormones, you may have enough sperm to cause pregnancy. You should continue to use protective barriers (as described in Chapter 1) to decrease the risk of unwanted pregnancy, HIV, and other sexually transmitted infections.

Transgender People and Pregnancy

If they want to, transgender women and men can have children. Transgender women can use their own sperm to impregnate their partner, donate their sperm to a surrogate, or save their sperm in a sperm bank for a future time when they're ready to have a baby. If they are taking hormones, they may need to stop taking them for a few months in order to make enough sperm to initiate pregnancy. Transgender men can save their eggs before having surgery to remove their ovaries and uterus, donate eggs to a female partner or friend to carry the pregnancy, or, if they have their own uterus and ovaries, use their own eggs to carry the pregnancy. For transgender people living with HIV, it's important to follow all of the same advice about HIV and pregnancy listed in this chapter.

Aging and HIV

HIV medications have improved and now most people with HIV are living a normal lifespan.

Growing older affects all of us in different ways. As you age with HIV, you will start to notice changes in your general health due to aging, as well as changes due to HIV. Together these changes may present specific challenges, which we discuss in this section.

As you read through the material in this section, it is important to keep in mind that all chronic health conditions, not just HIV, can be managed using the strategies discussed in this book. Exercising can prevent and improve heart disease, diabetes, depression, memory loss, as well as other health problems. Eating healthy, not smoking, reducing stress, and having a strong support system in place can also improve most chronic conditions and are critical to living well with HIV. These topics are presented in more detail in other chapters, so be sure to check the table of contents.

Multiple Chronic Health Conditions

As you age, you may be diagnosed with additional chronic conditions, such as heart disease (high blood pressure, peripheral vascular disease), diabetes, cancer, arthritis, osteoporosis, and others. Studies indicate that these diseases occur more frequently and earlier in people with HIV. It has also been shown that learning to manage HIV helps you to lead a healthier and fuller life. Managing HIV includes taking your medication, working closely with your doctor, exercising, eating right, and other tasks that are discussed throughout this book. Additional chronic health conditions add to this work. Let's consider some of these special challenges:

Multiple Doctors

Often, when you are diagnosed with an additional chronic health condition, such as heart disease or diabetes, your primary care doctor refers you to a specialist. This specialist will examine you, run tests, and prescribe the best course of treatment. The specialist will then follow up with your primary care doctor.

If you see specialists regularly for other conditions, it is your job to find out which provider is in charge of coordinating your care. Ask each provider who that is. Usually it is your primary care doctor, which is most likely your HIV doctor, but ask to confirm. When working with different providers, your job is to keep your primary care doctor informed about any tests and new medications ordered by the others. This is especially important if any of your providers are not in the same clinic or health care system and do not share your electronic medical record. Although people like to think that doctors all communicate with each other, the truth is that often you are the only person who has all the pieces of the puzzle. Do not assume that doctors talk to each other or read each other's notes. Be proactive about sharing information.

Multiple Medications

You must take your HIV medications every day. This is the case for many of the medications prescribed for other chronic conditions as well. Taking more medications creates more challenges: finding the best time and place to take all of your medications as prescribed every day; remembering to take them; watching for possible side effects and interactions; and managing these negative effects.

To better manage your medications, it is helpful to develop a system to track all of your medications and the times that you take them. Options include marking a calendar, keeping a journal to note difficulties or problems, getting a medication tracking app for your smartphone, or organizing them daily in a medication sorter (pill box).

If managing your medications is a problem for you, talk to your health care team and work together to devise a personalized plan for you. They have a lot of experience working with people taking multiple medications and can share what they have learned from working with others. Also, they may be able help make your medication regime simpler.

You may also want to talk to a pharmacist. These unsung heroes of the medical community can be very helpful. They are often easier to reach by phone than your doctor, and they can answer almost all your questions about medications. If you walk into a pharmacy when it is not busy, you can expect to receive plenty of personal attention to your questions and concerns.

When you are taking HIV medications and other medications, there is always a chance that they will interact with each other in a way that can make them less effective. This interaction can also lead to symptoms or side effects that can be unpleasant or dangerous. To help prevent this, make sure all of your doctors know all the medications you are taking and how much (dose) you take each day. Although electronic medical records can make this process easier, records may contain errors. Carrying an up-to-date list of all your medications with you is still the best way to ensure that your doctors have current information. Ask your health care providers if they have a medication card for you to complete. If not, make your own card detailing this information, or get a medication app for your smartphone. Some medical groups allow you to make your own list in your online medical record. Keep your medication card or latest list in your purse or wallet. You can also take a photo of your list with your smartphone and store the photo on your phone for easy reference.

Also, take the lead when telling your new doctors about your medications. Let them know that you have HIV, when you were diagnosed, and your HIV doctor's name and contact information, and give them a list of all your current medications. This should alert your doctor to consider the possible interactions that sometimes occur between HIV and other, non-HIV medications. You can find more information about managing medications in Chapters 8 and 9.

Memory Problems

Many people worry about changes in their memory, particularly as they age. Although all of us are sometimes forgetful, there are other illnesses that cause memory loss, including HIV. This is discussed in Chapter 3, "Health Problems of People with HIV," in the section on Neurocognitive Disorders, pages 39–40. Unfortunately, because HIV can affect the brain, this may lead to difficulty remembering events, words, or people. If you notice you are having memory problems, please let your HIV doctor know as soon as possible. Also, tell your family or friends when you start to experience any trouble remembering things. Even if you are as young as 50, others should remind you to write it down when they notice your forgetfulness. They, too, should write this down. Notify your doctor right away with this record of events so they can determine if you need additional treatment and help you find strategies to manage these memory problems.

People with memory problems need a support system. Friends and partners can help with things like remembering when to take HIV medications. Many people keep cues around them (such as notes, calendars, or alarms) to remind themselves about medicines, appointments, and other important things. Treatment with HIV medications may help control mild memory problems and prevent them from developing into dementia by reducing HIV in the nerve tissues.

Depression, Anxiety, and Other Difficult Emotions

Everyone goes through periods of depression and anxiety; this is normal. However, as you age, you may start to feel sadder or more anxious than when you were younger. Both HIV and aging can lead to increased feelings of depression, anxiety, and other difficult emotions. Although these emotions can be signs of serious mental health conditions, like physical conditions, they are treatable and manageable. Depression often affects people's ability and desire to take their HIV medications. Therefore, it is important to find ways to treat it, which can range from practicing self-management techniques such as those suggested in Chapter 11, "Understanding the Symptom Cycle" on pages 136–137, and Chapter 12, "Using Your Mind to Manage Symptoms."

Sexual Health and Aging

Many older adults continue to enjoy an active sex life. This is great news! However, it is important that everyone with HIV practice safe sex to prevent HIV infection no matter their age. Approximately 40 percent of sexually active older adults have sex without condoms. Using safer sex practices helps to prevent the spread of HIV and other sexually transmitted infections whether you are 15 or 90. Postmenopausal women may have an increased risk of HIV infection and should continue to use protective barriers such as condoms or dental dams every time they have sex.

Older men with erectile dysfunction and older women with vaginal dryness may experience decreased sexual satisfaction. If this occurs, you can talk with your doctor about medications to decrease these symptoms. These medications should only be obtained with a prescription to ensure your safety as well as to give your doctor an opportunity to examine the causes and potential seriousness of these symptoms. Many doctors might not ask about your sexual health. If they do not, don't be shy. Bring up any questions or concerns you have about sex and aging with your HIV doctor.

Long-Term Survivors

HIV is one of the best success stories of modern medicine. When HIV was first identified in the 1980s, people who had HIV were not expected to live for very long. Today, people with HIV live almost as long as those who are not infected. In those early days, whole communities died from AIDS, leaving those left behind feeling guilt, sadness, relief, confusion, and apprehension, all at the same time. Losing friends and community members is hard for anyone to go through, and it is important to remember that grieving your losses is necessary and normal. It may help to remind yourself that you cannot change places with any of the people you lost, nor would they want you to. Rather, you can honor their memory by continuing to take care of yourself.

It is also helpful to find a positive way to channel your emotions. For example, you can contribute to the AIDS Memorial Quilt. By making a memorial patch, you can begin to accept that a loved one's passing is a reality. (This quilt travels around the world and is likely to come to a location near you. Check the website for the display schedule: www.aidsquilt.org). Other community events, such as the National HIV/AIDS Long-Term Survivor Awareness Day, help to bring together people to address the psychological and social effects of long-term HIV survival. The website can be found at http://nhaltsad.org/ and provides information for planning events and connecting with long-term survivors.

Another positive way to deal with your grief is to care for a sick friend or invest your energy in some other new and productive way. Also, try talking to someone about the loss or whatever has triggered your sad emotions. Sharing your feelings can help you process emotions in a healthy way. Talk to a trusted member of your support network, a religious leader, or a therapist. Whomever you choose, make sure it is someone who will help you deal with your emotions in a positive way.

While all people with HIV share many of the same problems and concerns, HIV can and does impact every individual in a unique way and at different times during the lifespan. In discussing some of the specific concerns for different groups, it is important to know that the self-management skills presented in this book can be useful for members of all age groups—children, teens, young adults, and older adults—at different times in their lives.

Additional Resources

Adolescent, Youth, and Young Adults

AIDS.gov: www.aids.gov/hiv-aids-basics/prevention/reduce-your-risk/mixed-status-couples and https://aids.gov/hiv-aids-basics/staying-healthy-with-hiv-aids/friends-and-family/having-children

AIDSinfo: www.Aidsinfo.nih.gov

Camp Sunrise: www.sunrisekids.org/what-we-do

HIV Clinical Resource: www.hivguidelines.org/clinical-guidelines/adolescents/transitioning-hiv-infected-adolescents-into-adult-care

The Laurel Foundation: www.laurel-foundation.org

OneHeartland youth camps: www.oneheartland.org/camps-and-programs/camp-heartland and http://www.oneheartland.org/camps-and-programs/camp-hollywood-heart

Project Kindle: www.projectkindle.org

Additional Resources (*continued*)

HIV Stigma

International Planned Parenthood Federation: www.ippf.org/our-work/what-we-do/hiv-aids/reducing-hiv-related-stigma

Lambda Legal: www.lambdalegal.org/publications/fs_hiv-stigma-and-discrimination-in-the-us

The Stigma Project: www.thestigmaproject.org/#!resources-links/c287

Women and HIV

AIDS.gov: https://www.aids.gov/hiv-aids-basics/staying-healthy-with-hiv-aids/taking-care-of-yourself/womens-health

The Well Project: www.thewellproject.org/hiv-information/women-children-family

What Women Need to Know—The HIV Treatment Guidelines for Pregnant Women: http://womenandhiv.org/sites/default/files/pdf/WhatWomenKnow_En_Booklet_2013_FXB.pdf

Transgender Health

Centers for Disease Control and Prevention: www.cdc.gov/lgbthealth/index.htm

Human Rights Campaign: www.hrc.org/resources/entry/transgender-people-and-hiv-what-we-know

UCSF Center of Excellence for Transgender Health: http://transhealth.ucsf.edu

Older Adults and HIV

Age Is Not a Condom: www.ageisnotacondom.org/facts.html and www.ageisnotacondom.org/sexuality-and-aging.html

AIDS InfoNet: www.aidsinfonet.org/fact_sheets/view/616

AIDSMeds: www.aidsmeds.com/articles/hiv_exercise_aging_1667_20989.shtml

American Heart Association: http://www.heart.org/HEARTORG/Conditions/More/HIVandYourHeart/HIV-Medications_UCM_315426_Article.jsp

The Body—The Complete HIV/AIDS Resource: www.thebody.com/content/art54795.html

HIV-Age: http://hiv-age.org/

The Well Project: www.thewellproject.org/hiv-information/health-and-medical-issues

CHAPTER 5

Barriers to HIV Self-Management

MOST OF US SOMETIMES MAKE lifestyle choices and health-related decisions that are not good for us. For everyone, those choices can affect our overall health. So it is no surprise to learn that if you have HIV, there are habits and behaviors that can make it more difficult to maintain your health in the face of your illness. In this chapter, we look at how people with HIV can benefit from changing some of the most common unhealthy behaviors.

Risky Sexual Behaviors

For all people with HIV, there are times when sex is not safe. For example, it is not safe to have sex when you do not use barriers (such as condoms or dental dams) or are under the influence of drugs or alcohol (see below). If you engage in these activities, you can give HIV to someone else or you can get HIV from someone else. Even though you already have HIV, you can still get a different strain or a more drug-resistant strain of HIV from someone who's HIV positive.

For people with HIV, the only safe way to have sex is to always use protection, such as a latex condom or a latex or plastic barrier for oral sex. Recall from Chapter 1 that oral sex involves some risk of transmitting HIV, especially if sexual fluids enter the mouth and if there are sores in the mouth or bleeding gums. Whereas condoms make sex safer during intercourse, pieces of latex or plastic wrap placed over the vagina, or condoms over the penis, can be used as barriers during oral sex. By using protective barriers, in addition to preventing the spread of HIV, you also help prevent the spread of other sexually transmitted infections and prevent unwanted pregnancy as well.

In addition to using protection, you are also much less likely to transmit HIV if you take your HIV medications every day, and if your HIV viral load is suppressed or undetectable. This means the doctor cannot find any virus in your blood. (You can read more about viral load tests in Chapter 7, "Making Treatment Decisions.")

Many people with HIV have spouses or sexual partners who do not have HIV. These partners can stay HIV negative by practicing safe sex. Recently, it has also been shown that an HIV-negative partner of an HIV-positive person can take HIV medications daily to help prevent HIV infection; this is called pre-exposure prophylaxis (PrEP). If you and your sexual partner are interested in this, talk with your HIV doctor.

Sex is a decision between two people. Both you and your partner must consent to sex with each other. By disclosing your HIV status to your partner, together you have the opportunity to discuss safer sex options and can decide what is right for both of you. Talking about this can be scary because there is a chance your partner will reject you, but often it can open up a deeper communication between you. It is also important to know what the laws are in your state or country regarding partner notification about HIV. Your health care team is a good source of information about the legal obligations in your area, as well as how those obligations apply to you.

Tobacco*

Did you know that people with HIV have a much higher rate of tobacco use than the general population? This is the case even though tobacco use is more dangerous for people with HIV than for those without the virus. If you are HIV positive and you smoke (or use alternative tobacco products such as chewing tobacco, e-cigarettes, hookahs, or cigars), this section is for you. Our intention is not to scold you—we just want to give you some tools to add to your self-management tool kit. Consider the following facts about tobacco use:

---

*With acknowledgment and thanks to the U.S. Department of Veterans Affairs. Much of the material in this section was adapted from its excellent publication, *HIV Provider Smoking Cessation Handbook*. See the Additional Resources section for more information.

- Smokers are at greater risk of experiencing conditions caused by the HIV virus. (See HIV-Related Opportunistic Infections in Chapter 3, "Health Problems of People with HIV.")

- Antiviral (ART) medications (the most common drugs used for HIV; see Chapter 8, "Managing Medications for HIV") do not work as well in smokers as they do in people who do not smoke.

- Smokers with HIV have a higher death rate from all causes than people with HIV who do not smoke.

- Simply being in a room with someone who smokes, has recently smoked, or even only smokes once in a while can be almost as bad as being a heavy smoker.

All in all, smoking and being around smokers is not good for your health, and this is especially true if you are HIV infected.

Of course, everyone knows that tobacco is not good for us, but we also know that quitting can be hard. Nicotine, the main ingredient in tobacco, is as addictive as heroin. The good news is that you *can* quit, just as many people have. And you can quit even if you have not been successful at quitting in the past. In fact, every time you try to quit tobacco, your chance of success increases! Before we tell you about the tools to help you quit, let's tell you what we know about quitting:

- The most successful way for most people to quit is to combine counseling or quitting classes with one or two types of medications such as nicotine patches. To find classes in your area, see the list of resources at the end of this chapter.

- Only a few people can quit cold turkey (fewer than 5 in 100)—that is, they are able to just stop smoking and never smoke again. Most people need more support; it is normal to need help.

- Hypnosis and e-cigarettes have about the same success as going cold turkey. They are not very effective ways of quitting.

- If alcohol has been a problem in your life and you are no longer drinking, stopping smoking does not need to affect your sobriety.

The following active, healthy steps can help you set yourself up for success when you make the decision to quit using tobacco:

- Set a start date within the next two to three weeks. Give yourself enough time to prepare.

- Make an action plan. Review Chapter 2, "Becoming an HIV Self-Manager."

- Tell your friends and family about what you plan to do and ask for their support.

- Remove all tobacco products and e-cigarettes from your home.

- If you live with smokers, ask them to smoke elsewhere. Make your house and car smoke-free zones.

- Sign up for help to quit smoking—counseling, classes, a support group, or a workshop.

- Expect some challenges in the first tobacco-free weeks, including nicotine withdrawal. Symptoms of withdrawal may include irritability, anxiety, restlessness, hunger, depression, tobacco cravings, and trouble sleeping.

- Talk to your health care provider and ask about nicotine-replacement therapy or other medications that can help you quit smoking. (See below for more on this.)

- Most importantly, remain a nonsmoker through the first few months of the quitting process. Once you get past the first few months, your chances of long-term success increase dramatically!

Nicotine-Replacement Medications

Nicotine-replacement medications can help you quit smoking and remain a nonsmoker. The most common medications work by replacing the nicotine you no longer get from tobacco once you quit using. You might wonder why medications containing nicotine are better than cigarettes. Cigarettes have bad chemicals in them in addition to nicotine. By not smoking, you are not getting all these harmful chemicals even though your body is still getting reduced doses of nicotine. And nicotine replacement can be tapered, which means you can take less medicine gradually over time. This tapering process ensures that you are getting less and less nicotine as your body adjusts to being nicotine-free.

You might think that e-cigarettes or "vaping" could accomplish the same thing as nicotine-replacement medications. E-cigarette makers often market their products as a way to cut down on smoking. True, e-cigarettes do not have as much of the other harmful chemicals in cigarettes, but they also do not contain a consistent amount of nicotine. That means that you cannot control the amount of nicotine you are getting when you vape. The only way to cut down on tobacco use is to use all smoking, smokeless, and electronic tobacco products less. Unfortunately, there are no reliable scientific research studies (as of this writing) that indicate that e-cigarettes help people to become nonsmokers.

Nicotine-replacement medications come in many forms: patches, lozenges, gum, nose spray, and inhalers. Not all of these are the same. Consider the following information when you choose a product:

- Patches take 3 to 12 hours to reach their highest dose. Once they reach their peak, and if used as directed, patches deliver a steady dose of nicotine for as long as they are on the skin.

- Nicotine gum takes about 30 minutes to reach peak nicotine level, and then levels drop slowly over 2 to 3 hours. You should not eat or drink 20 minutes before chewing the gum, while you are chewing it, and for 15 minutes after you are done chewing it.

- Nicotine lozenges work about the same way as gum. You should suck the lozenge until dissolved. Your body gets about 25 percent more nicotine from lozenges than from gum.

- Nasal sprays or oral inhalers work faster than gum and are an option for those who react poorly to patches or do not like the taste of the gum or lozenges. The inhalers are shaped like cigarettes, so they provide a familiar substitute for smokers trying to quit.

Although you can buy nicotine-replacement medications without a prescription, we strongly recommend that you talk to your health care provider before using these products. There are two reasons for doing this:

- It is often useful to use more than one nicotine-replacement therapy. Some medications that can help you quit smoking can only be obtained by prescription, and they can be helpful. Only you and your health care provider can make the best decision about what is right for you.

■ Your insurance may pay for nicotine replacement if prescribed by your doctor.

Dealing with Withdrawal and Preventing Relapse

If you are a former smoker, whether you smoked for six hours or six years, there will be times when you want to smoke. These urges become less and less over time, but there is no denying that they do occur. When this happens, think DEADS (delay, escape, avoid, distract, substitute):

Delay. The urge will usually go away in 5 to 10 minutes if you wait. Use some positive thinking and self-talk (see pages 178–180 in Chapter 12, "Using Your Mind to Manage Symptoms"). Tell yourself, "This urge *will* go away, and I am not going to have a cigarette because I don't need one."

Escape. Sometimes urges hit during times of stress or if someone else is smoking around you. In either case, leave the environment that is triggering your craving. Go outside and take a short walk, or just leave the room. You will probably soon feel ready to go back to the situation.

Avoid. Avoid places and situations where you are tempted to smoke. If you always smoke when you take a coffee break, take your break somewhere that is smoke-free. This is especially true in the first couple of days. You may find it easier to quit when you are away from your regular routine.

Distract. If an urge hits, find something else to do right away. Choose an activity that you must do in a place where you cannot smoke, such as taking a shower or reading a book in a place where smoking is not allowed.

Substitute. Chew on a toothpick, eat a piece of fruit, chew sugarless gum. Use something to substitute for the cigarette. But be careful not to eat empty calories such as candy or chips.

Chewing Tobacco

Some people think that chewing tobacco is not as bad for your health as smoking is. Unfortunately, this is not true. Chewing tobacco causes all the same problems that smoked tobacco causes. In addition, it can cause mouth and throat cancer. The good news is that you can use all the advice in this chapter to stop using chewing tobacco.

Alcohol and Other Recreational Drugs

It is important to note that just because alcohol is legal does not mean it is safe. For many people alcohol use is not a problem, but for many others it is. Look at the chart on page 63. If you have any of these symptoms, there is a good chance you are abusing alcohol. These symptoms indicate that, even if you may not be addicted to alcohol, it is causing problems in your life.

Similar to tobacco, substances (alcohol and/or recreational drugs) can be dangerous to people living with HIV. The term "substance use" refers to the use of recreational drugs and/or alcohol in a way that causes problems for yourself or others. Sometimes people use these substances as a way to deal with the stress of having HIV, or to relieve depression or loneliness. Substance use does not address the root cause of your stress or loneliness. It often does not help you feel better even in the short term, and it can increase your risk of HIV transmission, interfere with taking your HIV medications, and increase your risk of becoming infected with another strain of HIV or such other conditions as hepatitis C. For healthy ways to deal with stress, depression, or loneliness, see Chapter 12, "Using Your Mind to Manage Symptoms."

Substance use can lead to the transmission of HIV in two ways. First, if you are injecting drugs, you can transmit HIV to others by sharing your needles ("works"). This is also a way to infect and be infected with hepatitis C. Second, when you use alcohol and/or recreational drugs, you are more likely to engage in other risky behaviors. This can include having sex without a condom or other barrier, and trading sex for drugs, alcohol, food, shelter, or money. These behaviors increase the chance that you will transmit HIV to others and that you may get another sexually transmitted disease yourself.

Substance use can also lead to poor HIV outcomes. It can do this by interfering with your ability to remember to take your medications. Taking your medications every day as prescribed

is one of the most important things you can do to help your body fight the virus and improve your immune system. See Chapter 8, "Managing Medications for HIV," for more details about why taking your medications daily is so important to becoming and staying healthy.

Substance use can also lead to circumstances that make it difficult for you to take your medications, including staying in unstable housing, losing your job, losing your support network, losing your driving privileges, or landing in jail. All of these circumstances can make it hard to take your HIV medications and engage in the other healthy behaviors that we describe throughout this book (eating well, sleeping, exercising, managing your stress), which can make you feel better and live a longer, stronger life. Certain drugs, such as methamphetamine, can also directly weaken your immune system.

Substance use can lead to abuse and addiction, which is a preventable and treatable disease. People recover from substance abuse and addiction every day and are able to lead the lives they want to. If you, or someone you care about, seems to have any of the symptoms listed in the box on page 63, talk with a health professional about getting help. You can also look at the information on the Substance Abuse and Mental Health Services Administration (SAMSHA) website at www.samhsa.gov/treatment. They have a useful tool to locate treatment centers in your area and a lot of good information about the different types of substance abuse treatment.

There is no one right way to treat a substance use problem. Treatment works best when it is individualized to your needs. The ultimate goal is to stop using substances and start your

Symptoms of a Substance (Alcohol and/or Drug) Disorder

- Problems with attendance and performance at work or school
- Instances of getting into trouble (fights, accidents, illegal activities)
- Substance use in hazardous situations such as while driving
- Secretive or suspicious behaviors
- Changes in appetite or sleep patterns
- Unexplained changes in personality or attitude
- Sudden mood swings, irritability, or angry outbursts
- Periods of unusual hyperactivity, agitation, or giddiness
- Lack of motivation
- Appearing fearful, anxious, or paranoid, with no reason

- Bloodshot eyes and abnormally sized pupils
- Sudden weight loss or weight gain
- Deterioration of physical appearance
- Unusual smells on breath, body, or clothing
- Tremors, slurred speech, or impaired coordination
- Sudden change in friends, habits, and hobbies
- Legal problems related to substance use
- Unexplained need for money or financial problems
- Continued use of drugs and/or alcohol even though it is causing problems in relationships

journey toward recovery. This takes time. As with tobacco use, some people may be able to stop cold turkey, but not many; for most people this is a lifelong process.

Work with a treatment specialist that you trust, who understands you, and who shares your recovery goals. Some options for treatment include individual or group counselling, medications that reduce the urge to use substances or block the reward from using them, and support services. Sometimes people are nervous about taking medications to help with their substance use recovery. However studies have shown that these medications can help people sustain their recovery journey and can be an important part of the treatment "toolbox." Substance use

treatment can be delivered in an outpatient setting (in other words, in the community where you live while you stay in your own home) or in a residential treatment facility. Work with your team to figure out which "tools" work best for you in each stage of your recovery.

Marijuana

Marijuana is a drug that is legal in some places and not in others. If marijuana use is causing any of the symptoms listed in the Symptoms of a Substance (Alcohol and/or Drug) Disorder box above, then you should consider its continued use to be a problem for you. The content in this chapter applies equally to people who have a marijuana abuse problem.

Physical and Emotional Trauma

People living with HIV report higher rates of past and current traumatic experiences (e.g. intimate partner violence, sexual, physical and emotional abuse) than the general population. It can be an issue with anyone, but women and girls are disproportionally affected. Reasons for this may include structural issues such as racism, sexism, classism, homophobia and transphobia. Traumatic experiences lead to negative health outcomes for people living with HIV, including increased depression, fatigue and anxiety, antiretroviral viral therapy failure, faster development of opportunistic infections, and death.

Many HIV providers will ask you about your current relationships and if you are being hurt. If this happening, you can work with someone in your clinic to develop a plan to ensure your safety, and that of your family, if that is a concern.

Some people living with HIV may also have lasting impacts from previous trauma. These experiences can impact how you feel now and how you care for yourself. While not all HIV clinics will ask about your past experience, if you feel like this is impacting you, ask someone at the clinic for counselling or for a referral to services that could help you to change the impact trauma has in your life and may be getting in the way of how you care for yourself.

Self-management can be increasingly challenging for those living with these issues. If your ability to care for yourself is being affected by present or previous trauma, it is essential that you include addressing these as part of your self-management plan.

Additional Resources

Risky sex

AIDS.gov: www.aids.gov/hiv-aids-basics/prevention/reduce-your-risk/mixed-status-couples

Centers for Disease Control and Prevention: www.cdc.gov/hiv/basics/prevention.html and
   www.cdc.gov/hiv/riskbehaviors/index.html

Office on Women's Health:
   www.womenshealth.gov/hiv-aids/preventing-hiv-infection/practice-safer-sex.html

Planned Parenthood: http://plannedparenthood.org/learn/stds-hiv-safer-sex/safer-sex

Tobacco

Centers for Disease Control and Prevention: www.cdc.gov/tobacco and www.cdc.gov/tobacco/
   data_statistics/sgr/2010/consumer_booklet

Additional Resources (*continued*)

Healthfinder.gov: www.healthfinder.gov/scripts/SearchContext.asp?topic=860

My HealtheVet: www.myhealth.va.gov

National Cancer Institute: www.cancer.gov or 1-877-44U-QUIT (1-877-448-7878), 8 a.m.–8 p.m., Monday–Friday (EDT)

Office of the Surgeon General: www.surgeongeneral.gov/priorities/tobacco

Office on Women's Health: www.womenshealth.gov/aging/wellness/quitting-smoking.html

Quit Now national hotline: 1-800-QUIT-NOW (1-800-784-8669), 24 hours a day, 7 days a week

Smokefree Women: www.women.smokefree.gov

Smokefree.gov: www.smokefree.gov

U.S. Department of Health and Human Services: www.ahrq.gov/professionals/clinicians-providers/guidelines-recommendations/tobacco/clinicians/tearsheets/helpsmokers.html

U.S. Department of Veterans Affairs, general information: www.publichealth.va.gov/smoking

U.S. Department of Veterans Affairs, *My Smoking Cessation Workbook—A Resource for Patients*: www.va.gov/vhapublications/ViewPublication.asp?pub_ID=2827 and *HIV Provider Smoking Cessation Handbook*: www.va.gov/vhapublications/ViewPublication.asp?pub_ID=2826

UCanQuit2.org: https://ucanquit2.org

Alcohol

National Institute on Alcohol Abuse and Alcoholism: www.niaaa.nih.gov/alcohol-health/overview-alcohol-consumption

Substance Abuse and Mental Health Services Administration (SAMSHA): www.samhsa.gov/treatment/substance-use-disorders

Recreational Drugs

AIDS.gov: www.aids.gov/hiv-aids-basics/staying-healthy-with-hiv-aids/taking-care-of-yourself/substance-abuse-issues/index.html

MentalHealth.gov: www.mentalhealth.gov/what-to-look-for/substance-abuse

National Institute on Drug Abuse: www.drugabuse.gov/publications/research-reports/hivaids/how-does-drug-abuse-affect-hiv-epidemic

Substance Abuse and Mental Health Services Administration (SAMSHA): www.samhsa.gov/treatment/substance-use-disorders

Additional Resources (*continued*)

Physical and Emotional Trauma

Untangling the Intersection of HIV & Trauma: Why It Matters and What We Can Do
http://www.poz.com/pdfs/gmhc_treatmentissues_2013_9.pdf

National HIV/AIDS Strategy for the United States for 2015–2020:
www.aids.gov/federal-resources/national-hiv-aids-strategy/nhas-update.pdf

Addressing the Intersection of HIV/AIDS, Violence against Women and Girls, & Gender–
Related Health Disparities: www.whitehouse.gov/sites/default/files/docs/vaw-hiv
_working_group_report_final_-_9-6--2013.pdf

CHAPTER 6

Working with Your Health Care Team

With all the new medications and research coming out, it might seem that HIV care is impossibly complicated, and that patients should just go to the doctor, listen, and do as the doctor says. But that's not the way chronic diseases work. Patients with chronic diseases spend only a little time with their health care providers. Patients, not doctors, therefore must act as their own "first-line" caregivers—taking medications on their own, and monitoring their daily activities and symptoms on their own or with family members. No matter how complicated or technical your HIV treatment is, no one knows better than you do what problems are arising on a day-to-day basis, or how the care plan fits into your routine.

At the same time that you take care of yourself, you work closely with a health care team. The help of doctors, nurses, and other experts is critical to doing that. To live well with HIV you need to be able to work with your doctor; that means being able to choose doctors and to talk with them about treatments and about how you're doing, and about what you should keep doing and might need to consider changing. These are the topics we will discuss in this chapter.

Choosing a Doctor

Finding the right doctor is a concern for most people, and it is even more important for a person with HIV. There are many different kinds of doctors out there, and sometimes it is difficult to know which type of doctor is right. Although many HIV doctors have specialty training in infectious diseases, no one single type of specialty training is always necessary for treating HIV. Usually, you will want to find an internal medicine specialist ("internist") for adults, or a pediatrician for children.

Not every internist, pediatrician, or even infectious disease specialist is experienced in treating HIV. It is best to find a doctor who is familiar with treating HIV and has taken care of many people with HIV, not just a few. Look for a doctor who has experience, preferably one who has many HIV patients as part of his or her practice.

Another factor to consider when choosing a doctor is finding one that you like and can get along with. The sooner it's possible to find such a doctor, the sooner you can begin to build a partnership and develop the best HIV treatment plan. Being able to establish and maintain this relationship, though, means learning effective ways to communicate with the doctor, especially given the time constraints you must work with during visits.

Communicating with Members of Your Health Care Team

Communicating with health care providers can be a challenge. During an appointment, you may be afraid to talk freely, or you may feel that there is not enough time to discuss everything you would like to. Health professionals may use words you do not understand, or you might not want to share personal and possibly embarrassing information. These fears and feelings can block communications with providers and harm your health.

Providers share the responsibility for poor communication. They sometimes feel too busy or important to take the time to talk with and know their patients. They may ignore or tune out your questions. Their actions or inaction might confuse or offend you.

Although you do not have to become best friends with your providers, you should expect them to be attentive, caring, and able to explain things clearly. This is especially important with chronic HIV, because many people have lots of misconceptions about HIV, and you may be anxious or scared to ask questions to get accurate information. You may think that you can only get the best care by going to specialists. But if you are only seeing specialists, they may not really get to know you and may not be aware of what your other care providers are doing, thinking, or prescribing. These are good reasons to have a primary provider, or a medical "home." A relationship with a provider is much like a business partnership or even a marriage. Establishing and maintaining this long-term relationship may take some effort, but it can make a large difference to your health.

Your provider probably knows more intimate details about you than anyone else, except perhaps your spouse, partner, or parents. You should feel comfortable expressing your fears, asking questions that you may think are "stupid," and negotiating a treatment plan to satisfy you both.

Poor communication is the number one threat to a good relationship with your health care providers. To keep the lines of communication open, make sure you are being realistic and clear about what you want from your providers. Many of us would like our physicians to be like warmhearted computers—gigantic brains, stuffed with knowledge about the human body and mind (especially ours). We want our providers to analyze the situation, read our minds, make a perfect diagnosis, come up with a treatment plan, and tell us what to expect. At the same time, we want them to be warm and caring and to make us feel as though we are their most important patient.

Most providers wish they were just that sort of person. Unfortunately, no one provider can be all things to all patients. Providers are human. They have bad days, they get headaches, they get tired, and they get sore feet. They have families who demand their time and attention, and they may get frustrated by paperwork, electronic record keeping, and large bureaucracies.

Most doctors and other health care professionals endured grueling training. They entered the health care system because they wanted to help sick people, so naturally they can become frustrated when they cannot cure someone with a chronic condition. Many times they must take their satisfaction from improvements rather than cures, or even from slowing the decline of some conditions. Undoubtedly, you have been frustrated, angry, or depressed about your illness

from time to time. Bear in mind that your doctors have probably felt similar emotions about their inability to make you well. In this, you are truly partners.

Time is the second threat to a good patient-provider relationship. If you or your provider could choose the best way to improve your relationship, it would probably involve more face-to-face time. When time is short, the resulting anxiety can bring about rushed communication, and misunderstandings are common.

Most doctors and other providers are on very tight schedules and are often only given 20–30 minutes to spend with each patient. This becomes painfully clear when you have to wait in the doctor's office because of an emergency or a late patient that has delayed your appointment. Doctors try to stay on schedule. This sometimes causes both patients and doctors to feel rushed.

One way to get the most from your visit is to take P.A.R.T. This acronym stands for **Prepare, Ask, Repeat, Take action**. In the following section, we explain more about taking P.A.R.T.

Take P.A.R.T.

Prepare

Ask

Repeat

Take action

Prepare

Before visiting or calling your health care provider, prepare an agenda. What are the reasons for your visit? What do you expect from your doctor? Take the time to make a written list of your concerns or questions. Have you ever thought to yourself, after you walked out of the doctor's office, "Why didn't I ask about . . . ?" or "I forgot to mention . . ." Making a list beforehand helps ensure that your main concerns get addressed. Be realistic in your agenda. If you have 13 different problems, your provider probably cannot deal with all of them in one visit. Star or highlight your two or three most important items.

Give the list to your doctor at the beginning of the visit, and explain that you have starred your most important concerns. By giving your doctor the whole list, you let the doctor see everything in case there is something medically important that is not starred and at the same time you let the doctor know which items are the most important to you. If you wait until the end of your appointment to bring up concerns, there will not be time to discuss them.

Here is an example. The provider asks, "What brings you in today?" and you might say something like, "I have a lot of things I want to discuss this visit [thinking of the day's appointment schedule, the doctor immediately begins to feel anxious], but I know that we have a limited amount of time. The things that most concern me are my shoulder pain, my dizziness, and the side effects from one of the medications I'm taking" [the doctor feels relieved because the concerns are focused and potentially manageable within the appointment time available].

There are two other things to prepare before your visit. Bring a list of all your medications and the dosages. If this is difficult, put all your meds in a bag and bring them with you. Do not forget vitamins and over-the-counter medications and supplements. Even if your provider uses an electronic medical record, your medication list may not be up to date, so be sure to always take your medication list to all of your appointments.

The final thing to prepare is your story. Visit time is short. When the provider asks how you are feeling, some people will go on for several minutes about this and that symptom. It is better to be brief and to the point and make clear statements such as, "I think that overall my anxiety is less, but now I have more trouble sleeping." Be prepared to describe your symptoms, including:

- When they started
- How long they last
- Where they are located
- What you do that makes them better or worse
- Whether you have had similar problems before
- Whether you have changed your diet, exercise, or medications in a way that might contribute to the symptoms
- What worries you most about the symptoms
- What you think might be causing the symptoms

If you have recently begun a new medication or treatment, be ready to report how it is going. If you have several providers, bring a list of all the tests and test results from the past six months.

In telling your story, talk about trends—in other words, are you getting better or worse, or are you the same? Also talk about tempo—are your symptoms more or less frequent or intense? For example, you might tell your doctor, "In general, I am slowly getting better, although last week I did not feel well."

Be as open as you can in sharing your thoughts, feelings, and fears. Remember, your provider is not a mind reader. If you are worried, explain why: "I am worried that I may not be able to work," or "My father had similar symptoms before he died." The more open you are, the more likely it is that your provider can help. If you have a problem, don't wait for the provider to "discover" it. State your concern immediately. For example, "I am worried about this mole on my chest."

The more specific you can be (without overdoing it with irrelevant details), the clearer a picture the doctor will have of your problem, and the less time will be wasted for both of you.

Share your hunches or guesses about what might be causing your symptoms, as they often provide vital clues to an accurate diagnosis. Even if it turns out that your guesses are not correct, it gives your doctor the opportunity to reassure you or address your hidden concerns.

Most importantly, when you doctor asks, "What's the matter?" you need to share what matters most to you.

Ask

Your most powerful tool in the doctor-patient partnership is the question. You can fill in vitally important missing pieces of information and close critical gaps in communication with your questions. Asking all your questions reflects your active participation in the process of care, and that participation is a critical ingredient to managing your health. Getting answers and information you understand is a cornerstone of self-management. Be prepared to ask questions about diagnosis, tests, treatments, and follow-up.

- **Diagnosis.** Ask what's wrong, what caused it, is it contagious, what the future outlook (prognosis) is, and what can be done to prevent or manage it.

- **Tests.** If the doctor wants to do tests, ask how the results are likely to affect your treatment and what will happen if you are not tested. If you decide to have a test, find out how to prepare for the test and what the test will be like. Also ask how and when you will get the results.

- **Treatments.** Ask if there are any choices in treatments and the advantages and disadvantages of each. Ask what will happen if you do not receive treatment.

- **Follow-up.** Find out if and when you should call or return for a follow-up visit. What symptoms should you watch for, and what should you do if they occur?

Repeat

One way to check that you have really understood everything your doctor tells you is to briefly report back key points. For example, "You want me to take this three times a day." This gives the provider a chance to quickly correct any misunderstandings and miscommunications.

If you don't understand or remember something the provider said, admit that you need to go over it again. For example, "I'm pretty sure you told me some of this before, but I'm still confused about it." Don't be afraid to ask what you may consider to be a stupid question. Such questions are important and may prevent misunderstanding.

It can be difficult to remember everything that you discuss in an appointment. Take notes, or bring another person to important visits. You can even record the visit if the medical professional grants permission.

Take Action

At the end of a visit, you need to clearly understand what to do next. This includes treatments, tests, and when to return. You should also know how to recognize any danger signs and what you should do if they occur. If necessary, ask your provider to write down instructions, recommend reading material, or indicate other places you can get help.

If for some reason you can't or won't follow the provider's advice, let her or him know. For example, "I didn't take the Sustiva. It gives me crazy dreams and I can't sleep," or "My insurance doesn't cover that medication. I can't afford it," or "I've tried to quit smoking, but everyone in my house smokes, and I can't seem to stay off cigarettes." If your providers know why you can't or won't follow advice, they may be able to make other suggestions. If you don't share the barriers to taking actions, it's difficult for your providers to help.

Using E-mail to Communicate with Your Doctor

If your providers offer a patient "portal" online, you can send and receive secure e-mail through that system. This is one of the best features of the "electronic medical record" (EMR). E-mail can provide a convenient and effective way to communicate with your doctor and health care team . . . if used with care. Here are some tips:

- **Find out if your doctor uses e-mail** and if you can use a special secure e-mail system. E-mails sent through regular channels do not provide adequate confidentiality and security. Some e-mail systems allow you to attach photos, which is very helpful for communicating about certain types of problems such as rashes.

- **Do not use e-mail in emergencies.** You cannot be sure when your doctor will receive and read your message. Phone your doctor or, if it is a life-threatening emergency, call 911 (in the United States) or its equivalent in your country, or go to a hospital emergency department.

- **Only send e-mail messages to your doctor when necessary.** Use e-mail appropriately and only for issues directly related to your medical condition and care. Don't contact your doctor for routine administrative matters. Many health systems have ways for you to view lab results, request prescription refills, make appointments, and inquire about insurance issues without contacting your doctor directly.

- **Use descriptive subject headers.** This ensures that your doctor can be clear what your message is about. And usually it is best to avoid discussing more than one subject in an e-mail.

- **Keep it short and sweet.** Make your messages clear, direct, and concise. Describe your question or problem as specifically as you can (see tips on describing symptoms on pages 70 and 71). Carefully worded messages prevent a lot of back-and-forth exchanges. If you find that you can't sum up your question or issue in a short paragraph, it's a sign that e-mail is not the best forum for this topic and you probably need to make an appointment.

- **Don't expect an immediate response.** You can request a response in one to three days in your message, but if you don't hear back, pick up the phone and call.

Asking for a Second Opinion

Sometimes you may want to see another provider or get a second opinion. Asking for this can be awkward or uncomfortable. This is especially true if you have had a long relationship with your provider. You may worry that asking for another opinion will anger your provider, or that your provider will take your request in the wrong way.

Providers are seldom hurt by requests for a second opinion. If your condition is complicated or difficult, the doctor may have already consulted with another doctor (or more than one). This is often done informally. However, if you find yourself asking for third, fourth, and fifth opinions, this may be unproductive.

Asking for a second opinion is perfectly acceptable, and providers are taught to expect such requests. Ask for a second opinion by using a nonthreatening "I" message:

"I'm still feeling confused and uncomfortable about this treatment. I feel that another opinion might reassure me. Can you suggest someone I could see?"

In this way, you have expressed your own feelings without suggesting that the provider is at fault. You have also confirmed your confidence in your provider by asking for his or her recommendation. However, you are not bound by this suggestion; you may choose to see anyone you wish. Second opinions may sometimes be more useful if they are from an independent source.

Giving Positive Feedback to Your Providers

Let your provider know how satisfied you are with your care. If you do not like the way you have been treated by any of the members of your health care team, let them know. Likewise, if you are pleased with your care, let your providers know. Everyone appreciates compliments and positive feedback, especially members of your health care team. They are human, and your praise can help nourish and console these busy, hardworking professionals. Letting them know that you appreciate their efforts is one of the best ways to improve your relationship with them!

Your Role in Medical Decisions

Many medical decisions are not clear-cut, and often there is more than one option. The best decisions, except in life-threatening emergencies, depend on your values and preferences and should not be left solely to your doctor. For example, if you have high blood pressure in addition to your HIV, you might say, "I'm very conservative about taking medications, and I'm not sure I want to take even more. Could I try exercise, diet, and relaxation first, before I start taking this medication?"

No one can tell you which choice is right for you. But to make an informed choice, you need information about the treatment options.

Informed choice, not merely informed consent, is essential to quality medical care. The best medical care for you combines your doctor's medical expertise with your own knowledge, skills, and values.

To make an informed choice about any treatment, you need to know what the cost and risks of the proposed treatment are. This includes the likelihood of possible complications such as drug reactions, side effects, bleeding, infection, injury, or death. It also includes the personal costs, such as absences from work, and financial considerations, such as how much of the proposed treatments your insurance will cover.

You also need to understand how likely it is that the proposed treatments will benefit you in terms of prolonging your life, relieving your symptoms, or improving your ability to function. Sometimes the best choice may be to delay a decision about treatment in favor of "watchful waiting."

Making decisions about treatments can be difficult. For some suggestions on how to make decisions, see pages 22–23, and see Chapter 7, "Making Treatment Decisions," for help on how to evaluate new treatments.

Sometimes it is difficult to come up with the right words to communicate with providers. For tips on how to communicate more effectively, see Chapter 16, "Communicating with Family, Friends, and Anyone Else."

Talking to Your Provider about Medications

It is common for people with HIV to be taking several medications: HIV antiviral medications, cholesterol-lowering medications, antidepressants, antacids, plus a handful of over-the-counter (OTC) remedies. *Remember, the more medications you are taking, the greater the risk of drug side effects.* Fortunately, you may be able to reduce the number of medications and the associated risks if you forge an effective partnership with your doctor. Such a relationship requires your participation in determining the need for the medication, selecting the medication, properly using the medication, and reporting back to your doctor the effects of the medication.

An individual's response to a particular medication varies depending upon age, metabolism, activity level, and the waxing and waning of symptoms caused by most HIV diseases. Many medications are prescribed on an as-needed (PRN) basis, so you need to know when to begin and end treatment and how much medication to take. You need to work out a plan with your doctor to suit your individual needs.

For most medications, *your doctor depends on you* to report what effect, if any, the drug has on your symptoms and what side effects you may be experiencing. On the basis of that information, your doctor may continue, increase, discontinue, or otherwise change your medications. A good doctor-patient partnership requires a continuing flow of information. There are important things you need to let your doctor know and critical information you need to receive in return.

Unfortunately, this vital exchange of information is too often shortchanged. Studies indicate that fewer than 5 percent of patients receiving new prescriptions ask their physicians or pharmacists any questions. Doctors tend to interpret patient silence as understanding and satisfaction with the information received. Mishaps often occur because patients either do not receive adequate information about medications and don't understand how to take them, or fail to follow instructions given to them. Safe, effective medication use depends on your understanding of the proper use, the risks, and the necessary precautions associated with each medication you take. *You must ask questions.*

The goal of treatment is to maximize the benefits and minimize the risks. Whether the medications you take are helpful or harmful often depends on how much you know about your medications and how well you communicate with your doctor.

What You Need to *Tell* Your Doctor About Medication

Even if doctors don't ask about your medications, there is certain vital information you should mention to them. The answers to the following questions should be part of your regular communication with your doctor.

Are you taking any medications?

Report *all* the prescription and nonprescription medications you are taking, including experimental medicines, herbs, birth control pills, vitamins, aspirin, antacids, laxatives, eye drops, suppositories, and ointments. This information is especially important if you are seeing more than one health care provider because one may

not know what the others have prescribed. Knowing all the medications you are taking is essential for correct diagnosis and treatment. For example, symptoms such as nausea, diarrhea, sleeplessness, drowsiness, dizziness, memory loss, impotence, and fatigue may be due to a drug side effect rather than your disease.

It is critical for all of your doctors to know what medications you are taking to help prevent problems from drug interactions. This is very important because HIV medications often interact with other common medications. Carry an up-to-date list with you, or at least know the names and dosages of all the medications you are taking. Saying that you are taking "the little green pills" usually doesn't help identify the medication.

Get into the habit of doing a "brown bag" medicine check at least once every six months. The idea is simple: Put all the medicines you're taking into a bag, and bring them with you when you see your doctor. Review *all* the medicines with your doctor, and make sure you know which to continue and which to stop or discard. Don't forget the over-the-counter and the "as-needed" medications!

Are you taking all your prescribed medications?

There are lots of different reasons that people miss taking their medications, at least once in a while. It can be hard to tell your doctors about it when you skip doses. You might feel as if they will be disappointed, or just scold you, rather than telling you anything to help you.

Especially for HIV antiretroviral medications, taking them as prescribed is crucial. But again, people can miss doses for all sorts of reasons.

Sometimes you just forget a dose. Sometimes you get out of your routine—maybe you stayed at a friend's house over the weekend and forgot to bring your medication. It might be hard to find a place to take the medication in private. Maybe you were out partying and got drunk or high, and that led to a missed dose. Whatever the reason, it's important to tell the health care team about it, so together you can problem-solve and come up with solutions.

Have you had allergic or unusual reactions to any medications?

Describe any symptoms or unusual reactions to medication you have taken in the past. Be specific: Which medication and exactly what type of reaction? A rash, fever, or wheezing that develops after you take a medication is often an actual allergic reaction. If any of these symptoms develops, call your doctor at once. Nausea, ringing in the ears, light-headedness, and agitation are likely to be side effects rather than signs of drug allergies.

Do you have any major chronic diseases or medical conditions other than HIV?

Many diseases can interfere with the action of a drug or increase the risk of using certain medications. Diseases involving the kidneys or liver are especially important to mention, because these diseases can slow the metabolism of many drugs and increase toxic effects. Your doctor may also tell you to avoid certain medications if you have or have had such diseases as hypertension, peptic ulcer disease, asthma, heart disease, diabetes, or prostate problems. Be sure to let your doctor know if you could be pregnant or are breastfeeding, since many drugs are not safe to use in those situations.

What medications were tried in the past to treat your disease?

If you have a chronic symptom or symptoms, it is a good idea to keep your own written record of all the medications you have ever taken for the condition and what the effects were. Your past responses to various medications can help guide the doctor's recommendation of any new medications. However, just because a medication did not work well in the past does not necessarily mean that it shouldn't be tried again today or in the future. Diseases change and may become more responsive to treatment.

What You Need to *Ask* Your Doctor About Medication

Make sure to ask the following questions when you talk to your doctor about medication:

Do I really need this medication?

Some physicians decide to prescribe medications not because they are really necessary, but because they think patients want and expect drugs. Don't pressure your physician for medications. If your doctor doesn't prescribe a medication, consider that good news rather than a sign of rejection or indifference. Ask about nondrug alternatives. Many conditions can be treated in a variety of ways, and your physician can explain your options. In some cases, lifestyle changes such as exercise, diet, and stress management should be considered before other choices. When any treatment is recommended, ask what the likely consequences are if you postpone treatment. Sometimes the best medicine is none at all.

What is the name of the medication?

When a medication is prescribed, it is important that you know its name. Write down both the brand name and the generic (chemical) name. (For example, Motrin® is the brand name of the common over-the-counter pain reliever; its generic or chemical name is ibuprofen.) If the medication you get from the pharmacy doesn't have the same name as the one your doctor prescribed, ask the pharmacist to explain the difference.

What is the medication supposed to do?

Your doctor should tell you why the medication is being prescribed and how it is expected to help you. Is the medication intended to prolong your life, completely or partially relieve your symptoms, or improve your ability to function? For example, if you are given an anti-HIV drug combination such as Kaletra® and Truvada®, the purpose is primarily to reduce the HIV in your blood and prevent damage to your immune system. It probably won't stop all of your symptoms, and it might have side effects. On the other hand, if you are given a skin cream, the purpose is to help ease your skin condition.

You should also know how soon you should expect results from the medication. Drugs that treat infections or inflammation may take several days to a week to show improvement, whereas antidepressant medications typically take several weeks to begin working.

How and when do I take the medication, and for how long?

Understanding how much of the medication to take and how often to take it is critical. Does "every six hours" mean "every six hours while awake"? Should the medication be taken before meals, with meals, or between meals? What should you do if you miss a dose? Should you skip it, take a double dose next time, or take it as soon as you realize you missed it? Should you continue taking the medication until the symptoms go away or until the medication is completely used up?

The answers to such questions are very important. For example, if you are taking an antibiotic for a lung infection, you may feel better within a few days, but you should continue taking the medication as prescribed to completely eliminate the infection; otherwise, the infection may come back, perhaps in a stronger, drug-resistant form. If you are using an inhaled medication for breathing problems, the way you use the inhaler determines how much of the medication actually gets into your lungs. Taking medication properly is vital. Yet when patients are surveyed, nearly 40 percent report that they were not instructed by their physicians how to take the medication or told how much to take. If you are not sure about your prescription, call your doctor, nurse, or pharmacist. Such calls are never considered a bother.

What foods, drinks, other medications, or activities should I avoid while taking this medication?

Having food in your stomach can help protect the stomach from some medications, whereas it can render other drugs ineffective. For example, milk products or antacids can decrease the absorption of some drugs (such as Nizoral®) but may increase the absorption of others. Some medications, like Bactrim®, may make you more sensitive to the sun, putting you at increased risk for sunburn. Ask whether a medication will interfere with driving. Other drugs you may be taking, even OTC drugs and alcohol, can either amplify or lessen the effects of the prescribed medication. The more medications you are taking, the greater the chances of undesirable drug interactions.

What are the most common side effects, and what should I do if they occur?

All medications have side effects. You need to know what symptoms to be on the lookout for and what action to take if they develop. Should you seek immediate medical care, discontinue the medication, or call your doctor? Your doctor cannot be expected to list every possible adverse reaction, but the more common and important ones should be discussed. Unfortunately, a recent survey showed that 70 percent of patients starting a new medication did not recall being told by their physicians or pharmacists about precautions and possible side effects. So it may be up to you to ask.

Are tests necessary to monitor the use of this medication?

Some medications are monitored by the improvement or worsening of symptoms. However, many medications used to treat people with HIV can disrupt body chemistry before any telltale symptoms develop. Sometimes these adverse reactions can be detected by laboratory tests such as blood counts or liver function tests. In addition, the levels of some medications in the blood need to be measured periodically to make sure you are getting the right amount. Ask your doctor if the medication being prescribed has any of these special requirements.

Can a generic medication that is less expensive be prescribed?

As mentioned, every drug has at least two names: a generic name and a brand name. The generic name is the nonproprietary, or chemical, name of the drug (e.g., acetaminophen). The brand name is the manufacturer's unique name for the drug (e.g., Tylenol®). When a drug company develops a new drug in the United States, it is granted exclusive rights to produce that drug for 17 years. After the 17-year period has expired, other companies may market chemical equivalents of that drug. These generic medications are generally considered as safe and effective as the original brand-name drug but often cost half as much.

Because many of the single-pill HIV medications (such as Atripla®) are relatively new, often no generic equivalent is available. But costs do differ even between brand-name drugs. If cost is a concern, ask your doctor if there is a lower-cost but equally effective medication. Sometimes you can save money by purchasing medications through the mail. Many health care organizations and mail-order pharmacies offer prescription services.

Is there any written information about the medication?

Realistically, your doctor may not have time to answer all of your questions in detail. Even if your physician carefully answers your questions, it can be difficult for anyone to remember all this information. Fortunately, there are many other valuable sources you can turn to: pharmacists, nurses, package inserts, pamphlets, books, and the Internet. Some useful sources to consult are listed in the "Additional Resources" section at the end of Chapter 8, "Managing Medications for HIV."

A Special Word About Pharmacists . . .

Pharmacists are experts on medications. You can often call them on the phone or walk into a pharmacy without an appointment to find out about medications and how they work. In addition, many hospitals, medical schools, and schools of pharmacy have medication information services you can call to ask questions. As a self-manager, don't forget pharmacists. They are important and helpful consultants.

Working with the Health Care System

So far we have only discussed communication with health care providers. Today most providers work in larger systems such as clinics. Appointments, billing, and telephone and e-mail contact are often decided by someone other than your provider.

If you are unhappy with your health care system, don't just suffer in silence. Do something about it. The problem is that the people who make the decisions tend to isolate themselves. It is easier to express our feelings to the receptionist, nurse, or doctor. Unfortunately, these people have little or no power in the system. But they can tell you who to contact. Find out who is running the organization and who makes decisions. Share your feelings in a constructive way by letter, phone, or e-mail. Most health care systems want to keep you as a patient and therefore usually respond. The more closely you can form a partnership with your providers, the better able all of you together will be to make the system more responsive.

If you do decide to write or e-mail, keep your letter short and factual. Describe what actions you would find helpful. For example:

Dear Mr. Brown:

Yesterday I had a 10:00 A.M. appointment with Dr. Zim. She did not see me until 12:15 P.M., and my total time with the doctor was eight minutes. I was told to make another appointment so I could get my questions answered.

I know that sometimes there are emergencies. I would appreciate being called if my doctor is running late or told when to return. I would also like 15 or more minutes with my doctor.

I would appreciate a reply within two weeks.

The following are a few hints for managing common complaints about the health care system. Not all of these problems and suggestions apply to all systems, but many do.

■ **"I hate the automated phone system."**
Often when you call for an appointment or information, you reach an automated system. This is frustrating. Unfortunately, you cannot change this. However, such phone

systems do not change often. If you can memorize the numbers or keys to press, you can move more quickly from one part of the system to another. If you have trouble memorizing the sequence of numbers or keys, write it down and keep it handy. Sometimes pressing the pound key (#) or 0 will get you to a real person. Once you do get through, ask if there is a way to move through the phone systems faster next time.

■ **"It takes too long to get an appointment."** Ask for the first available appointment. Take it. Then ask how you can learn about cancellations. Some systems are happy to call you when they have an empty spot. In others, you may have to call them once or twice a week to check on cancellations. Ask the person making the schedule what you can do to get an earlier appointment. Ask for a telephone number so you can reach the person making appointments directly. Some organizations set time aside each day for same-day appointments. If this is available, know when to call to request one of these appointment times. The time to call is usually early in the morning. If you are in pain or believe that you must see a doctor soon, tell the scheduler. If nothing is available, ask about the best way to get in to see someone soon. No matter how frustrated you are, be nice. You want the person who schedules appointments to be on your side and want to help you if they can, and you will feel better if you speak pleasantly and do not lose your temper.

■ **"I have so many providers; I do not know whom to ask for what."** One of those providers has to be in charge. Your job is to find out which one. Ask each provider who is in charge of coordinating your care. When you get a name, it is most likely your primary care doctor or general practitioner (GP). Call your doctor's office to confirm that they are coordinating your care. Ask how you can help. Always be sure to let your primary doctor know when someone else orders a test or new medication. Keeping the doctor informed is especially important when your providers are not in the same system and are not sharing their electronic medical records (EMRs).

■ **"What is an electronic medical record (EMR) anyway?"** Most of your medical information is stored on a secure central computer. Your information can be seen by any provider in the same system, and in some cases with other systems in your geographic area. You should know what information about you is on the system. Sometimes the EMR includes just test results, other times it has test results and medication information, and sometimes it has everything that your providers know about you. An electronic medical record is just like a paper record: it does no good if your providers don't read it. For example, when you have a test, the doctor ordering the test will know when the results are ready. However, your other doctors will not know anything about the test unless you tell them to read the results. In short, learn about the medical records system so you can help all your providers use it more effectively.

In the United States and many other countries, you have the right to a copy of almost everything in your record. Ask for copies of all your test results so that you can carry them with you from one provider to the next. In this way, you know they will not get lost.

Today, many health care systems have patient "portals." These give the patient access to the electronic medical record. If your system has a patient portal, sign up for an account. You will most likely gain access to your tests and, more importantly, a message system where you can write to your provider if you have questions or concerns between visits. These systems also may allow you to request prescription refills.

■ **"I can never reach my doctor on the phone."** It is difficult to get a provider on the phone, but you might be able to message them through your patient portal. If it is a medical emergency, however, do not waste time trying to contact your doctor. Rather, call 911 (in the United States) or its equivalent in your country, or go to a hospital emergency department.

■ **"I have to wait too long in the waiting room or the examination room."** Emergencies happen sometimes, and this can cause a wait. More often the system is just inefficient. If your schedule is tight and it may cause a problem if you are delayed at your appointment, call your doctor's office before you are scheduled to arrive. Ask if there is a delay and, if so, how long you will have to wait. If you learn that your doctor is running late, you can decide whether to go with a book to read or ask to reschedule. You can also show up with your book and ask about the wait. Rather than getting upset, let the receptionist know that you are going to step out for a little while to run a short errand nearby or for a cup of coffee or some shopping and that you will return within a specified amount of time.

■ **"I don't have enough time with the provider."** This may be a system problem since someone other than your provider often decides how many patients to schedule and for how long. The decision is sometimes based on what you tell the scheduler. If you say you need a blood pressure check, you will be given a short visit. If you say you are very depressed and cannot function, you may be given a longer appointment.

When making the appointment, request the amount of time you want, especially if this is more than 10 or 15 minutes. Be prepared to make a case for more time. You can also ask for the last appointment in the day. You may have to wait awhile, but at least the provider will not be pressured because there are more patients to see after you.

Remember, though, just like most of us, doctors sometimes have to be somewhere at the end of the day (pick up children at school or day care, for example). Once you are with a provider and you request more time than is allotted, you make other people wait. An extra five minutes may not seem like much. However, a doctor often sees 30 patients a day. If each one takes five extra minutes, this means that the doctor has to work an extra 2½ hours that day! Those little bits of extra time add up.

Parting Words of Advice

- If something in the health care system is not working for you, ask how you can help make it work better. Very often, if you learn how to navigate the system, you can solve or at least partially solve your problems.

- Be nice, and be reasonable. If the system or your provider sees you as a difficult patient, getting what you want out of the system could become more difficult for you.

If you think that you should not need to learn to manage the system and that it is not fair to place this burden on the patient, we wholeheartedly agree. Health systems should change to be more responsive and patient-friendly. A few health care systems are already doing this. In the meantime, the suggestions in this chapter should help you manage your health care system.

Additional Resources

ACT (Canada): www.actoronto.org/home.nsf/pages/choosedoctor

AIDS InfoNet: www.aidsinfonet.org/fact_sheets/view/202

AIDS.gov:
www.aids.gov/hiv-aids-basics/staying-healthy-with-hiv-aids/taking-care-of-yourself/doctor-clinic-and-dental-visits

AIDS.org: www.aids.org/topics/choosing-an-hiv-care-provider

American Academy of HIV Medicine: www.aahivm.org/ReferralLink/exec/default.aspx

The Body: The Complete HIV/AIDS Resource: www.thebody.com/index/choosing.html

Health Resources and Services Administration: http://hab.hrsa.gov/gethelp

HIV Medicine Association Provider Directory: www.hivma.org/cvweb/cgi-bin/memberdll.dll/OpenPage?WRP=hivma_member_search.htm&wmt=none

Medline Plus: www.nlm.nih.gov/medlineplus/talkingwithyourdoctor.html

U.S. Department of Health and Human Services, Office of Women's Health:
www.womenshealth.gov/hiv-aids/living-with-hiv-aids/finding-your-hiv-care-team.html

Suggested Further Reading

To learn more about the topics discussed in this chapter, we suggest that you explore the following resources:

Cichocki, Mark. *Living with HIV: A Patient's Guide.* Jefferson, N.C.: McFarland & Company, Inc., 2009.

Jones, J. Alfred, Gary L. Kreps, and Gerald M. Phillips. *Communicating with Your Doctor: Getting the Most Out of Health Care.* Cresskill, N.J.: Hampton Press, 1995.

McKay, Matthew, Martha Davis, and Patrick Fanning. *Messages: The Communication Skills Book.* Oakland, Calif.: New Harbinger, 2009.

CHAPTER 7

Making Treatment Decisions

MOST PEOPLE WITH HIV KNOW A LOT ABOUT how important it is to take antiretroviral therapy (ART) drugs. HIV medication today is excellent, with many options. But taking the right medications is just one of many treatment decisions people with HIV make. You hear about new treatments, new drugs, nutritional supplements, and alternative treatments all the time. Drug and nutritional supplement companies run commercials during the television news and place large ads in newspapers and magazines. Your e-mail box may be filled with promises of new treatments or cures from spammers. In the market and pharmacy, you are bombarded with signs and packaging for over-the-counter immune boosters. Not only that, your health care providers may recommend new procedures, medications, or other treatments for any of the health challenges you are facing.

What can you believe? How can you decide what might be worth a try?

An important part of managing your own care is being able to evaluate these claims or recommendations so that you can make an informed decision about trying something new. There are some important questions that you should ask yourself when making a decision about any treatment, whether it is a mainstream medical treatment, or a complementary or alternative treatment.

HIV treatment has come a very long way since the days when HIV medications were first developed. There are now many medications available to treat HIV. If they're started at the right time and monitored, the virus can be controlled and people with HIV can live long, full, healthy lives. In this chapter, we first discuss questions to think about as you consider treatment. In the following sections, we discuss important tests you need for HIV treatment. See Chapter 8, "Managing Medications for HIV," for more information about HIV medications and treatment options.

Questions to Think About When Making Treatment Decisions

Recall that making decisions is an important tool in your self-management toolbox. In order to make good decisions, you need to ask good questions. When you are considering a treatment option, begin by asking the following questions:

Where did I learn about this treatment?

Was it reported in a scientific journal, a supermarket tabloid, a print or TV ad, a website, or a flyer you picked up somewhere? Did your doctor suggest it?

The source of the information is important. Results that are reported in a respected scientific journal are more believable than those you might see in a supermarket tabloid or in advertising. Results reported in scientific journals such as the *New England Journal of Medicine*, *Lancet*, or *Science* are usually from research studies. These studies are carefully reviewed for scientific integrity by scientists, who are very careful about what they approve for publication. Many alternative treatments and nutritional supplements, in contrast, have not been studied scientifically, so they are not as well represented in the scientific literature as medical treatments are. If you are considering an alternative treatment or supplement, you need to be extra careful and critical about analyzing what you read or hear.

Were the people who got better from this treatment like me?

In the past, many studies were done with people who were easy for the medical profession to find, so older studies were often done on college students, nurses, or white men. This has changed, but it is still important to find out if the people that benefitted from the treatment are similar to you. Are they the same age as you? Do they lead similar lifestyles? Do they have the same health problems as you? Are they the same gender and race? If the people aren't like you, the results may not be the same for you.

Could anything else have caused the positive changes from this treatment?

A woman returns from a two-week stay at a spa in the tropics and reports that her fatigue improved dramatically thanks to the special diet and supplements she received. But is it correct to attribute her improvement to the treatment when the warm weather, relaxation, and pampering may have had even more to do with her improvement?

If you start a new treatment and you think it is causing positive changes, it is important to look at everything that has changed since you started this particular treatment. People commonly adopt a generally healthier lifestyle when they are starting a new treatment—could that be playing a part in the improvement? Did you start another medication or diet or exercise program at the same time? Has the weather improved? Are you under less stress than before you started the treatment? Can you think of anything else that could have affected your health?

Does taking the treatment mean that I have to stop other medications or treatments?

If a new treatment requires that you stop taking another basic medication because of dangerous interactions, this requires a discussion with your health care provider before making the change.

Does a proposed new treatment suggest not eating a well-balanced diet?

If a new treatment requires that you eliminate any important nutrients or stresses only a few nutrients, it may not be a good idea. Maintaining a balanced diet is important for your overall health. Be sure that you're not sacrificing important vitamins if you change your eating habits. Also be sure to avoid putting excessive stress on your organs by concentrating on only a few nutrients to the exclusion of others.

Can I think of any possible dangers or harm that might result from this treatment?

Some treatments take a toll on your body. All treatments have side effects and possible risks. Discuss these matters thoroughly with your health care provider. Only you can decide if the potential problems are worth the possible benefit, and you must have all the information in order to make that decision.

Many people think that if something is natural, it must be good for you. This may not be true. "Natural" isn't necessarily better. Just because something comes from a plant or animal doesn't make it good for you. For example, the powerful heart medication digitalis comes from the foxglove plant. It is "natural," but the dosage must be exact or it could be dangerous. Similarly, hemlock comes from a plant, but it is a deadly poison. Some treatments may be safe in small doses but dangerous in larger doses. Be careful.

It is important to know that nutritional supplements don't have the same safeguards as medications. In most countries, including the United States, no regulatory agency is responsible for determining if what is listed on the label of a nutritional supplement is actually what's inside the bottle. Do some research about the company selling the product before you try it. A good place to start is ConsumerLab (www.consumerlab.com).

Can I afford it?

Some treatments may cost a great deal of money, and sometimes it's money that you will have to pay yourself because the treatment is not covered by insurance. Do you have the money to give this treatment the chance it needs to produce an improvement? In addition to costing money, some treatments can involve other sorts of challenges or costs. Is your health strong enough to maintain this new regimen? Will you be able to handle it emotionally? Will it put a strain on your relationships at home or work?

Am I willing to go to the trouble or expense?

Some treatments may involve travel, disruption of daily routines, and other inconveniences. Do you have a clear understanding of what might be involved in the treatments, and are you prepared to accept that? Do you have the necessary support in place?

If you ask yourself all of these questions and decide to try a new treatment on your own, it is very important to inform your health care professional about it. After all, you are partners, and you need to keep your partner informed on your progress during the time you are taking the treatment.

The Internet can provide information about new treatments very quickly and is therefore a resource for up-to-date information about these treatments. But be cautious. Not every piece of information on the Internet is correct or even safe. Seek out the most reliable sources by noting the author or sponsor of the site and the site's URL (Internet address). Addresses ending in .edu, .org, and .gov are generally more objective and reliable; they originate from universities, nonprofit organizations, and governmental agencies, respectively.

Some .com or .biz sites can also be good, but because they are maintained by commercial or for-profit organizations, their information may be biased in favor of their own products, or they may sell advertising space on their site. One source of useful information about questionable treatments is Quackwatch, a nonprofit group whose purpose is to combat health-related frauds, myths, fads, and fallacies (www.quackwatch.org). Other useful sites are accessible from the Quackwatch site.

Sometimes it is wise to say no to conventional medical treatments as well. For example, after reviewing the medical evidence, various medical specialty organizations have recommended that nearly 50 common treatments and procedures should generally *not* be done. (See www .choosing wisely.org.) For more information on finding resources on the Internet and elsewhere, see Chapter 18, "Finding Resources."

Making decisions about new treatments can be difficult, but a good self-manager uses the questions presented in this chapter and the decision-making steps in Chapter 2, "Becoming an HIV Self-Manager," to achieve the best personal results.

Monitoring HIV and Your Immune System

People with HIV may get lots of different blood tests, but two blood tests are particularly important for monitoring HIV and helping you and your doctor to make treatment decisions. The first key blood test is the HIV viral load test, also called the HIV plasma RNA test or the PCR test. Many people just refer to it as the "viral load." This test measures how active the HIV virus is in your blood. The second important blood test is the T-cell or CD4 cell test. The terms CD4 cell and T cell both refer to the same type of cell—a CD4 T lymphocyte—and are often used interchangeably. CD4 cells or T cells are white blood cells that help protect your body from infection by activating your body's immune response. When a person is infected with HIV, the virus attacks and destroys CD4 cells. The T-cell or CD4 test measures the damage HIV has done to your immune function. It is important that you know the basics of these tests to understand and consider treatments for HIV.

HIV Viral Load

The HIV virus is constantly multiplying in a person infected with HIV, but whether it multiplies quickly or very slowly depends on the immune system and on the medications being used. Measuring the level of HIV in the blood is a way of telling how active the virus is. The more HIV in the blood, the more quickly the virus can damage the immune system. People with a high level of HIV activity in their blood (high viral load) and more immune system damage are the people who most need to take anti-HIV medications, including antiretrovirals. People with very low HIV in their blood (low viral load) and little immune system damage can also benefit from antiretroviral, but they may be advised to wait to start certain treatments.

There are different viral load tests that measure HIV in the blood, but they all count the number of HIV particles (HIV RNA) in the blood. Measurements are usually reported as the number of virus copies in each milliliter of blood. The virus may be undetectable (usually fewer than 50 copies per milliliter), it may

be detectable but low (fewer than 10,000 to 30,000 copies per milliliter), or it may be quite high (over a million copies per milliliter). The numbers range widely, and a very large drop in viral levels is possible with effective treatment. This means that someone with 100,000 or even a million HIV copies per milliliter before treatment can drop to less than 50 copies per milliliter with effective HIV antiretroviral treatment. When that happens, the virus is still in the body, and it could come back if antiretroviral medications stop, but when the virus is undetectable, it can't damage the immune system.

T-Cell or CD4 Cell Count

Whereas the viral load test tells how active the virus is, the T-cell count is the best way to monitor how much HIV has affected the immune system, and how strong your immune system is. The T-cell count is a blood test that measures the number of T cells (also called T helper cells and CD4 cells) in each microliter of blood. Because T-cells are important in fighting infections and cancers, having a low T-cell count increases the risk of illness. But T-cell counts change quite a bit, even in healthy, HIV-negative people. Many things affect the T-cell count, such as stress, sleep, time of day, the lab where the test was done, and whether the patient has other infections. The T-cell count is a bit like your blood pressure. It's important, but it goes up and down, and the overall trend is more important than any single reading. You should measure your T-cell count every three to six months.

Generally speaking, a T-cell count between 500 and 1800 is normal for adults. A count between 200 and 500 indicates that the immune system is weakened. People who have counts in this range can sometimes get certain infections, but they are usually not at high risk of getting the most serious AIDS illnesses. HIV-related opportunistic infections usually do not affect people with a T-cell count over 200. Kaposi's sarcoma (KS), tuberculosis (TB), and lymphoma are exceptions, but when a person's T-cell count is over 200, these diseases are less dangerous. Problems such as oral candidiasis (thrush) and skin problems might also appear when the T-cell count is over 200.

A T-cell count between 50 and 200 indicates that the immune system is severely weakened. Recall from Chapter 1 that when HIV infection becomes AIDS, the disease is serious and can cause many symptoms. The line between having symptomatic HIV and having "full-blown AIDS" is a matter of degree of damage to the immune system. One of the ways health care providers decide that a person who has HIV is sick with full-blown AIDS is if the T-cell count is 200 or less. Many opportunistic infections (the infections that develop when the immune system is weak, but not when it's strong—see Chapter 3, "Health Problems of People with HIV") occur when the T-cell count is 200 or lower. People with T counts lower than 200 definitely should take a special medication to prevent *Pneumocystis* pneumonia (PCP). Still, even though they are at risk and need to take medication, many people with T cells lower than 200 can feel healthy and have no symptoms.

A T-cell count below 50 indicates that the T-cell part of the immune system is not functioning. Good, comprehensive medical care is vital, and treatment with medicines to prevent opportunistic infections is very important. Most people who die of AIDS have a T-cell count below 50. Both the HIV viral load and the T-cell count must be considered in order to monitor how an individual person is doing.

With the strong and effective HIV antiretroviral medications that are available, why would a person have a low T-cell count below 200, or even below 50? The simple answer is that there are always some people that either can't take or don't take HIV medications, even though they need them. Or if they do take them, they might do it erratically—missing pills sometimes by mistake, or maybe intentionally. In these circumstances, the medications can't work properly, and sometimes the virus can develop resistance to the medications. Another reason that people can have very low T cells and get very sick is that many people with HIV have never been tested, so they don't know that they have the virus. In fact, about one quarter of all the people with HIV in the United States are like this. They don't get treatment and may not be using condoms or having safe sex, because they don't know they have the virus in the first place.

Now that you understand the importance of your involvement in treatment decisions, as well as the two tests used to help inform those decisions, in the next chapter we will explore the critical role of medications in controlling HIV infection.

Additional Resources

American Board of Internal Medicine Foundation's Choosing Wisely: www.choosingwisely.org

ConsumerLab: www.consumerlab.com

National Center for Complementary and Integrative Health: https://nccih.nih.gov

Quackwatch: www.quackwatch.org

CHAPTER 8

Managing Medications for HIV

SUCCESSFULLY MANAGING HIV INVOLVES TAKING the right medications at the right time. Therefore, a very important self-management task is to understand your medications and use them appropriately. In this chapter, we discuss general issues relating to the role of medications in fighting HIV, and specific medications that may be prescribed to you, including antiretroviral therapy (ART) drugs and preventive and treatment medications. Our goal in this chapter is to empower you with some of the basic information you'll need to effectively self-manage your medications for HIV as an active partner in your care.

HIV treatment is complicated. Even experienced doctors and other health care workers need all their professional skills and knowledge to do it well. To help make sure you are getting the best treatment you can, you need to know the basics about medication, too.

A Few General Words About Medications and HIV

Almost nothing is as aggressively advertised as medications. When we read a magazine, listen to the radio, log onto e-mail, visit websites, or watch TV, we are bombarded with a constant stream of ads aimed at convincing us that if we just take this pill or that tablet, our symptoms will be cured. "Recommended by 90 percent of doctors surveyed!" "Shouldn't *you* try Lyrica®?"

Almost as a backlash to this advertising, we have been taught to avoid taking excess medications. We have all heard about or experienced some of the ill effects of medications. The media also tell us, "Just say 'no' to drugs" and "Drugs can kill." It is all very confusing.

Medications are a very important part of managing HIV. So far, medications cannot completely cure the disease, but they can do many things to help people live well:

- Medications that fight HIV directly (such as antiretroviral therapy, or ART medications) reduce the level of virus and can *slow or stop the disease process*. Drug combinations such as Atripla® (efavirenz/emtricitabine/tenofovir), for example, can reduce the effects of HIV and improve the immune system.

- Medications help *prevent problems from starting*. For example, people at high risk for *Pneumocystis* pneumonia can take medicines to keep from ever getting the disease. In pregnant women with HIV, ART medications can prevent the baby in the womb from getting HIV.

- Medications *reduce symptoms* through their chemical actions. For example, pain medications decrease activity in nerve cells, which can decrease pain sensations. Nausea medications decrease stomach hyperactivity, which relieves stomach upset.

- Finally, there are medications that *replace substances that the body is no longer producing adequately*. Hormones such as testosterone and epoetin (Procrit®) are medications of this type.

In all cases, the purpose of medication is to lessen the consequences of disease or to slow its course. However, many of the drugs doctors prescribe will not have an immediate positive effect that you can feel instantly when you take them. Sometimes a drug will stabilize a condition that would have gotten worse without the drug. Sometimes a drug may only slow down a deterioration that would have been more rapid without the drug. It can be easy to think that a drug isn't doing anything. Except for drugs that are taken just for symptoms, it's hard to judge by how you feel whether medications are working.

This is why it's important to talk openly with your doctor about your medications and discuss any changes you may want to make. This is *especially* true with ART medications. If you stop taking some of them, or if you skip doses, you may make the HIV in your body resistant. This could make your HIV stronger rather than weaker and cause the disease to get worse instead of better.

What Medications Are Available to Treat HIV/AIDS?

The main treatments used for HIV/AIDS are medications that act in one of three ways:

- *Antiretrovirals* (also referred to as antiretroviral therapy, or ART drugs) fight the HIV itself by preventing the virus inside the body from reproducing. That is why these drugs are called "inhibitors." Protease inhibitors, reverse-transcriptase inhibitors, integrase inhibitors, entry inhibitors, and all the other ART drugs work this way.

- *Preventive medicines* prevent specific opportunistic infections (see Chapter 3, "Health Problems of People with HIV," for more about these infections). People with HIV are carefully monitored to find out when they are at high risk for certain specific diseases (see Chapter 7, "Making Treatment Decisions"). If they move into a high-risk group, they can start taking preventive medicines. Preventive strategies for *Pneumocystis* pneumonia, tuberculosis, toxoplasmosis, and *Mycobacterium avium* complex (MAC) are effective and well established.

- *Treatment medicines* are used to treat specific opportunistic infections and diseases once they are identified.

In this chapter, we discuss some of the more common medications used in HIV care. However, new medications for HIV are being developed all the time, and much more extensive and detailed descriptions of older and newer HIV medications are widely available in books or on the Internet (see "Additional Resources"

on page 104). Because research and experience with these medications is changing rapidly, we strongly suggest that you consult your physician, provider (NPs and PA's prescribe ART in the US and internationally), pharmacist, and a recent online or print drug reference book for the latest information.

Taking Antiretroviral (ART) Medications

Many different types of medications are prescribed for people with HIV (see Table 8.1 on pages 106–110), including antibiotics that fight a variety of infections and medications that treat symptoms such as pain and depression. But anti-HIV (antiretroviral) drugs are the ones that specifically attack HIV itself. These drugs are the main treatment for HIV, and improvement in these types of drugs in recent years has made a dramatic difference in many people's lives.

Antiretroviral medications get the most attention of the medications used by people with HIV. Again, ART stands for "antiretroviral therapy" and refers to combinations of three or more antiretroviral drugs that are taken together. These are often referred to as "cocktail" drugs. ART drugs are powerful and effective. In many people, they lower HIV in the blood so much that it can't be detected by blood tests. With the help of ART, many people who were very sick with HIV improve and can often return to active, healthy lives. Others can take the medications to keep from ever getting sick, or from even becoming HIV-infected in the first place.

That's the good part. The downside is that these drug combinations do not work well for everyone. Sometimes there can be drug interactions, resistance, or side effects. And taking ART can be difficult. Being on ART means always taking at least three different HIV medications at the same time. However, today these three medications are often put into one pill that is taken once a day. When you decide to be on ART, it is very important that you take the medication regularly, as discussed with your doctor, without missing any doses.

People who do well with ART medications are those who understand that they won't always be easy to take, but who decide to take them anyway. All medications can have side effects in at least some of the people who take them, and ART medications are no exception. In Chapter 7, "Making Treatment Decisions," we discuss issues to consider when making the decision to start on any treatment plan. In this chapter we describe the basics of HIV medications. We discuss side effects in Chapter 9, "Managing Side Effects of Medications."

The number of anti-HIV ART drugs available is growing every year. Once there were only a few different ART medication combinations. Now there are many drugs, and hundreds of combinations. Guidelines for treating HIV all recommend that at least three anti-HIV drugs be used in combination (often in one pill) whenever ART is given.

The table at the end of this chapter lists the different HIV medications available when this book was published. There is more information out there about medications and treatment, much of it on the Internet. Our goal here is to give you a good starting point for talking with your doctor and doing more of your own research.

How ART Medications Work

HIV lives in the body by making copies of itself, in a complicated series of chemical steps. If the virus *can't* copy itself, the immune system keeps the virus under control so that no HIV is detectable in the blood. As long as HIV isn't circulating in the blood, it can't damage your body. ART medications work by blocking the different steps the virus uses to copy itself. Here we discuss some of the different types of drugs that are part of ART, what each of them does in the body, and the importance of taking them in combination.

Reverse transcriptase is one of the chemicals that HIV uses to copy itself. Reverse transcriptase occurs naturally in the body. Many HIV drugs work by blocking reverse transcriptase. This is how nucleoside drugs such as zidovudine (Retrovir®), lamivudine (Epivir®), and abacavir (Ziagen®) work. The drugs "fool" the reverse transcriptase into trying to use them (instead of the virus) as raw material to make HIV copies, and so they block the copying. Non-nucleoside reverse-transcriptase inhibitors (NNRTIs), such as nevirapine (Viramune®), efavirenz (Sustiva®), and rilpivirine (Edurant®), work by binding to reverse transcriptase and blocking its action.

Protease is another naturally occurring chemical that HIV uses fairly late in the process of copying itself. Drugs that block the protease—called protease inhibitors—are very powerful anti-HIV drugs and have become a crucial part of ART combinations. Medications such as nelfinavir (Viracept®), atazanavir

(Reyataz®), and darunavir (Prezista®) are all protease inhibitors.

In order to copy itself and multiply in the body, HIV first has to *get inside* the human cell. Entry inhibitors block the virus from ever getting into cells in the first place. Maraviroc (Selzentry®) and enfuvirtide (Fuzeon®) are entry inhibitors.

The newest class of HIV drugs are the integrase inhibitors. These drugs stop the virus from integrating into DNA. In this way, they stop HIV from copying itself and taking over more immune cells. There are currently three approved integrase inhibitors—dolutegravir (Tivicay®), elvitegravir (Vitekta®), and raltegravir (Isentress®)—as well as two combination drugs co-formulated with integrase inhibitors in a single pill.

Drug Resistance and HIV

If all these drugs block the copying of HIV, why is it important to use two, three, or four different drugs at the same time? The reason is that HIV has the ability to become resistant to drugs. People who take only one HIV drug can develop resistant HIV within months—or even weeks, in some cases. Once a person develops resistance to an HIV drug, that drug won't work against that person's resistant HIV. Because drug-resistant HIV can then be passed on to other people, it is a big problem not only for the person who has it, but also for people who may catch it from that person.

HIV becomes resistant to a drug when the virus itself changes its structure so the drug can no longer attach to it, or otherwise can't do its work against the virus. How HIV does this is pretty complicated, but the good news is this: even though HIV can become resistant to *one* drug, it can't become resistant to three, four, or

more drugs *when they are taken at the same time*. It's almost as if the virus can only do its special "structure-changing" trick for one drug "enemy" at a time. When facing many drugs, HIV just can't defend itself. This is why multidrug ART is so effective, and why you shouldn't take only one HIV drug or skip taking your medications.

Like the viral load and T-cell tests discussed in Chapter 7, "Making Treatment Decisions," blood tests for resistance to HIV drugs are important tools. Doctors use them to find out if a patient has drug-resistant HIV. Whether the person develops drug resistance or catches a virus that is resistant from the start, these tests help doctors tell which ART medications an individual's HIV can respond to.

There are two main types of resistance tests. Genotype tests detect mutations directly on the HIV genes that cause drug resistance. Genotype-resistance tests give quick results, but they can be difficult to interpret and understand. In contrast, phenotype tests measure the HIV virus's ability to grow when exposed to different ART drugs. It takes longer to get the results of phenotype tests, and they cost more than genotype tests, but they can still be helpful in some situations.

In general, HIV-drug-resistance tests are most useful if you have been taking ART medications but the HIV is not responding. The tests may help tell you and your doctor *why* the HIV is not responding, and help you and your health care team to choose a new, better ART combination.

The Importance of Adherence

"Adherence" means that after you and your doctor have agreed on what medications to try, *you stick to taking the medications exactly as they are prescribed by the doctor.* If it is impossible for you to stick to the medications because of side effects or for some other reason, you need to talk about the problem with the doctor right away. It's very important to not miss any pills—whether by forgetting, intentionally skipping, lowering the dose, or changing the schedule.

There is so much information about ART medications, and so many details to think about, that sometimes it's hard to see the big picture. Antiretroviral medications have transformed HIV care, and they are very effective for many people. They may be effective for you—but they also require a big commitment. Taking ART is work. When patients take ART they must take it consistently, without missing any doses. ART can lead to side effects or drug resistance if not taken correctly. On the other hand, the benefits are real: people who take ART correctly are much less likely to get AIDS-related infections and are much less likely to die. The sooner that people start taking HIV medicines after they are infected with the virus, the less chance they have of developing other chronic health conditions (such as cardiovascular disease and osteoporosis). People who take HIV medications typically feel a lot stronger and healthier, too. ART has revolutionized the lives of people with HIV.

Adhering to ART regimens can be difficult for all sorts of reasons. For one thing, HIV treatment plans can be complicated. Research with people who have diseases that are much simpler than HIV (high blood pressure, for example) indicates that many people have difficulty adhering to even the simplest treatment plans. And HIV treatment plans are *not* simple. ART therapy sometimes involves taking many pills

each day. Some HIV medications must be taken on an empty stomach, while others must be taken with meals. All this can be difficult, especially for people who are sick, weak, or experiencing severe HIV symptoms. To make it even more difficult, people with HIV usually need to continue their treatments for the rest of their lives. That can seem like a daunting task.

Side effects also can make it hard to stick with HIV treatment. Medications can cause problems such as nausea, headaches, diarrhea, tiredness, or dizziness. Although it's much harder to stay on a medication that is causing side effects, it's not impossible. Many side effects ease off with time or can be managed using simple techniques. Some of these techniques are discussed in Chapter 9, "Managing Side Effects of Medications."

For many people, the major problem with taking the medicines is that they don't fit well into some daily routines. The medications aren't convenient, so doses are forgotten. You may sleep through a dose, you may be away from home or be too busy at work, or you may simply forget.

Whether you're about to start HIV medications or you're already on ART drugs, the following are some helpful things that you can do to make your ART treatment successful.

If you are considering starting ART . . .

1. *Play an active role in the treatment plan.* Ask your doctor to describe all your options, including the potential benefits and risks of starting treatment now instead of later. Also ask your doctor to explain side effects or other problems that could be associated with the medication. If you're going to make

the effort necessary to take these medications correctly, you need to understand the goals of treatment and exactly how to achieve them.

2. *Let your doctor know about personal issues that may make it hard for you to take the medications.* Be honest. Some things, such as cost, use of recreational drugs or alcohol, or problems with housing or mental illness are not easy to talk about, but they should be discussed. It's also important to let your doctor know if you don't want other people in your house knowing you take HIV medications. Studies have shown that adherence to a treatment plan can be more difficult—but not impossible—for people dealing with drugs or alcohol or other personal problems. Adherence also may be more difficult for people who have very complex regimens or who have had problems taking medications in the past.

 You can't always be sure what the problems are going to be. Some people do a "dry run" before they begin taking the actual medications, practicing the treatment using jellybeans or other candy instead of real pills. This can help you anticipate what problems could arise.

3. *Ask for a written or digital copy of your treatment plan.* It's helpful to have a list that shows each medication, when and how much to take each time, and whether it must be taken with food or on an empty stomach. Many doctors can give you a list that has pictures of the pills so you won't get them confused. At the end of this chapter, we'll refer you to one such guide

that is current at the time of this book's publication.

4. Most importantly, *talk to your doctor about how to make your treatment fit your lifestyle.* For example, you might discuss how you can link the taking of medicines to certain things that you do each day—waking up in the morning, brushing your teeth, taking a child to school, leaving work, or watching a certain TV show. People who arrange their medication schedule around their daily routine adhere to their treatment plans better than those who don't.

5. *Make sure you can make a personal commitment to the treatment plan.* Talk to your doctor about all your concerns. Ask as many questions as you need to in order to feel good about committing to a treatment plan. You may need to talk things over more than once before you feel comfortable about starting the anti-HIV drugs.

If you are already on ART drugs and want to do better at taking them . . .

There are lots of strategies you can try, and it's vital that you find one that works for you. Here are some ideas:

1. *Keep your medications where you'll see them.* Some people find it helpful to keep their first morning dose next to the alarm clock or the coffeepot. Others keep backup medication supplies at work or in a briefcase. However, if children are around, be careful to store your medications safely to prevent accidental access.

2. *Use daily or weekly pillboxes to organize your medications.* Some people count and set out

a week's medications at a time, with one box or space for each part of the day. It often works well to count out pills at the same time each week, like every Sunday night at bedtime.

3. *Plan ahead for weekends, holidays, trips, and changes in routine.* Many studies have shown that weekends are a big problem for adherence. Decide ahead of time how you will remember to take all of your doses. Make a plan for remembering your medications, and write it out.

4. *Use timers, alarm clocks, pagers, or other tools to remind you when to take your medication.* There are a lot of tools out there, and one might work for you. For example, almost all cell phones have a reminder system, and you can download apps to remind you to take your medicine. Take each medication at the same time every day.

5. *Keep a medication diary.* You can write the names of your drugs on a small card or in your daily planner, and then check off each dose as you take it. Again, there are many free apps to help you track your medication routine, such as care4today (www.care4today.com).

6. *Get help and support from your family and friends.* You don't always have to go it alone. If you can, ask family members, friends, or loved ones to remind you to take your medication. Some people also find it helpful to join an HIV support group.

7. *Don't run out of medication.* Be sure to call your doctor or clinic if your supply won't last until your next visit. Many pharmacies offer mail service for a three-month supply of your medication. If your particular plan allows it, you can sign up for automatic refills, and a new supply of medication arrives automatically at your home toward the end of the three-month period. This type of service can help ensure you always have enough medications on hand.

ART Medications for Pregnant Women with HIV

Women with HIV who are pregnant can pass the virus to their babies. But if they take ART medications while they are pregnant, the chance that the baby will get HIV is very low. It is very important for all women to get tested for HIV early in pregnancy, so that any woman who does have HIV can take antiretroviral medications to protect the baby.

Several different medication combinations can prevent passage of HIV from mother to child. Zidovudine and lamivudine has been used widely in the past and may be combined with a protease inhibitor mix such as atazanavir and ritonavir. But many other combinations may also work well. If you are pregnant and know you have HIV, it is very important to talk to your doctor and your obstetrician to get good advice. And women who don't know their HIV status should always be sure to be tested very early in pregnancy.

After the baby is born, the baby must also take anti-HIV medications for a while. By administering medication to both the pregnant mother and the new baby, HIV in newborn babies has been almost eliminated in the United States, Canada, and much of Europe. This is one of the biggest successes in HIV treatment worldwide.

Taking Preventive Medications

Even with good ART medications available, specific antibiotics are still important for preventing opportunistic infections. (For more on opportunistic infections see Chapter 3, "Health Problems of People with HIV.") Here we list some of the major AIDS opportunistic infections, along with descriptions of the medicines used to prevent and treat them. For more on the side effects of these medications, see Chapter 9, "Managing Side Effects of Medications."

Pneumocystis Pneumonia (PCP)

Examples: trimethoprim/sulfamethoxazole (TMP/SMX; Bactrim®, Septra®), aerosolized pentamidine, dapsone (and dapsone + pyrimethamine + leukovorin). Atovaquone may also be an appropriate preventive medication for some people.

How they work: These medications work by giving a steady, low dose of antibiotic to kill *Pneumocystis jiroveci* (formerly known as *Pneumocystis carinii*), a common fungus that causes pneumonia, before there are enough organisms to create a true pneumonia.

Possible side effects: The most common side effect of TMP/SMX is an allergic skin reaction resulting in rashes, which can be successfully managed. Fair-skinned people on TMP/SMX are also sensitive to sunlight and should wear sunscreen and protective clothing when they are outdoors. Other side effects include minor fevers, nausea, low white blood cell count, decreased

platelet count, and liver irritation. Dapsone is associated with less severe occurrence of nausea, vomiting, rashes, lowered red and white cell counts, and liver function problems. People with low levels of G6PD (a liver function indicator) can develop rapid loss of blood cells on dapsone, so a G6PD test should be done before starting dapsone treatment. Aerosolized pentamidine is inhaled into the lungs rather than taken as a pill, so its most common side effect is a cough or raspy, dry throat, which can be minimized or eliminated by using inhaled medicines such as albuterol. Other side effects include a burning sensation in the back of the throat, an unpleasant taste, brief lung spasms, and (rarely) a mild decrease in blood sugar. Atovaquone has fewer side effects, but it is expensive.

Comments: TMP/SMX works extremely well for preventing PCP and is the recommended therapy; almost no one who takes it regularly (daily or three times per week) comes down with the disease. The problem is that some people experience toxic reactions to TMP/SMX. These people may be able to take the medication if they take a gradually increasing dose so that their bodies can get used to it. Otherwise, they should use one of the other medications.

Toxoplasmosis ("Toxo")

Examples: trimethoprim/sulfamethoxazole (TMP/SMX; Bactrim®, Septra®), dapsone + pyrimethamine + leukovorin, and atovaquone are all used to prevent toxoplasmosis.

How they work: As with *Pneumocystis*, the idea is to kill the *Toxoplasma gondii* organisms when they are present at microscopic levels, before they have started to actually invade the body. These medications work by giving a steady low dose of antibiotic. Steady low doses are particularly important for people with a low CD4 cell count (see Chapter 7, "Making Treatment Decisions") and with a positive blood *Toxoplasma* antibody test.

Possible side effects: The side effects of TMP/SMX and dapsone are the same whether these drugs are used for toxoplasmosis or *Pneumocystis* prevention. Atovaquone has fewer side effects but can include nausea, vomiting, diarrhea, rash, or headache. Pyrimethamine can cause loss of red blood cells in some people but is well tolerated in most.

Comments: People who need toxoplasmosis prevention almost always need *Pneumocystis* prevention, too, so taking either TMP/SMX or dapsone can accomplish both goals. The other medications are less well proven but can be considered for a person who is taking aerosolized pentamidine to prevent *Pneumocystis* and therefore needs another medicine to prevent toxoplasmosis.

People need medications to prevent PCP and toxo when their CD4 cell count (T-cell count) is lower than 200 per microliter. With ART medications, many people can boost their immune systems so that their counts get above 200 and stay there. When this happens, they and their doctors may decide that they no longer need to take medicines to prevent PCP or toxo. But of course they still need to stay on the ART medications to keep the immune system strong, and they need to be tested regularly to make sure that the CD4 cell count hasn't dropped back down below 200.

Tuberculosis (TB)

Examples: Isoniazid (also known as isonicotinylhydrazide, or INH) is the most common medicine for preventing TB disease in people who have a positive TB skin or blood test. Rifampin or rifabutin and pyrazinamide may also be used. Still other drugs may be used if your doctor thinks you have been exposed to a drug-resistant form of TB. Depending on which medication or combination of medications is used, a person who has a positive TB skin test may need as little as four months or as much as 12 or more months of treatment to avoid getting TB disease.

How they work: If you're around someone with TB, a small number of organisms may get into your lungs and create a tiny infection. This is enough to make your immune system react and make your skin test positive, but it's not enough to cause disease. This is called latent TB infection. You've been *exposed* to TB, but you don't have the disease yet. The TB medications listed above, if taken correctly, can kill the TB organisms before they become active.

Possible side effects: INH can occasionally cause liver damage. It can also cause neuropathy (nerve damage in the arms and legs), but this problem can be prevented by taking vitamin B6 while you're on the INH.

Comments: The test for TB is very important because it can detect TB before it becomes active. Taking one medication to prevent TB disease is much better than waiting until the TB has spread to the lungs or other parts of the body. If TB becomes active in a person with HIV, usually at least four TB medications are needed to treat it. If the TB progresses too far without being treated, sometimes it can't be cured.

Mycobacterium Avium Complex (MAC)

Examples: Azithromycin (Zithromax®, Zmax®) and clarithromycin (Biaxin®) are effective for preventing MAC, and rifabutin (Mycobutin®) is also sometimes used.

How they work: MAC differs from TB in that there is no blood or skin test that can "catch" MAC when you've been exposed but are not yet actively infected. But we do know that the risk of MAC goes up sharply when the T-cell count is below 100, and the risk is highest when the count is below 50. If a person has a low T-cell count (below 50 cells per microliter), taking azithromycin or clarithromycin can reduce the chances of getting MAC. These medicines work by killing the MAC before it gets a foothold in the body. As with PCP and toxo, a strong immune system is the best protection—it is possible to stop taking the MAC medication if ART treatment makes the T-cell count go above 100 and stay there.

Possible side effects: Clarithromycin and azithromycin can cause stomach upset or diarrhea, but generally they are well tolerated. Rifabutin may cause rashes, stomach upset, or a drop in the white blood cell count.

Taking Treatment Medications

Many of the medications described in the previous section for *preventing* opportunistic infections in HIV/AIDS are also used for *treating* those problems when they occur. But treating an infection is always more difficult. It requires higher doses, more medicines, and more complicated combinations, and it has more side effects. Many, many medications are used to treat different acute infections, so we will not discuss all of them here. Generally speaking, all these medications exert their toxic effects to kill the invading virus, bacteria, parasite, or fungus, and all attempt to do this with minimal damage to the cells of the human body. Your treatment team should be your first source for information about medicines used to treat acute infections, but there are also other resources you can use. See the "Additional Resources" on the next page for more information.

Deciding When to Try a New Medication Regimen

Just like deciding when to start anti-HIV medications, deciding when to switch to a new combination of medicines is something that must be done very carefully, and always with the help of your doctor. Jumping from one set of medications to another too often can use up all your medication options, due to problems of resistance that we discussed earlier in this chapter.

But often, changing medications is necessary, and this is an important time for you to talk carefully with your doctor.

Although there are many factors to consider (see Chapter 7 to learn more about making treatment decisions), in general there are two reasons why you might stop one set of anti-HIV medications and start another:

1. *Your current medications aren't working.* The job of your medications is to suppress the HIV in your blood, to boost or maintain your T-cell count, and to keep you from getting HIV-related infections. If some of these things aren't being done well enough, it may be time to switch. This sounds pretty obvious, but what isn't so obvious is where to draw the line. How low should the viral load number be for your medicines to be considered successful? If your numbers have been low, how much of an increase should cause you to decide to make a change? How much of a drop in the T-cell count should make you change? The main point to keep in mind is that if the numbers are going in the wrong direction (up for viral load, down for T cells) and they're consistent on consecutive blood tests, then you and your doctor should talk about it. Depending on your situation, either staying on your medication or switching to a new combination may be the right decision.

2. *Your current medications are too toxic.* It could be that your anti-HIV drugs are suppressing HIV very well and boosting your T cells, but that one or more of the drugs is making you so sick that you have to change. If you find this happening to you, talk with your doctor right away. Otherwise, you may unintentionally skip or "forget" doses and put yourself at risk for resistance. Only you know what your side effects are like and whether they're severe enough to warrant a change of medications. Although there are more treatment options now than ever before, the choices are still limited in many cases, so it's important to balance side effects against benefits when you make your decision.

In Chapter 9, "Managing Side Effects of Medication," we discuss some additional common side effects of the medications we introduced here.

Additional Resources

AIDS Info: https://aidsinfo.nih.gov/hiv-aids-health-topics/topic/51/treatment-resources

The Body—The Complete HIV/AIDS Resource: www.thebody.com/index.shtml

Care4Today medication adherence app: www.care4today.com

Suggested Further Reading

To learn more about the topics discussed in this chapter, we suggest that you explore the following resources:

Bartlett, John G., and Ann K. Finkbeiner. *The Guide to Living with HIV Infection*, 6th ed. Baltimore, Md.: Johns Hopkins University Press, 2006.

Grodeck, Brett. *The First Year—HIV: An Essential Guide for the Newly Diagnosed.* New York: Marlowe, 2003.

Rybacki, James J. *The Essential Guide to Prescription Drugs.* New York: Collins Reference, 2007.

Silverman, Harold. *The Pill Book*, 15th ed. New York: Bantam, 2012.

Table 8.1 **Antiretroviral Therapy (ART) Drugs[3]**

		Nucleoside Reverse Transcriptase Inhibitors (NRTIs)		
Generic Name (Abbreviation)	**Formulations**	**Usual Adult Dose**	**Food Effects**	**Common Side Effects**
Abacavir (ABC)	Ziagen Trizivir (with ZDV + 3TC) Epzicom	300 mg 2 times/day; or 600 mg once daily	Take with or without food	Nausea, vomiting, headache, fatigue. A small number of people develop hypersensitivity, with flu-like symptoms. If this happens, stop the drug immediately and contact your doctor.
Emtricitabine (FTC)	Emtriva Truvada (with TDF)	200 mg once daily	Take with or without food	Rash, diarrhea, headache, nausea, vomiting
Lamivudine (3TC)	Epivir Combivir (with ZDV) Epizicom (with ABC) Trizivir (with ZDV + ABC)	150 mg 2 times/day; or 300 mg once daily	Take with or without food	Headache, nausea, sense of feeling ill, diarrhea, anemia, hair loss
Tenofovir Disoproxil Fumarate (TDF)	Viread Truvada (with TDF)	300 mg once daily	Take with or without food	Nausea, diarrhea, vomiting, flatulence, rash
Zidovudine (AZT, ZDV)	Retrovir Combivir (with 3TC) Trizivir (with 3TC + ABC)	300 mg 2 times/day	Take with or without food	Headache, nausea, sense of feeling ill, anemia

[3]Adapted from *Guidelines for the Use of Antiretroviral Agents in HIV-1-Infected Adults and Adolescents*, developed by the panel on Clinical Practices for Treatment of HIV Infection convened by the Department of Health and Human Services (DHHS), May 1, 2015.

Non-Nucleoside Reverse Transcriptase Inhibitors (NNRTIs)

Generic Name (Abbreviation)	Formulations	Usual Adult Dose	Food Effects	Common Side Effects
Delavirdine(DLV)	Rescriptor	400 mg 3 times/day; avoid taking within an hour of taking buffered didanosine or antacids	Take with or without food	Rash, which usually appears within first 3 weeks of starting medication
Efavirenz (EFV)	Sustiva	600 mg daily at or before bedtime	High-fat/high-calorie food can make drug levels too high in the blood; take on an empty stomach	Neurological symptoms such as dizziness, drowsiness, and problems with concentration
Nevirapine (NVP)	Viramune XR	200 mg once daily for 14 days; thereafter, 400 mg per day by mouth	Take with or without food	Rash, which usually appears within first 3 weeks of starting medication
Rilpivirine (RPV)	Edurant	25 mg once daily	Take with meal containing fat	Insomnia, rash
Etravirine (ETR)	Intelence	200 mg 2 times/day	Take with food	Rash, peripheral neuropathy

Continues ▶

107

Table 8.1 **Antiretroviral Therapy (ART) Drugs** (*continued*)[3]

		Protease Inhibitors (PIs)		
Generic Name (Abbreviation)	**Formulations**	**Usual Adult Dose**	**Food Effects**	**Common Side Effects**
Atazanavir (ATV)	Reyataz	400 mg once daily; or 300 mg ATV + 100 mg RTV once daily	Take with food; avoid taking with antacids	Nausea, headache, rash, vomiting, diarrhea, jaundice
Fosamprenavir (f-APV)	Lexiva	1400 mg 2 times/day; or 700 mg f-APV + 100 mg RTV 2 times/day	Take with or without food	Diarrhea, headache, nausea, vomiting, depression, abdominal pain, rash
Indinavir (IDV)	Crixivan	800 mg every 8 hours; may boost with RTV (IDVr)	For RTV-boosted IDV, take with or without food; for unboosted concentrations, take 1 hour before or 2 hours after meals	Kidney stones. Drink at least 8 glasses of water per day to reduce this risk. Diabetes
Lopinavir + Ritonavir (LPV/r)	Kaletra	LPV 400 mg + RTV 100 mg 2 times/day	Moderate-fat meal increases concentration; take with food	Diarrhea, nausea, high blood lipids, headache
Nelfinavir	Viracept	1250 mg 2 times/day; or 750 mg 3 times/day	Take with food	Diarrhea and nausea
Ritonavir (RTV)	Norvir	600 mg every 12 hours (when ritonavir is used as sole PI; rarely). When used to boost blood levels of other PI: 100–400 mg per day, in 1–2 divided doses.	Take with food	Diarrhea and nausea, which are usually worse in the first few weeks of starting medication

[3]Adapted from *Guidelines for the Use of Antiretroviral Agents in HIV-1-Infected Adults and Adolescents*, developed by the panel on Clinical Practices for Treatment of HIV Infection convened by the Department of Health and Human Services (DHHS), May 1, 2015.

Protease Inhibitors (PIs)

Generic Name (Abbreviation)	Formulations	Usual Adult Dose	Food Effects	Common Side Effects
Saquinavir (SQV)	Invirase	Boosted SQV with RTV (1000 mg SQV + 100 mg RTV), 2 times/day	Take within 2 hours of a meal	Diarrhea and nausea
Tipranavir	Aptivus	500 mg + 200 mg RTV 2 times/day	Take with food	Nausea, dizziness, headache, liver problems
Darunavir	Prezista	800 mg + 100 mg RTV once daily, or 600 mg + 100 mg RTV 2 times/day	Take with food	Nausea, vomiting, diarrhea, headache, skin rash

Fusion and Entry Inhibitors

Generic Name (Abbreviation)	Formulations	Usual Adult Dose	Food Effects	Common Side Effects
Maraviroc (MVC)	Selzentry	Dose varies dependingon other medications, but generally 150 mg, 300 mg, or 600 mg 2 times/day	Take with or without food	Upper respiratory tract infections, cough, rash, dizziness

Integrase Inhibitors

Generic Name (Abbreviation)	Formulations	Usual Adult Dose	Food Effects	Common Side Effects
Dolutegravir	Tivicay	50 mg once daily	Take with or without food and 2–6 hours after taking antacids with calcium, aluminum, magnesium, or iron	Rash, which usually appears within first 3 weeks of starting medication
Raltegravir (RAL)	Isentress	400 mg 2 times/day	Take with or without food	Headache, nausea, diarrhea, trouble sleeping

Continues ▶

109

Table 8.1 **Antiretroviral Therapy (ART) Drugs (*continued*)**[3]

		Integrase Inhibitors		
Generic Name (Abbreviation)	**Formulations**	**Usual Adult Dose**	**Food Effects**	**Common Side Effects**
Efavirenz/ Emtricitabine/ Tenofovir	Atripla	1 tablet once daily	Take on empty stomach, preferably at bedtime	Headache, insomnia dizziness, diarrhea, vomiting, unusual dreams
Elvitegravir/Emtricitabine/ Tenofovir/Cobicistat	Stribild	1 tablet once daily	Take with food	Nausea, vomiting, diarrhea, headache, fatigue, dizziness, insomnia, rash, fatigue
Dolutegravir/Abacavir/ Lamivudine	Triumeq	1 tablet once daily	Take with or without food	Insomnia, headache, fatigue. If you are at risk for a serious allergic reaction, contact your doctor if you have a rash, shortness of breath, fever, extreme tiredness.
Rilpivirine/Emtricitabine/ Tenofovir	Complera		Take with food; take antacids 12 hours before or 4 hours after taking Complera	Insomnia, unusual dreams headache, dizziness, diarrhea, nausea, rash, fatigue, depression

[3]Adapted from *Guidelines for the Use of Antiretroviral Agents in HIV-1-Infected Adults and Adolescents*, developed by the panel on Clinical Practices for Treatment of HIV Infection convened by the Department of Health and Human Services (DHHS), May 1, 2015.

CHAPTER 9

Managing Side Effects of Medications

MEDICATION SIDE EFFECTS ARE AN IMPORTANT ISSUE IN HIV treatments. Sometimes, managing the side effects of antiretroviral therapy (ART) and other medications used for HIV can be almost as large a part of your treatment as managing HIV itself. But there are many good ways to manage side effects, and managing them is crucial because ART medications control the HIV virus in your body. This chapter provides you with information that will help you identify, cope with, and self-manage these side effects.

Most side effects are predictable and minor, but some can be serious and on rare occasions even require hospitalization. By knowing all of the medications you're taking, knowing what (and what not) to expect, and getting proper checkups and tests, you can maximize your benefit and reduce the chances of serious side effects.

What Is a Side Effect?

A side effect is any effect a medication has other than the one you want. Usually, it is an undesirable effect. Examples of undesirable side effects are stomach problems, constipation, diarrhea, insomnia, sleepiness, and dizziness. You should be aware of the common side effects of your medications. When people start taking HIV medications, they usually experience mild side effects for the first month or so. This is common and means that the medications are starting to work.

Patients and doctors have to figure out how to manage side effects and how to decide when side effects are dangerous, when they will improve on their own, and when they are so bothersome that the medications should be changed. Luckily, many side effects can be managed, so you don't have to stop using a medication and give up its benefits.

Questions to Ask about Side Effects

Sometimes people say they can't or won't take a drug because of its possible side effects. This is understandable. However, before you decide to stop taking a drug or refuse to take it in the first place, you should ask yourself and your doctor the following questions.

Are the benefits from this medication more important than the side effects?

ART drugs are a good example of medications whose benefits should be weighed against their undesirable side effects. Although these drugs have side effects, many people still take them because of their life-saving qualities. To start or not start the drugs is your decision. However, you should always ask yourself, "*Even with* the side effects, will I be better off with the drugs than I would be without them?"

With ART, it's also important to remember that a decision you make today may be different from the decision you make later on. For example, if you don't think you could take the medications every day, you and your doctor may decide that starting ART now isn't worth it. But later on, you might make a very different decision if you're not feeling as well and your T-cell counts are lower. See Chapter 7, "Making Treatment Decisions," for more guidance on making decisions about this important treatment option.

Is the problem I'm having really a medication side effect?

Sometimes it is easy to tell whether a symptom you're having is a side effect from a medication, but other times it can be difficult. You might think, for example, that a new headache, pain in your leg, or other symptom is being caused by your medication. But the symptom may be temporary, or it may be caused by something different. Before you make a permanent change, it's important to discuss these issues with your provider. Many symptoms get better on their own, so continuing the medication and watching the symptoms can be a good choice.

Are there ways of avoiding the side effects or making them less severe?

Many times, the *way* you take the drug—for example, with or without food—can make a difference. Several self-management strategies for side effects are included in this book. Ask your doctor or pharmacist for advice, too.

Are there other medications that have the same benefits, but fewer side effects?

Several different drugs may be designed to treat the same medical problem, and they may have different side effects in different people. Unfortunately, you cannot know how you will react to a drug until you have taken it. Therefore, your doctor may have you try several different medications before finding the ones that are best for you.

Common Side Effects of HIV Medications

The effects and side effects of HIV medications can be complicated. It may be challenging to figure out how to minimize the side effects and still get the benefits you need from the medications. Your doctor, nurse, and pharmacist are your main resources for advice about your medications, and you need to talk to them whenever you think of making a change. There are lots of other places to get helpful information, too. Some information about lipodystrophy, high blood sugar, and high cholesterol is included here. See Table 8.1, "Techniques for Managing Side Effects," for more on other common side effects.

You will also find information about medication-specific side effects in Table 9.1 in Chapter 8, "Managing Medications for HIV." That table lists some of the other side effects that have been associated with HIV medications and gives some self-management tips to lessen side effects. Even if you have success in managing your side effects, remember to keep your doctors and nurses informed about new side effects—especially any severe ones. You should also check the symptom action charts in Chapter 10, "Evaluating Symptoms of HIV," which can help you determine whether a symptom is a side effect or a sign of a serious illness.

Fat Redistribution (Lipodystrophy)

Some people getting treatment for HIV experience changes in the way fat is distributed on their bodies. Their bodies may gradually start to look different. Doctors call this lipodystrophy. The changes are difficult to describe exactly, but usually *more* fat appears in the central part of the body (the stomach, the breasts, the upper back), and *less* fat remains in the face, rear end, and arms and legs. Women's breasts may get larger due to fatty deposits, which may cause problems with comfort and clothing fit.

People with lipodystrophy may start to see prominent veins on their legs, or they may notice that their face thins as a result of the fat loss. These changes can be accompanied by changes in cholesterol and blood sugar levels, so they should not be ignored. In some cases, lipodystrophy can make people feel uncomfortable and self-conscious, and may reduce their quality of life. In other cases it is pretty mild and feels like a good trade-off for the big benefits of HIV treatment.

Doctors are not certain exactly what causes lipodystrophy. It may be a side effect from taking some HIV medications, it may be related to the HIV virus, or there may be some other reason (age, race, time living with HIV, and T-cell count).

Whatever the cause, the changes in appearance can be disturbing for some people, and some may even decide to stop taking their HIV medications because of the changes. Before discontinuing ART medications, you must first discuss the possible causes of fat accumulation with your doctors.

Exercise and gradual, healthy weight loss may help reduce lipodystrophy in some people. Exercise to build muscle has been found effective in studies. Please see Chapter 13, "Physical Activity for Fun and Fitness," for more about how exercise can help you deal with this condition. Some people have cosmetic surgery to remove fat or to fill in places where fat has been lost, but this is a costly approach and is not available to everyone. There are also new medications that can help reduce fat accumulation caused by lipodystrophy.

High Cholesterol and High Blood Sugar

High levels of cholesterol and sugar in the blood are conditions that may be caused by a person's diet, or they can run in some families. These conditions are a problem for many people, and that's why you often see ads on TV, in magazines, and on websites for cholesterol and blood sugar treatments.

People with HIV can also have higher cholesterol and blood sugar levels. In addition, ART increases the risk of high blood sugar and cholesterol. Because of this, people taking ART may have a higher risk of heart disease. People living with HIV need to take steps to lower blood sugar and cholesterol to reduce the risk of heart disease.

If a person on ART has large enough increases in blood sugar, they may develop diabetes. If diabetes develops, it may be necessary to use prescription medications to reduce cholesterol or lower the blood sugar. Chapter 14, "Healthy Eating," provides some tips on how to cut back on sugar and carbohydrates in the diet. People with high blood cholesterol or blood sugar can use these tips to change their eating habits.

If you smoke, the best way to lower your heart disease risk is to stop smoking. You will also want to keep your blood pressure at a healthy level, eat a healthy diet, and exercise. All these things will lower your chances of heart disease.

While ART medications can cause side effects, remember: these medications can prevent complications with HIV and save lives. And most side effects improve and can be managed.

Additional Resources

AIDSinfo:
   https://.aidsinfo.nih.gov/education-materials/fact-sheets/22/63/hiv-medicines-and-side-effects

U.S. Department of Veterans Affairs:
   www.hiv.va.gov/patient/drug-dosing-toolkit/side-effects-tips.asp

Table 9.1 **Techniques for Managing Side Effects**

These are very common side effects, especially in the first few weeks of taking a new medication. They often go away on their own as your body adapts to the treatment.

Diarrhea	Nausea	Dizziness
■ Eat frequent, small meals. ■ Eat plenty of fiber (vegetables) and drink lots of liquids (water, juice, caffeine-free beverages). ■ Eat rice and other starches, oatmeal, potatoes, apples (peeled and allowed to brown), pears, bananas. ■ Avoid dairy products (milk, ice cream, cheese), caffeine, fast foods, fried foods. ■ Consider adding acidophilus (from a health food or drugstore) to your diet. Share your plan to take acidophilus with your doctor or nurse beforehand to make sure it does not interfere with the rest of your treatment plan. ■ When traveling away from home, make sure bathrooms will be available. ■ Consider taking extra underpants with you if you will be away from home for a long time. ■ Ask your doctor about Metamucil®, Lomotil®, Imodium®, or tincture of opium.	■ Eat bland crackers, or sip ginger ale or soda water ■ Eat cold or room temperature foods and liquids. ■ Avoid strong odors, sights, or sounds that trigger the nausea. ■ Breathe in fresh air or pleasant smells such as lemon, lime, or ginger. ■ Try Mylanta® or Maalox®. ■ Avoid spicy or acidic foods (oranges, tomatoes). ■ Try distraction or relaxation techniques.* ■ Ask your doctor about ondansetron, prochlorperazine, or benzodiazepines.	■ Since dizziness can be serious, have any new dizziness evaluated by your doctor or nurse. ■ Sit down and put your head between your knees, or lie down with your feet higher than your head. ■ Drink plenty of liquids (water, juice, caffeine-free beverages). ■ Rise slowly when waking up—sit up first. ■ Eat high-energy foods. ■ When indoors, make sure you have enough fresh air. ■ Loosen tight-fitting clothing. ■ Avoid alcohol and other drugs.

*Relaxation techniques are described in Chapter 12, "Using Your Mind to Manage Symptoms."

Keep your doctor or primary care provider informed
of any side effects you may be experiencing.

Headache	Fatigue	Numbness or Tingling	Rash
■ Take an over-the-counter medication such as acetaminophen, aspirin, or ibuprofen. ■ Try relaxation techniques.*	■ Take frequent, short naps and try to sleep longer at night. ■ Limit caffeine, sugar, and alcohol. ■ Limit work hours, if possible. ■ Try relaxation techniques.* ■ Exercise every day (e.g., a brisk 15–30 minute walk).	■ Eat a balanced diet and take a multivitamin each day. ■ Do passive flexibility exercise with your hands, arms, legs, or feet; ask a family member to help. ■ Massage your hands, arms, legs, or feet. ■ Wear loose-fitting, comfortable shoes with padded soles.	■ Talk to your doctor immediately to get urgent care for new rashes ■ Air- or pat-dry your skin after bathing. ■ Apply moisturizing creams or lotions that do not contain alcohol or scent. ■ Wear light, nonirritating clothing and a hat when in the sun. ■ Keep sheets and blankets off sensitive skin (e.g., use a pillow at the foot of the bed to hold sheets off your feet). ■ Try not to scratch. Keep your fingernails short and clean. ■ Report increasing rash, fever, headache, flu-like symptoms, or any sores in your mouth or vagina. ■ Diphenhydramine (e.g., Benadryl®) may help with itching (but use it only with your doctor's approval).

*Relaxation techniques are described in Chapter 12, "Using Your Mind to Manage Symptoms."

Keep your doctor or primary care provider informed of any side effects you may be experiencing.

CHAPTER 10

Evaluating Symptoms of HIV

Symptoms are the body's signals that something unusual is happening. They cannot always be seen by others, are often difficult to describe, and are usually unpredictable. If you have HIV, you are going to have symptoms that need to be managed.

Although chronic symptoms are difficult to live with, there are many things you can do to deal successfully with them. Many symptoms that people with HIV get are very similar to symptoms of other chronic conditions such as heart disease, arthritis, diabetes, depression, and asthma, as well as other physical and mental health problems. Like all people who experience symptoms due to a medical condition, people with HIV need to know how to evaluate symptoms, and decide whether a new symptom needs immediate medical attention. If you have not had the symptoms in this chapter, this information will help prepare you if one of these symptoms begins. In Chapter 11, "Understanding the Symptom Cycle," we discuss other common chronic symptoms that many people get, and how to manage them. In Chapter 12, "Using Your Mind to Manage Symptoms," we discuss suggestions and techniques that involve using your mind to deal with symptoms.

Symptom Types

In general, people living with HIV can view their symptoms as falling into three broad groups. First, many chronic conditions (including HIV) cause chronic symptoms themselves. People with HIV may have fatigue or body aches or other symptoms, people with arthritis may get joint or back pains, and people with chronic lung disease may feel short of breath. Chronic symptoms may wax and wane, but they can be managed. Since today's treatments for HIV are very good, people with HIV grow older and, like all older people, they acquire other chronic conditions over time.

Second, some symptoms are medication side effects—i.e., symptoms caused by medications themselves. We discuss side effects and some management strategies in Chapter 9, "Managing Side Effects of Medications," and you will find additional medication-specific information in Table 8.1 at the end of Chapter 8, "Managing Medications for HIV."

Third, some symptoms can be caused by HIV-related infections. This is a particular worry if a person is not on treatment for HIV or hasn't seen an HIV doctor for some time. For example, a new cough with a fever could be a symptom of pneumonia. This is why every person with HIV must be linked to good HIV medical care, and should stay in regular care after they begin seeing a doctor. If you have a symptom that might be from a new infection, you need to see the doctor right away, because finding the problem and starting treatment early is vital. Everyone with HIV should see their doctor routinely, but the symptom action charts later in this chapter can help people decide when it's important to see the doctor right away.

Evaluating Your Symptoms

One of the difficult things about living with HIV is that you can develop an AIDS-related infection or other condition. New symptoms, especially if they are your first symptoms, are distressing in and of themselves. They are also distressing because they could be signals of a new or more serious problem. Symptoms can sometimes be signals that a serious illness is starting, for which you should see your doctor. However, just as often, the symptoms are part of the cycle of chronic disease, for which self-management may be the best approach (see Figure 1.1, The Vicious Cycle of Symptoms, on page 5).

To be a confident self-manager, you need to know when it's time to call the doctor. But how can you tell? Some of it is common sense. If it's clear you're having a medical emergency, see a doctor immediately or call 911 or its equivalent in your country. On the other hand, if you're having symptoms similar to what you've often had in the past, you can probably use self-management techniques confidently.

Another important factor in evaluating symptoms is knowing your T-cell count (also called CD4 cell count). T-cell counts are one way to measure the strength of your immune system (as we discuss in detail in Chapter 7, "Making Treatment Decisions"). People with T-cell counts below 200 are at higher risk for getting infections, so they have to be very careful. Your doctor will try to get your T-cell count as high as possible with HIV medications. You should measure your T-cell count every three to six months, and it's a good idea to know the result of your most recent measurement. Of course, T cells aren't the only measure of how healthy you are, but they are useful. You can read more information about T-cell counts in Chapter 7, "Making Treatment Decisions."

FAST Check Your Symptoms

One quick way to judge whether you should see your doctor for a symptom is to do a "FAST" check. The initials in the acronym "FAST" stand for *Fever*, *Altered mental status*, *Severe*, and *Typical*. Ask yourself the four simple questions listed in the chart below. If the answer to any of the questions is yes, you should see your doctor promptly. Your provider will be able to tell you if the symptom is due to a new AIDS-related infection or cancer.

Fever

Fever can be an important clue, especially when it occurs with another symptom. A temperature of 101°F (38.3°C) or higher is more likely to be associated with infection. Everyone with HIV needs to own, and know how to use, a good thermometer. It is important to measure your temperature when you think you have a fever. Write down your temperature so you will be able to tell the doctor exactly how high it is if necessary.

Altered Mental Status

"Altered mental status" is a term doctors use to describe a person whose brain functioning is not normal. This can mean confusion, excessive sleepiness, or "I can't put my finger on it, but they just aren't themselves." It can also take a much more dramatic form, such as a coma (the most extreme decrease in mental function) or a seizure. All of these conditions represent altered mental states. Anyone who develops altered mental status over a short period of time, particularly in association with other symptoms, should see a doctor promptly.

You may not be able to recognize a serious alteration in mental function yourself, but you

Do a F.A.S.T. Check on All New or Worsening Symptoms

Fever	Is the new symptom associated with a fever (a temperature of 101°F or more)?
Altered	Is the new symptom associated with a change in your mental status (e.g., confusion, sleepiness, seizures)?
Severe	Is the new symptom much more severe than anything you've had in the past?
Typical	Is the new symptom not typical for you? Is it unusual or out of the ordinary?

If the answer to any of these questions is **yes**, you should see your doctor promptly.

can teach those close to you how to easily diagnose such a change. If they suspect you may be subject to an altered mental status, they should simply see how well you answer questions such as what is your name, what day of the week is it, what city are you in, etc. If you can't answer such questions coherently or can't wake up enough to answer them, urgent action is needed.

Severe

Chronic symptoms will often increase and decrease depending on whether you're having a good day or a bad day. However, any symptom that is much more severe than it has ever been before should be evaluated by your health care team.

Typical

Any symptom that is completely new for you (that is, *not* typical) should be discussed with your medical team. This is a very general guideline that you probably use already when deciding whether to go to the doctor.

Depending on what the new symptom is, you may want to consult one of the symptom action charts that follow for more guidance. But remember that when in doubt, it's better to be safe than sorry. If you're experiencing a symptom you've never had before and you're not sure whether self-care is the right thing to do, it's best to consult your doctor to be sure.

Using Symptom Action Charts

Another way to evaluate your symptoms is to use the action charts in this chapter. These charts guide you in evaluating several common HIV-related symptoms that sometimes require a doctor's rapid attention. Not every symptom is included here, but if you have one of the symptoms listed, the chart will help you decide what to do.

If you have more than one symptom, you may need to look at more than one of the charts. If the advice in the two charts doesn't agree, follow the most "conservative" (that is, the safest) advice. For example, if one chart says to call the doctor and the other recommends home treatment, you should call your doctor.

To use the charts properly, follow the steps below. They will guide you through the key questions you should consider in deciding whether you need the help of your health care team right away.

1. *Determine your "chief complaint" or main symptom*, and then find the correct chart. (They are listed alphabetically in the material that follows.)

2. Before you look at the chart, *read the general text information on the symptom that accompanies the chart*. This information will help you understand the questions in the chart. If you ignore the general information, you may not understand the questions in the chart correctly, and you could do the wrong thing.

3. *Read the action chart*. Start at the top and follow the arrows. Skipping around may result in errors. Each question assumes that you have answered all of the previous questions.

Note: These charts are intended only to help you decide whether you urgently need to see your doctor for certain symptoms. Regardless of symptoms, you should always get the routine checkups that you and your doctor have scheduled, and you should have a checkup at least every six months.

Cough

The cough reflex is a defense mechanism used by the body to clear abnormal material from the lungs. When the cough is bringing up infected material, such as pus, from the lungs, coughing is beneficial and shouldn't be suppressed. However, anything that irritates the lungs will cause a cough, and many of these stimuli do not produce pus, or even anything that's particularly easy to clear from the lungs. This type of cough will continue but not produce anything, which can be quite aggravating.

A cough can also be a medication side effect. The medications most commonly associated with cough are for blood pressure or the heart (fosinopril, lisinopril, enalapril, benazopril, ramipril). For most people with HIV, a new cough is related to something else.

People with HIV get coughs for all the same reasons other people do. Smoking is a very common cause (see page 58–61 for more information about tobacco and HIV). The toxins in smoke irritate and kill cells in the lining of the bronchial tubes (breathing tubes) and stimulate the cough. This can happen even to those who don't smoke themselves but have to breathe other people's smoke. Viral infections ("colds") are the next most common cause of a cough. These

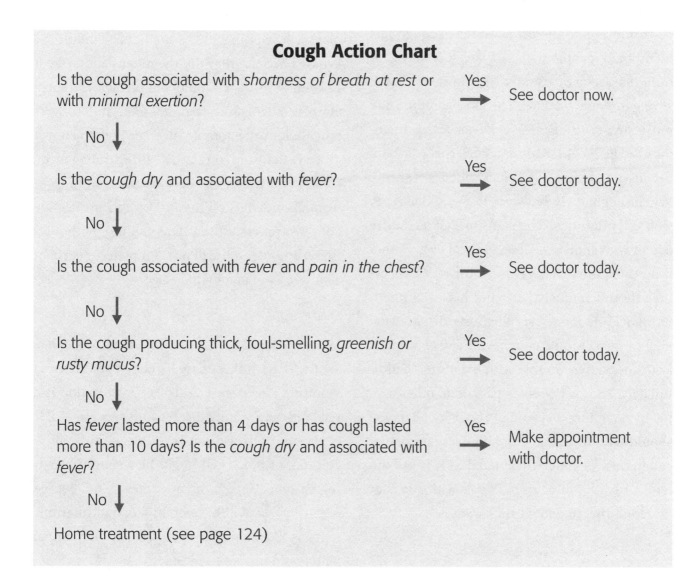

Cough Action Chart

Is the cough associated with *shortness of breath at rest* or with *minimal exertion*?   Yes → See doctor now.

No ↓

Is the *cough dry* and associated with *fever*?   Yes → See doctor today.

No ↓

Is the cough associated with *fever* and *pain in the chest*?   Yes → See doctor today.

No ↓

Is the cough producing thick, foul-smelling, *greenish or rusty mucus*?   Yes → See doctor today.

No ↓

Has *fever* lasted more than 4 days or has cough lasted more than 10 days? Is the *cough dry* and associated with *fever*?   Yes → Make appointment with doctor.

No ↓

Home treatment (see page 124)

coughs usually produce only yellow or whitish mucus, not the green or rusty stuff produced by a more serious bacterial infection. Cold viruses don't respond to antibiotics; the only treatment for them is to strengthen the body's immune system with rest, good food, lots of fluids, and time. Bacterial or opportunistic infections, which can also cause coughs, can be more serious and require a doctor's attention and antibiotics. Infection in the sinuses (sinusitis) doesn't affect the lungs directly, but it often causes coughing because mucus from the sinuses drips down the throat and into the lungs, irritating them. This is particularly a problem at night or in the morning just after awakening.

In addition to the usual causes of cough just mentioned, people with HIV are susceptible to lung diseases not usually seen in people with strong immune systems. The most common and most important of these is *Pneumocystis* pneumonia (PCP). Identifying PCP early is vital because it is very dangerous when advanced. When caught early, however, PCP responds very well to antibiotics. The signs of PCP are a dry cough with shortness of breath and fever. Other lung infections that people with HIV can get include tuberculosis (TB) and bacterial pneumonia. TB is a very serious lung disease that may cause a chronic cough with fevers, yet may not cause much trouble with breathing. Unfortunately, TB is very easy to pass on to other people by coughing. Because of the risk of TB, you should talk to your doctor about any persistent cough (lasting longer than ten days). See Chapter 3, "Health Problems of People with HIV," for more information about these illnesses.

Home Treatment of Cough

To calm a cough, the mucus in the bronchial tubes may be made thinner and less sticky by several means. Increasing the humidity in the air will help; a vaporizer and a steamy shower are two ways to add humidity. Drinking a lot of fluids is also helpful, particularly if a fever has dehydrated the body. Glyceryl guaiacolate (Robitussin®, Mucinex®) may help liquefy mucus so it can be coughed out of the lungs more easily. Decongestants (pseudoephedrine) and/or antihistamines (loratadine, citerizine, diphenhydramine) may help if the cough is caused by nasal or sinus material dripping down into the lungs. (Note: Unless the cough is caused by nasal or sinus dripping, these medicines should be avoided because they dry the mucus and make it thicker. Over-the-counter cold medicines almost always contain antihistamine—and/or decongestant and/or expectorant—in some combination.)

Dry, tickling coughs are often relieved by sucking on cough lozenges or hard candy. Dextromethorphan (Robitussin-DM®) is an effective cough suppressant that you can buy without a prescription, but it will not completely get rid of a cough, even at a high dosage.

Diarrhea

Many of the concerns associated with diarrhea are the same as those associated with nausea and vomiting (see page 129–130). Dehydration is a risk and may require intravenous medicines if it is severe. Diarrhea that is jet-black, burgundy-colored, or blood red might be a sign of bleeding in the stomach or intestines. Most people with diarrhea will have cramping and intermittent gas-like pains, but severe, steady abdominal pain could be more serious.

In people with HIV, diarrhea can be caused by viral, bacterial, or parasitic infection and may be caused by the effect of the virus itself on the intestines. In some cases, diarrhea is a side effect of a drug. Several antiretroviral HIV medicines can cause loose bowel movements or even diarrhea. Antibiotics and anticancer drugs also cause diarrhea in some people. If medications seem to be responsible for your diarrhea, it is important to discuss this side effect with your doctor. See Chapter 9 for more information on side effects.

Home Treatment of Diarrhea

Home treatment of diarrhea is about getting enough fluid into the body to prevent dehydration. Sip clear fluids, such as water or ginger ale.

If you are vomiting and nothing will stay down, suck on ice chips; this is usually tolerated and provides fluid. Gatorade, bouillon, and Jell-O are also good sources of liquid.

The next step is to eat foods that will slow your gut down. Follow the "BRAT" rule: *B*ananas, *R*ice, *A*pplesauce, and *T*oast. Dairy foods and fats will not absorb well—you should avoid them for a few days. Nonprescription remedies such as Kaopectate® will make the stool more solid, but they won't change the amount or frequency of the stools. Many cases of diarrhea get better on their own within five days, but if this doesn't happen, call your doctor. You may need tests, or eventually need stronger medication to slow down the intestinal tract.

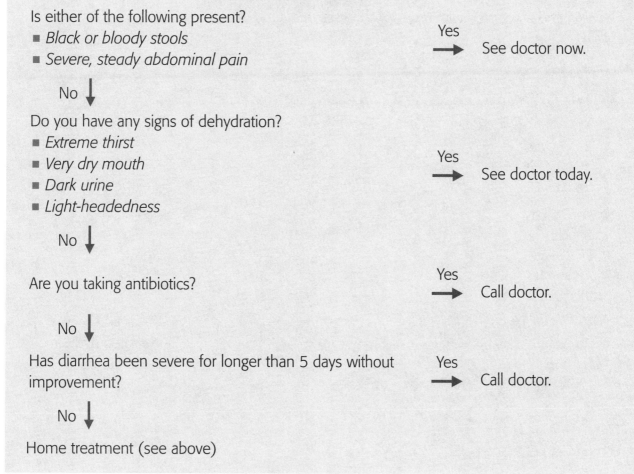

Fever

The most common cause of fevers in people with HIV is infection. When HIV is at high levels in the body, the virus itself causes fever. Fever can also be caused by other viral, bacterial, and parasitic infections, and is sometimes caused by cancers or medications. Fever is a distressing symptom, although it's rarely dangerous in itself. However, the infection that might be causing the fever could be very serious. Everyone needs to know how to measure a fever and how to decide when it's time to see the doctor.

If you have HIV, you should have a thermometer and know how to use it properly. Both Fahrenheit and centigrade thermometers are acceptable. If your temperature is greater than or equal to

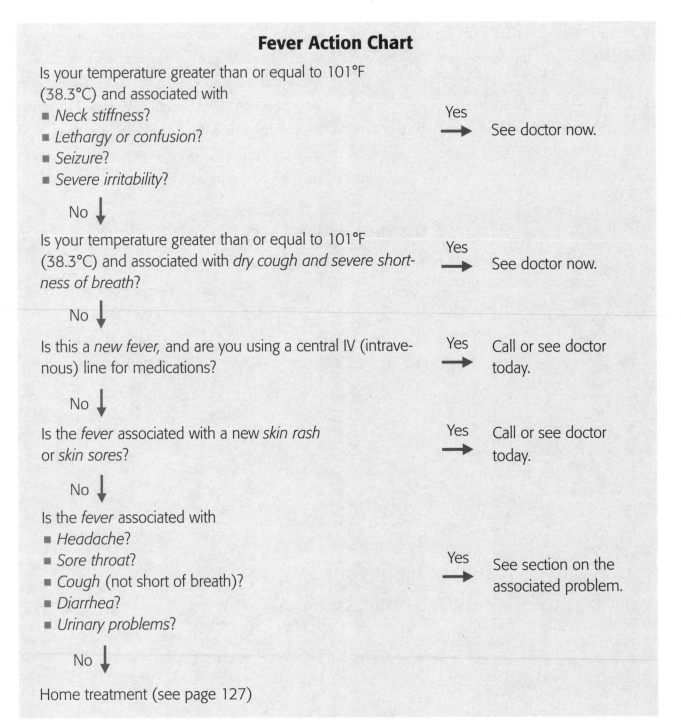

Fever Action Chart

Is your temperature greater than or equal to 101°F (38.3°C) and associated with
- *Neck stiffness?*
- *Lethargy or confusion?*
- *Seizure?*
- *Severe irritability?*

Yes → See doctor now.

No ↓

Is your temperature greater than or equal to 101°F (38.3°C) and associated with *dry cough and severe shortness of breath?*

Yes → See doctor now.

No ↓

Is this a *new fever,* and are you using a central IV (intravenous) line for medications?

Yes → Call or see doctor today.

No ↓

Is the *fever* associated with a new *skin rash* or *skin sores?*

Yes → Call or see doctor today.

No ↓

Is the *fever* associated with
- *Headache?*
- *Sore throat?*
- *Cough* (not short of breath)?
- *Diarrhea?*
- *Urinary problems?*

Yes → See section on the associated problem.

No ↓

Home treatment (see page 127)

101°F (38°C), it is important to consider whether you could have one of the serious HIV-related opportunistic infections or emergency AIDS-associated infections. These include meningitis, an infection of the lining of the brain that causes neck stiffness and confusion, and *Pneumocystis* pneumonia (PCP), an infection of the lungs that causes dry cough and shortness of breath, particularly when you're walking or climbing stairs.

If none of these problems are present, the fever could still be serious but probably doesn't require immediate attention in the emergency department. The important consideration is what symptoms are associated with the fever and how they should be managed.

Home Treatment of Fever

There are two ways to reduce a fever: sponging and medication. Sponging the skin with tepid water will bring the body temperature down as the water evaporates. Medications to lower fever include aspirin, acetaminophen (Tylenol®, Datril®), and ibuprofen (Motrin®, Advil®). Adults can take two aspirins every three to four hours as required. Acetaminophen is taken similarly and is often confused with aspirin, but it is a completely different medicine. It has the same temperature-lowering effect as aspirin but causes less stomach upset. On the other hand, acetaminophen can cause liver damage in high doses, and overdose can be fatal. Because aspirin and acetaminophen are different drugs, they can be given together to control fever when one or the other alone is not effective. When you do this, stagger the doses every three hours, alternating doses of aspirin and acetaminophen.

If you have a fever, make sure to increase your fluid intake to prevent dehydration. You may need as much as a glass of water taken in sips every hour or two. The signs of dehydration include extreme thirst, very dry mouth, dark urine or infrequent urination, and light-headedness.

Headache

Headache is the single most frequent complaint of modern times. The most common causes of headache are tension, eyestrain, and muscle spasms. Medications can also lead to headaches; headache can be a side effect of zidovudine (AZT), for example.

While headaches are common, they are not always harmless. There are several opportunistic diseases that can start out as headaches in people with HIV. Headache associated with fever and a neck so stiff that the chin cannot be touched to the chest suggests the possibility of meningitis, a serious infection of the lining of the brain. Headaches can be caused by infection or a tumor in the brain itself if they are associated with neurological problems such as slurred speech, weakness or paralysis in the arms or legs, or new visual problems. Any headache after a severe head injury can be serious.

Home Treatment of Headache

The usual over-the-counter drugs (aspirin, acetaminophen, ibuprofen, naproxen) are typically quite effective in relieving headache. Headache also responds very well to techniques that help reduce stress and tension. Try massage or heat applied to the back of the upper neck, or simply rest with your eyes closed and your head supported. Meditation can also be effective. Headaches that don't respond to these measures should be brought to the attention of a doctor.

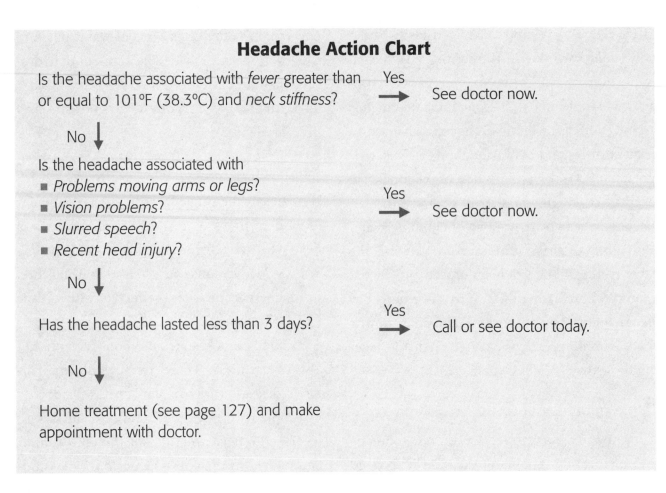

Headache Action Chart

Is the headache associated with *fever* greater than or equal to 101°F (38.3°C) and *neck stiffness*?

Yes → See doctor now.

No ↓

Is the headache associated with
- *Problems moving arms or legs?*
- *Vision problems?*
- *Slurred speech?*
- *Recent head injury?*

Yes → See doctor now.

No ↓

Has the headache lasted less than 3 days?

Yes → Call or see doctor today.

No ↓

Home treatment (see page 127) and make appointment with doctor.

Impaired/Decreased Vision

Your vision is important, so see your doctor about any vision change that doesn't improve on its own. The most common causes of vision problems are nearsightedness (when you have trouble seeing things in the distance) and farsightedness (when you have trouble seeing things that are up close). Vision is also sometimes affected by medications, high blood sugar, headaches, eyestrain, or fatigue. When one of these things is causing vision problems, the change is usually gradual and about equal in both eyes. You should see a doctor if this is the case for you, although this isn't an emergency. But in people with low T-cell counts, HIV can lead to CMV (cytomegalovirus) retinitis, an infection of the back of the eye that can damage vision severely. It usually begins in one eye but can affect both eyes. In its worst forms, CMV retinitis can lead to blindness, but it can be arrested with medications. This is why you should see your doctor about any visual change, and see a doctor *promptly* about a rapid visual change or a change that affects one eye and not the other.

Home Treatment of Impaired/ Decreased Vision

If you experience temporary changes in vision caused by medications or fatigue, try resting with your eyes closed in a darkened room for a few minutes. Be sure to protect your eyes with sunglasses; this will decrease strain and allow your eyes to accommodate more easily. If you are on a computer or tablet a lot, it might help to cut

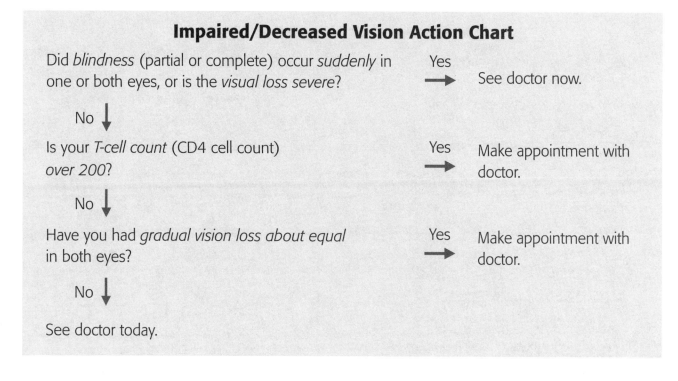

Impaired/Decreased Vision Action Chart

Did *blindness* (partial or complete) occur *suddenly* in one or both eyes, or is the *visual loss severe*?   Yes → See doctor now.

No ↓

Is your *T-cell count* (CD4 cell count) *over 200*?   Yes → Make appointment with doctor.

No ↓

Have you had *gradual vision loss about equal* in both eyes?   Yes → Make appointment with doctor.

No ↓

See doctor today.

the glare on your screen by closing the shades or rearranging your desk. It's also important to look away from the screen frequently. Progressive or persistent changes in your vision should be discussed with your doctor.

Nausea and Vomiting

Many of the concerns associated with nausea and vomiting are the same as those associated with diarrhea (see page 124–125). Medications are the most common cause of nausea in people with HIV, although viral infections can also cause problems. Dehydration presents the greatest risk of vomiting; as with diarrhea, intravenous medicines may be needed when it gets severe. People with severe dehydration often experience dizziness, severe thirst, dry mouth and tongue, decreased amounts of urine, dark urine, and wrinkled, dry skin. Vomit that is bloody or black may indicate that severe stomach or intestinal bleeding is present. This prob-

lem is particularly an issue in people with liver disease. An infection of the brain can sometimes lead to nausea and vomiting, so if you are nauseous and vomiting and have a headache and a stiff neck, see your doctor right away. Women who are sexually active should always consider the possibility that their nausea is due to pregnancy. The best way to know for sure is to get a pregnancy test, either over the counter at your local drugstore or in your doctor's office.

Some medications for HIV can cause nausea as a side effect. Some of the HIV drugs that can cause stomach upset include zidovidune (AZT; Retrovir®), didanosine (ddI; Videx®), lamivudine (3TC; Epivir®), nelfinavir (Viracept®), ritonavir (Norvir®), and amprenavir (Agenerase®). But in truth, many medications can upset your stomach. For example, antibiotics and anticancer drugs also can cause stomach issues. If nausea begins soon after you start a new medicine, call your doctor to discuss this side effect.

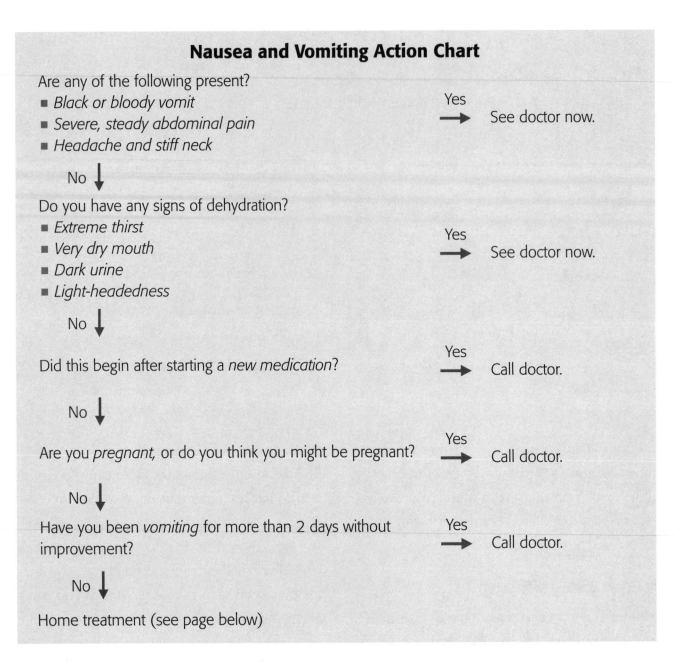

Nausea and Vomiting Action Chart

Are any of the following present?
- *Black or bloody vomit*
- *Severe, steady abdominal pain*
- *Headache and stiff neck*

Yes → See doctor now.

No ↓

Do you have any signs of dehydration?
- *Extreme thirst*
- *Very dry mouth*
- *Dark urine*
- *Light-headedness*

Yes → See doctor now.

No ↓

Did this begin after starting a *new medication*?

Yes → Call doctor.

No ↓

Are you *pregnant,* or do you think you might be pregnant?

Yes → Call doctor.

No ↓

Have you been *vomiting* for more than 2 days without improvement?

Yes → Call doctor.

No ↓

Home treatment (see page below)

Home Treatment of Nausea and Vomiting

The goal of home treatment of nausea is to get as much fluid as possible into your body without further upsetting your stomach. Sip clear fluids, such as water or ginger ale. Suck on ice chips if nothing else will stay down. Don't drink too much at any one time, as this will aggravate the stomach. Add Gatorade, bouillon, soups, and Jell-O as your condition improves. If the vomiting does not go away within two days, call the doctor.

Shortness of Breath

Shortness of breath is normal during hard activity or when you're exercising. But if you get "winded" at rest or with only minimal exertion, or if you wake up at night short of breath, you may have a serious symptom that should be evaluated by a doctor. In people with HIV, the major concern is pneumonia, most often caused by *Pneumocystis* pneumonia (PCP). PCP almost always causes a dry cough and a fever, so if you

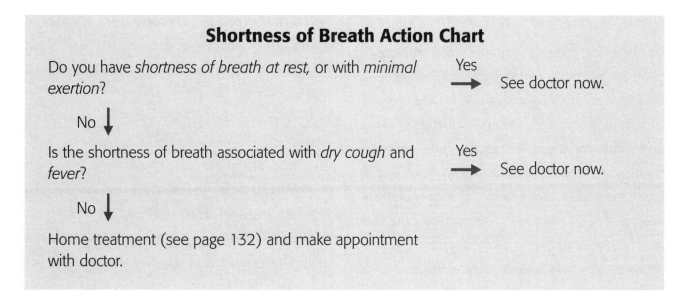

Shortness of Breath Action Chart

Do you have *shortness of breath at rest,* or with *minimal exertion?*   Yes → See doctor now.

No ↓

Is the shortness of breath associated with *dry cough* and *fever?*   Yes → See doctor now.

No ↓

Home treatment (see page 132) and make appointment with doctor.

have shortness of breath and these other symptoms you may need to be treated for PCP. There are several other causes of chronic shortness of breath, including lung damage caused by previous lung infections, anemia, and smoking-related lung disease. Several suggestions that are often helpful for people with chronic shortness of breath are given in Chapter 11, "Understanding the Symptom Cycle."

Sore Throat

A sore throat is almost never a life-threatening problem, but it can be painful. Sore throats can be caused by several infections. Cold viruses are the most common cause and cannot be treated successfully with antibiotics; they must be allowed to run their course. Mononucleosis ("mono") is a viral infection that causes a severe, prolonged illness with painful swelling and soreness in the throat. Even though it sounds like a major problem, mono rarely causes complications and usually gets better with rest and time. As with colds, antibiotics won't combat the symptoms of mononucleosis.

Streptococcal bacteria ("strep throat") are another common cause of sore throat. Strep throat should be treated with antibiotics in order to prevent the small chance of an abscess forming and to prevent the heart and kidney damage that it can sometimes cause. It's hard to tell when a sore throat might be strep throat, but it's unlikely that you have strep throat if the sore throat is a minor part of a typical cold (runny nose, stuffy ears, etc.). A high temperature, pus in the back of the throat, or swollen tonsils can be clues indicating that strep throat may be present. Sore throat in people with HIV can also be caused by infection with candidiasis (thrush) or by ulcers in the throat from herpes or CMV (cytomegalovirus) infections.

None of these conditions is an emergency (unless, of course, you are unable to swallow or breathe), but a sore throat should sometimes be looked at by a doctor. If your sore throat doesn't seem to be associated with usual cold symptoms or if it lasts longer than ten days, you should contact your doctor.

Home Treatment of Sore Throat

Cold liquids, aspirin, ibuprofen, and acetaminophen are effective for the pain and fever associated with some sore throats. If you have had oral thrush in the past and think you might have it now (look for white, cottage cheese–like material in your mouth), you should start the thrush medicine your doctor gives you (usually clotrimazole lozenges; Mycelex®)). Home remedies that may help include over-the-counter lozenges, salt-water gargles, and honey or lemon in tea.

Urinary Infection: Painful, Frequent, or Bloody Urination

Urinary infections are much more common in women than in men, but men can get them too, especially if they have HIV. The most common symptoms of urinary infection are pain or burning during urination, frequent urgent urination, and blood in the urine. But sometimes these symptoms are not caused by infection.

They can also be due to excessive use of caffeine-containing beverages (coffee, tea, or cola), bladder spasms, or even anxiety. Bladder infection in women is often caused by having sex.

If fever, vomiting, back pain, or teeth-chattering or body-shaking chills are present with urination problems, the urinary infection may have spread from the bladder to the kidneys and may be much more serious. Bladder infections are common during pregnancy, when the treatment is more difficult. For women who get repeated bladder infections, it is important to remember to wipe the toilet tissue from front to back after urinating. Most bacteria that cause bladder infections come from the rectum.

Irritation from the vagina can sometimes cause frequent urination or blood in the urine. When this happens, the infection may not be in the urinary system, but in the vagina or cervix. If there is pain in the abdomen along with vaginal discharge, this suggests a potentially serious

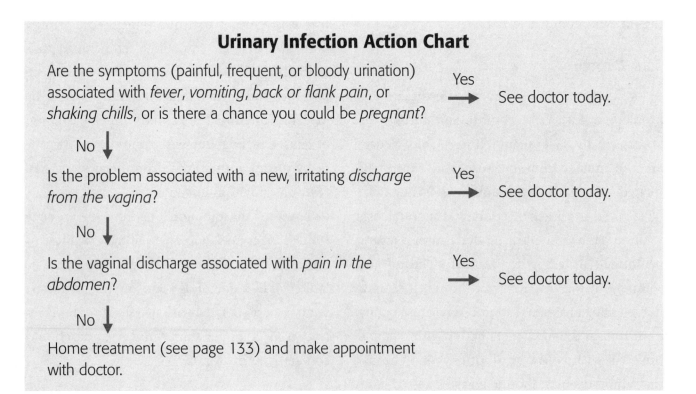

Urinary Infection Action Chart

Are the symptoms (painful, frequent, or bloody urination) associated with *fever, vomiting, back or flank pain*, or *shaking chills*, or is there a chance you could be *pregnant*?   Yes → See doctor today.

No ↓

Is the problem associated with a new, irritating *discharge from the vagina*?   Yes → See doctor today.

No ↓

Is the vaginal discharge associated with *pain in the abdomen*?   Yes → See doctor today.

No ↓

Home treatment (see page 133) and make appointment with doctor.

disease, ranging from gonorrhea to an ectopic pregnancy in the fallopian tube. These conditions are also suggested by bloody discharge that comes between periods, frequently or in large amounts. All these conditions should be evaluated by the doctor.

Candida yeast (the same thing that causes thrush) often causes discharge from the vagina—it looks like white, cheesy material. It may respond to over-the-counter anti-yeast medications (Monistat®, Mycolog®), but some women with HIV need stronger medicines available only by prescription.

The major concern in women with discharge from the vagina is the possibility of sexually transmitted disease (STD). All the organisms that cause STDs can cause severe infections in women with HIV. If sexual contact in the past few weeks may have led to an STD, you must see a doctor.

It's okay to start home self-management, but make an appointment with the doctor, too.

Home Treatment of Urinary Infection

Home treatment of urination problems involves drinking a lot of fluids because you need to flush your system out. Drink a gallon or more of fluid in the first 24 hours after symptoms start. Drink fruit juices to put more acid into the urine. Begin home treatment as soon as you notice the symptoms. Relief may well begin before you see the doctor.

Women who are taking antibiotics often get worse yeast infections in the vagina. To prevent these infections, some find it helpful to eat yogurt, buttermilk, or sour cream and to use less sugar and drink less alcohol. It may be helpful to call the doctor for advice on changing medications.

The symptoms described in this chapter may be minor and not worrisome, or they may be more serious and HIV-related. Use the descriptions and action charts to help you wisely decide when and how to home treat and when you should seek professional care.

Additional Resources

"Supplement: Evidence-Based Practice for HIV Symptom Management." *Journal of the Association of Nurses in AIDS Care* 24, no. 1 (January-February 2013): S1–S146, www.nursesinaidscarejournal.org/issue/S1055-3290%2812%29X0008-6

Suggested Further Reading

To learn more about the topics discussed in this chapter, we suggest that you explore the following resources:

Fries, James F., and Donald M. Vickery. *Take Care of Yourself*, 9th ed. Cambridge, Mass.: Da Capo Press, 2009.

Ward, Darrell E. *The AmFAR AIDS Handbook: The Complete Guide to Understanding HIV and AIDS*. New York: W.W. Norton & Company, 1998.

CHAPTER 11

Understanding the Symptom Cycle

CHRONIC HIV, LIKE ALL CHRONIC ILLNESSES, has symptoms. These may include fatigue, stress, numbness in hands and feet, skin rash, anger, depression, and sleep problems. Some symptoms cannot be seen by others, and some are very difficult to describe to others. Often you may not know when they will occur. Although some symptoms are common, the times when they occur and the ways in which they affect each person are very personal. What's more, these symptoms can interact, which may worsen existing symptoms or even lead to new symptoms or problems. This can create the "vicious cycle" of symptoms (Figure 11.1) we discussed in Chapter 1 and we include again in this chapter because we are discussing it in more detail here.

Regardless of the causes of these symptoms, the tools you can use to manage them are often similar. These tools are your basic self-management tools. This chapter discusses several of the chronic symptoms that you may have. It also discusses their causes and how you can use your self-management tools to address them. Additional cognitive tools—ways you can use your mind to help deal with many of these symptoms—are discussed in Chapter 12, "Using Your Mind to Manage Symptoms."

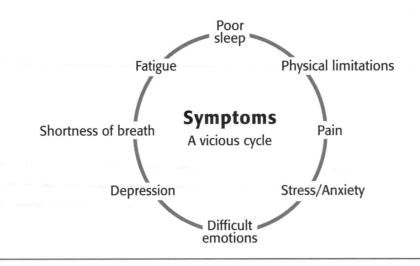

Figure 11.1 **The Vicious Cycle of Symptoms**

Dealing with Common Symptoms

Learning to manage symptoms is very similar to problem-solving, which we discuss in Chapter 2, "Becoming an HIV Self-Manager." First, it is important to identify the symptom. Next, determine why you might be having the symptom now. This may sound like a simple process, but it is not always easy. If you are not getting effective treatment for your HIV, then HIV-related problems may be causing your symptoms. If this is the case, you may want to review Chapter 10, "Evaluating Symptoms of HIV," before going on.

On the other hand, if you are like many people, all of your symptoms may not be directly linked to HIV. You can experience many different symptoms, and each symptom can have various causes, and may interact with other symptoms. The ways in which these symptoms affect your life can also be unique to you and vary over time. All of these factors can become very tangled, like the frayed threads of a cloth.

To manage your symptoms, it is often helpful to figure out how to untangle the threads.

One way to do this is to keep a daily diary or journal. This can be as straightforward as writing your symptoms on a calendar along with some notes about what you were doing before the symptom started or worsened, as shown in Figure 11.2, the Sample Calendar Symptom Journal. After a week or two, you may see a pattern in your entries. For example, you go out to dinner on Saturday evening and wake up in the night with stomach pain. Once you realize that you tend to overeat when you go out, you know to adjust what you order and eat in future visits to restaurants. Or you may notice that every time you go dancing, your feet hurt, but this does not occur when you walk. Could the different shoes you wear for each activity account for the difference? Recognizing patterns is the first step in symptom self-management for many people.

Sample Calendar Journal

Mon.	Tue.	Wed.	Thur.	Fri.	Sat.	Sun.
Grocery shop	Babysit grandkids Pain P.M.	Tired	Water exercise Feel great	Little stiff Clean house	Dinner out Poor sleep	Tired
Mon.	**Tue.**	**Wed.**	**Thur.**	**Fri.**	**Sat.**	**Sun.**
Grocery shop	Babysit grandkids Pain P.M.	Tired	Water exercise Feel great	Clean house	Feel great	Feel great Dinner out Poor sleep

Figure 11.2 **Sample Calendar Symptom Journal**

As you read this chapter, you will note that many symptoms have the same causes. In addition, one symptom may actually cause other symptoms. For example, pain may change the way you walk. This new way of walking may change your balance and cause a new pain or cause you to fall. As you gain a better understanding of the possible causes of your symptoms, you will be able to identify better ways to deal with them. You may also find ways to prevent or lessen certain symptoms.

Let's look at what you can do to lessen some of the more common symptoms experienced by people with particular chronic conditions. We hope you will find many tools in this book to help you with your symptoms.

Common Symptoms

The following common symptoms are discussed in this chapter:

- Fatigue (page 138)
- Pain or Physical Discomfort (page 140)
- Shortness of Breath (page 144)
- Sleep Problems (page 148)
- Depression (page 152)
- Anger (page 158)
- Stress (page 160)
- Itching (page 164)
- Urinary Incontinence (page 166)

Using Symptom-Management Tools

- **Choose a tool to try.** Be sure to give the method a fair trial. We recommend that you practice it for at least two weeks before deciding whether the tool is going to be helpful.

- **Try other tools, giving each a fair trial period.** It is important to try more than one tool because some tools may be more useful for certain symptoms, or you may find that you simply prefer some techniques over others.

- **Think about how and when you will use each tool.** For example, some tools may require more lifestyle changes than others. The best symptom managers learn to use a variety of techniques. These depend on your condition and what you want and need to do each day.

- **Place some cues in your environment to remind you to practice these techniques.** Both practice and consistency are important for mastering new skills. For example, place stickers or notes where you'll see them, such as on your mirror, on your cell phone, in your office, on your computer, or on the car's dashboard. Change the notes from time to time so that you'll continue to notice them. Also, ask a friend or family member to remind you to practice your techniques each day; they may even wish to participate.

- **Try linking the practice of each new tool with some other established daily behavior or activity.** Try to determine what behavior happens *right before* you want to try to develop a habit for using the new tool or behavior. For example, practice relaxation as part of your cool-down from exercise. Right before you take your HIV medications, you might want to try a new breathing exercise or stretching exercise. Right after your head hits the pillow, you might want to try a brief gratitude or relaxation exercise. Get the idea? Make action plans (see Chapter 2, "Becoming an HIV Self-Manager") to get started using the tools that work the best for you!

Fatigue

A chronic condition can drain your energy. Fatigue is a very real problem for many people. It is not, as some might say, "all in the mind." Fatigue can keep you from doing things you'd like to do. People who do not have a chronic illness often misunderstand fatigue. They might notice that your energy level is low, but they cannot feel what you are feeling inside. As a result, unfortunately, spouses, partners, family members, friends, doctors, and coworkers sometimes do not understand the unpredictable way in which the fatigue associated with your condition can affect you. They may think that you are simply not interested in certain activities or that you want to be alone. Sometimes even you may not recognize the negative ways that fatigue is affecting you.

To be able to manage fatigue, it is important to understand that your fatigue may be related to several factors, including the following:

■ **The disease itself.** When you have an illness or illnesses, whatever you do demands more energy of your body and mind than it requires of an illness-free person. When a chronic illness is present, the body uses energy less efficiently. This is because the energy that could be going to everyday activities is being used to help heal the body. Your body may release chemical signals to conserve energy and make you rest more. Some chronic conditions are also associated with anemia (low blood hemoglobin), which can contribute to fatigue.

■ **Inactivity.** Muscles that are not used regularly become deconditioned and less efficient at doing what they are supposed to do. The heart, which is made of muscle tissue, can also become deconditioned. When this happens, the ability of the heart to pump blood, which carries necessary nutrients and oxygen to other parts of the body, is decreased. When muscles do not receive these necessary nutrients and oxygen, they cannot function properly. Deconditioned muscles also tire more easily than muscles in good condition.

■ **Poor nutrition.** Food is your basic source of energy. If the fuel you take in is of inferior quality, is not consumed in the appropriate quantities, or is improperly digested, fatigue can result. Rarely are vitamin deficiencies a cause of fatigue. For some people, carrying excess weight results in fatigue. Extra weight causes an increase in the amount of energy a body needs to perform daily activities. Being underweight can also cause problems associated with fatigue. This is especially true for individuals with HIV. Many people with HIV experience weight changes because of a change in their eating habits, or stomach upset, or effects of the virus, and they experience fatigue as a result.

■ **Not enough rest.** For a variety of reasons, there are times when everyone does not get enough sleep or does not sleep well. This can also result in fatigue. We discuss how to manage sleep problems in more detail later in this chapter.

■ **Emotions.** Stress, anxiety, fear, and depression can cause fatigue. Most people are aware of the connection between stress and feeling tired, but fewer people are aware that fatigue is a major symptom of depression. Depression can be treated, so you should let your doctor know if you are feeling fatigue resulting from stress, depression, or anxiety.

■ **Medications.** Some medications can cause fatigue. If you think your fatigue is medication-related, talk to your doctor. Sometimes medications or the dose can be changed.

If fatigue is a problem for you, start by trying to determine the cause. Again, a journal may be helpful (see Figure 11.2). To address your fatigue, start with the things that are most within your control to improve. Are you eating healthy foods? Are you exercising? Are you getting enough good-quality sleep? Are you effectively managing stress? If your answer is no to any of these questions, you may be well on your way to finding one or more of the reasons for your fatigue.

Remember that things other than HIV can also cause fatigue. Therefore, to combat and prevent fatigue, you will want to address all of its possible causes. This may mean trying a variety of self-management tools.

If your fatigue is the result of not eating well, such as eating too much junk food or drinking too much alcohol, then the solution is to eat better-quality foods in the proper quantities or to drink less alcohol. For others, their problem may be a decreased interest in food, leading to a lack of calories and subsequent weight loss. Chapter 14, "Healthy Eating," discusses some of the problems associated with poor eating habits and provides tips for healthier eating.

People often say they can't exercise because they feel fatigued. Believing this creates a vicious cycle: people are fatigued because of a lack of exercise, and they don't exercise because of the fatigue. Believe it or not, motivating yourself to do a little exercise might be the answer to feeling too tired to exercise! You don't have to run a marathon. The important thing is to get outdoors and take a walk. If this is not possible, walk around your house or try some gentle chair exercises. See Chapter 13, "Physical Activity for Fun and Fitness," for more information and to get started on an exercise program.

If emotions are causing your fatigue, rest alone will probably not help. In fact, it may make you feel worse, especially if your fatigue is a sign of depression. We talk about how to deal with depression later in this chapter. If you feel that your fatigue may be related to stress, read the section on managing stress on pages 160–164.

Pain or Physical Discomfort

Pain or physical discomfort is a problem shared by many people with chronic illness, including those with HIV. As with most symptoms of chronic illness, pain or discomfort can have many causes. The following are some of the most common causes:

- **The disease itself.** Pain can come from inflammation in any part of the body, damage in or around joints and tissues, insufficient blood supply to muscles or organs, mouth or throat sores, or irritated nerves, to name just a few sources.

- **Tense muscles.** When a part of your body hurts, the muscles in that area become tense. This is your body's natural reaction to pain—to try to protect the damaged area. Stress can also cause you to tense your muscles. Tense muscles can cause soreness or pain.

- **Muscle deconditioning.** With chronic disease, it is common to become less active; this leads to weakening of the muscles, or muscle deconditioning. When a muscle is weak, it tends to "complain" anytime it is used. This is why, once you stop being active on a regular basis, even the slightest activity can sometimes lead to pain and stiffness.

- **Lack of sleep or poor-quality sleep.** Pain can interfere with your ability to get either enough sleep or good-quality sleep. But poor sleep can also make pain worse and lessen your ability to cope with it.

■ **Stress, anxiety, and emotions such as depression, anger, fear, and frustration.** These emotions are all normal responses to living with a chronic condition such as HIV, and they can affect your pain or discomfort. When we are stressed, angry, afraid, or depressed, everything, including pain, seems worse.

■ **Medications.** Medicines can sometimes cause abdominal or other discomfort, as well as pain, weakness, or changes in your thinking. If you suspect that medications are the cause of your pain, talk with your doctor.

Acute and Chronic Pain

There are two types of pain—acute and chronic. You experience acute pain when you have an injury, for example. Your pain is there to tell you "danger" is present and to warn you to protect yourself. If you twist your ankle, for example, acute pain tells you to stop what you are doing, rest, and let healing begin.

Sometimes the pain that we experience continues and doesn't go away. Your brain no longer regards the pain as "danger," but you continue to feel the pain. This is chronic pain. Chronic pain is pain that extends over months or years and is often difficult to explain. Most experts now believe that most unexplained chronic pain is originally caused by some type of physical problem such as damaged or inflamed nerves, blood vessels, muscles, or other tissues. These underlying physical problems simply can't be pinpointed.

Controlling the "Pain Gates"

Even though you may know the source of your pain in your body, it's important to realize that all pain is governed by the brain. Without your brain recognizing the pain signals from your body, you would not feel pain. That doesn't mean that your pain isn't real or is "all in your mind." It is absolutely real. Although it is real, that doesn't mean you can't do anything about your pain. Research suggests that we are not helpless in the face of pain. The brain can regulate the flow of pain messages by sending electrical and chemical signals that open and close "pain gates" along nerve pathways.

The brain can release powerful opiate-like chemicals—such as endorphins—that can effectively block pain. For example, when people are very seriously injured, they may experience very little pain while they are focused on survival. How you focus your attention, your mood, and the way you view your situation can open or close the pain gates. The techniques in Chapter 12, "Using Your Mind to Manage Symptoms," can be helpful as you work to manage your pain.

Your day-to-day pain level depends on how your mind and body respond to pain. For example, the body quickly attempts to limit the movement of a damaged area. This causes muscle tension, which can cause more pain. Chronic pain often leads to inactivity. Muscles often become weakened and may then hurt with the slightest use.

Feelings of anxiety, anger, frustration, and loss of control also amplify the experience of pain. Again, this doesn't mean that the pain is not real; it just means that emotions can make a painful situation worse.

Keep a Pain Diary

To better understand how your moods, activities, and conditions affect your pain, keep a pain diary. Begin by recording your activities and pain levels three times a day, at regular intervals. There are apps for your smartphone or tablet that will make this easy. For each entry:

1. Record the date and time.

2. Describe the situation or activity (watching TV, doing housework, arguing, etc.).

3. Rate the physical sensation of pain on a scale from 0 (no pain) to 10 (worst pain).

4. Describe the pain sensation (for example, "deep aching pain in left lower back").

5. Rate the emotional distress of pain on a scale from 0 (no distress) to 10 (terribly distressed).

6. Describe the type of emotional distress (for example, "felt very angry" or "needed to cry").

7. Describe what you did, if anything, to alleviate the discomfort (took medication, had a massage, did a relaxation exercise, took a walk, etc.) and its effect.

Look for patterns in your entries. For example, is your pain often worse after you sit for a long time? Is it less when you are engaged in a favorite hobby?

How much you notice pain can vary according to your mood, fatigue, and muscle tension. It's important to distinguish between physical pain sensations (stabbing, burning, and aching sensations) and emotional pain distress (the accompanying anger, anxiety, frustration, or sadness). This is useful because even if your physical pain cannot be reduced, you can learn to feel better about the pain and experience less distress, anxiety, helplessness, and despair.

Here are four examples of ways in which the mind and body interact:

- **Inactivity.** Because of the pain, you tend to avoid physical activity, which in turn causes you to lose strength and flexibility. The weaker and more out of condition you become, the more frustrated and depressed you feel. These negative emotions can open the pain gates and cause pain levels to rise.

- **Overdoing.** You may be determined to prove that you can still be active, so you overexert. This increases the pain and leads to more inactivity, more depression, and more pain.

- **Misunderstanding.** Your friends, family, boss, and coworkers may not understand that you are suffering and may dismiss your pain as "not real." This evokes frustration as well as more anger or depression.

- **Overprotection.** On the other hand, friends, family, and coworkers may coddle you and make excuses for you. This can lead you to feel and act more dependent and disabled.

Fortunately, this downward spiral of mind-body interaction can be interrupted. Since your brain governs your pain, learning ways to use your mind to stop the pain can help a great deal.

Being told you have to learn to live with pain doesn't have to be the end of the road. It can be a new beginning. You can learn techniques such as the following:

- Redirecting your attention to control pain

- Challenging negative thoughts that support pain

- Cultivating more positive emotions

- Slowly increasing your activity and reconditioning yourself

Tools for Managing Pain

There are many tools for managing pain. Just as one cannot build a house with one tool, one often needs several tools to manage pain.

Physical Activity

Exercise and physical activity can be excellent pain relievers. The benefits of exercise as well as tips for starting an exercise program are discussed in Chapter 13, "Physical Activity for Fun and Fitness." If you are not able to do the things you want and need to do because of physical limitations, a physical or occupational therapist may be helpful.

Mind-Made Medicine

As we discussed in this chapter and we cover in more depth in Chapter 12, you can use your mind to manage pain through relaxation, imagery, visualization, and distraction. Positive thinking is another powerful way to challenge pain. Learn how to monitor and challenge negative thinking or self-talk. If you find yourself waking up in pain and saying, "I'm going to be miserable all day; I won't get anything done," tell yourself instead, "I've got some pain this morning, so I'll start with some relaxation and stretching exercises. Then I'll do some of the less demanding things I want to get done today." You will find more about positive thinking in Chapter 12, "Using Your Mind to Manage Symptoms."

Ice, Heat, and Massage

For pain in a localized area such as the back or knee, the application of heat, cold, and massage have all been proven to be helpful. These three tools work by stimulating the skin and other tissues surrounding the painful area, which increases the blood flow to these areas or blocks transmission of pain in nerve fibers.

Apply heat by using a heating pad or by taking a warm bath or shower (with the water flow directed at the painful area). You can make a homemade heating pad by placing rice or dry beans in a sock, knotting the top of the sock, and heating it in a microwave oven for three to four minutes. Before use, be sure to test the heat so you don't burn yourself if it's too hot. Do not use popcorn!

Some people prefer cold to heat for soothing pain, especially if there is inflammation. A bag of frozen peas or corn makes an inexpensive, reusable cold pack. Ice and a little water in a zip-lock bag is another easy cold pack.

Whether using heat or cold, place a towel between the source and skin. Also, limit the application to 15 or 20 minutes at a time (longer can burn or freeze the skin).

Massage is one of the oldest forms of pain management. Hippocrates (c. 460–380 B.C.E.) said, "Physicians must be experienced in many things, but assuredly also in the rubbing that can bind a joint that is loose and loosen a joint that is too hard." Self-massage is a simple procedure that can be performed with little practice or preparation. Rubbing the painful area with a little applied pressure stimulates the skin, underlying tissues, and muscles. Some people like to use a mentholated cream with self-massage because it gives a cooling effect.

Massage, while relatively simple, is not appropriate for all sources of pain. Do not use self-massage for a "hot joint" (one that is red, swollen, and hot to the touch) or an infected area or if you are suffering from phlebitis, thrombophlebitis, or skin eruptions.

Medications for Pain

Acute pain usually responds to painkilling drugs, which range from mild over-the-counter analgesics for headaches (e.g., non-opioid drugs like acetaminophen, aspirin, or other anti-inflammatories) to powerful narcotic or opioid medications for postoperative and cancer pain (e.g., morphine and codeine-like drugs). Some medications open up blood vessels in the heart or muscles that can relieve pain.

Some types of chronic pain respond well to anti-inflammatory medications. Surprisingly, some medications originally used to treat depression have been found to relieve pain in lower doses without problems of addiction. Narcotic medications are rarely suitable for chronic pain, as they can become less effective over time and require increasing doses. They can also interfere with breathing, balance, and sleep and cause disturbances in mood and the ability to think clearly. Sometimes injections of a local anesthetic or a surgical procedure can block pain signals from a painful area. This provides temporary or sometimes lasting relief from chronic pain.

Two Important Final Notes about Pain

- If you have pain medication in the house, keep it in a place that is not accessible to young people or visitors. A locked box in a cabinet is a safe place for medications. The most common source of abused prescription drugs is the family medicine cabinet.

- If you or someone you care for is nearing the end of life (estimated to have six months or less to live) and pain is a problem, consider asking for palliative or hospice care. Hospice units are staffed by special teams of health professionals who are experts in relieving end-of-life pain while allowing the patient to remain alert. At this point in life, addiction is not a concern—comfort is.

If pain continues to be a major influence in your life, discuss your options with your doctor, including referral to a pain management clinic.

Shortness of Breath

HIV doesn't usually cause shortness of breath, but shortness of breath, like so many other symptoms, can have several other causes, all of which prevent your body from getting the oxygen it needs. Excess weight can cause shortness of breath because it increases the amount of energy you use and therefore the quantity of oxygen you need. Weight also increases the workload for the heart. Thus if excess weight is coupled with chronic lung or heart disease, it can be more difficult for the body to get the oxygen it needs.

Deconditioning of muscles can also lead to shortness of breath. This deconditioning can affect the breathing muscles as well as other muscles in your body. When muscles become deconditioned, they are less efficient at doing what they are supposed to do. They require more energy (and oxygen) to perform activities. In the case of deconditioned breathing muscles, the problem is complicated. If the breathing muscles are not strong, it becomes harder to cough and clear mucus from the lungs. When there is mucus in the lungs, there is less space for fresh air.

Just as there are many causes of shortness of breath, there are many things you can do to manage this problem. In this section we discuss some of the tools and techniques you can use if shortness of breath is a problem for you.

Breathing Self-Management Strategies

When you feel short of breath, don't stop what you are doing or hurry up to finish; instead, slow down. If shortness of breath continues, stop for a few minutes. If you are still short of breath, take medication if prescribed by your provider.

Shortness of breath can be frightening, and fear can cause two additional problems. First, when you are afraid, you release hormones such as epinephrine. This causes more shortness of breath. Second, you may stop activity for fear that it will hurt you. If this happens, you don't build up the endurance necessary to help your breathing.

The basic rule is to take things slowly and in steps. Increase your activity gradually, generally by not more than 25 percent each week. Thus, if you are now able to garden comfortably for 20 minutes, next week increase that time period by a maximum of 5 minutes. Once you can garden comfortably for 25 minutes, you can again add a few more minutes.

Don't smoke, and—equally important—avoid smokers. This may sometimes be difficult because smoking friends may not realize how they are complicating your life. Your job is to tell them. Explain that their smoke is causing breathing problems for you and that you would appreciate it if they would not smoke when you are around. Also, make your house and your car "no smoking" zones. At the house, ask people to smoke outside. With the vehicle, ask them to smoke before they get in, or to wait until after you've arrived at your destination. Most people will understand and comply with these reasonable requests to help improve your health.

If mucus and secretions are a problem, drink plenty of fluids (unless your doctor has told you to limit what you drink). This will help thin the mucus and make it easier to cough up. Using a humidifier may also be helpful.

Use your medications and oxygen as prescribed. We often hear that medications are harmful and should not be used. In some cases this is correct. However, when you have a chronic disease, they are often very helpful, even life savers. Don't skimp, cut down, or go without. At the same time, more is not better when it comes to medicine, so don't take more than the prescribed amount. If adjustments need to be made, let your health care provider make that decision.

Breathing Self-Management Techniques

Here are several tools you can use to help improve your breathing.

Diaphragmatic Breathing ("Belly Breathing")

Diaphragmatic breathing is also called "belly breathing" because when you do it properly, the diaphragm descends into the abdomen. One of the problems that cause shortness of breath, especially for people with emphysema, chronic bronchitis, or asthma, is deconditioning of the diaphragm and breathing muscles in the chest. When deconditioning occurs, the lungs are not able to function properly. That is, they do not fill well, nor do they completely get rid of old air.

Most of us use mainly our upper lungs and chest for breathing. Because diaphragmatic or belly breathing goes deeper, it requires a little practice to learn to fully expand the lungs. This deep breathing strengthens the breathing muscles and makes them more efficient, so breathing becomes easier. These are the steps for learning diaphragmatic breathing:

1. Lie on your back with pillows under your head and knees.

2. Place one hand on your stomach (at the base of your breastbone) and the other hand on your upper chest.

3. Breathe in slowly through your nose, allowing your stomach to expand outward. Imagine that your lungs are filling with fresh air. The hand on your stomach should move upward, and the hand on your chest should not move or should move only slightly.

4. Breathe out slowly, through pursed lips. At the same time, use your hand to gently push inward and upward on your abdomen. It should take about twice as long to breathe out as it does to breathe in.

5. Practice this technique for 10 to 15 minutes, three or four times a day, until it becomes automatic. If you begin to feel a little dizzy, breathe out more slowly.

You can also practice diaphragmatic breathing while sitting in a chair with the following technique:

1. Relax your shoulders, arms, hands, and chest. Do not grip the arms of the chair or your knees.

2. Put one hand on your abdomen and the other on your chest.

3. Breathe in through your nose, filling the area around your waist with air. Your chest hand should remain still and the hand on your abdomen should move.

4. Breathe out without force or effort.

Once you are comfortable with this technique, you can practice it almost anytime, while lying down, sitting, standing, or walking. Diaphragmatic breathing can help strengthen and improve the coordination and efficiency of the breathing muscles, as well as decrease the amount of energy needed to breathe. In addition, it can be used with any of the relaxation techniques that use the power of your mind to manage your symptoms (described in Chapter 12, "Using Your Mind to Manage Symptoms").

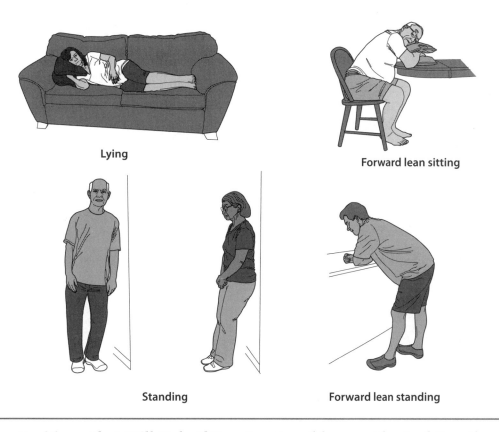

Lying

Forward lean sitting

Standing

Forward lean standing

Positions That Will Help If You Are Breathless or Short of Breath

Pursed-Lip Breathing

A second technique, pursed-lip breathing, usually happens naturally for people who have problems emptying their lungs. It can also be used if you are short of breath or breathless.

1. Breathe in, and then purse your lips as if to blow across a flute or into a whistle.

2. Using diaphragmatic breathing, breathe out through pursed lips without any force.

3. Remember to relax the upper chest, shoulders, arms, and hands while breathing out. Check for tension. Breathing out should take longer than breathing in.

By mastering this technique while doing other activities, you will be better able to manage your shortness of breath.

The next two techniques may be helpful for removing secretions (mucus, phlegm).

Huffing

This technique combines one or two forced "huffs" (puffs of breath) with diaphragmatic breathing. It is useful for removing secretions (phlegm) from small airways in your lungs.

1. Take in a breath as you would for diaphragmatic breathing.

2. Hold your breath for a moment.

3. Huff—keep your mouth open while squeezing your chest and abdominal muscles to force out the air. (This is a little like panting.)

4. If possible, do another huff before taking in another breath.

5. Take two or three diaphragmatic breaths.

6. Huff once or twice.

Controlled Cough

This technique helps remove secretions (phlegm) from larger airways.

1. Take in a full, slow diaphragmatic breath.

2. Keep your shoulders and hands relaxed.

3. Hold the breath for a moment.

4. Cough—tighten the abdominal muscles to force the air out.

Note: If you have a bout of uncontrolled coughing, the following may help:

- Avoid very dry air or steam.

- Swallow as soon as the bout starts.

- Sip water.

- Suck on lozenges or hard candy.

- Try diaphragmatic breathing, being sure to breathe in through your nose.

Sleep Problems

Sleep is a time during which the body can concentrate on healing and recovery. Little energy is required to maintain body functioning when we sleep. When we do not get enough sleep, we can experience a variety of other symptoms, such as fatigue, inability to concentrate, irritability, increased pain, and weight gain. Of course, this does not mean that all these symptoms are always caused by a lack of sleep. Remember, the symptoms associated with chronic disease can have many causes. Nevertheless, improving the quality of your sleep can help you manage many of these symptoms, regardless of the cause.

How Much Sleep Do You Need?

The amount of recommended sleep varies from person to person. Most people do best with seven and a half hours. Some feel refreshed with just six, but others need eight to ten to function well. If you are alert, feel rested, and function well during the day, chances are you're getting enough sleep. Sleep is a basic human need, like

food and water. Getting less sleep one night is not a big problem. But if you get less sleep than you require night after night, your quality of life and mood may suffer.

Getting a Good Night's Sleep

The self-management techniques we offer here are clinically proven, with a 75 to 80 percent success rate. They are not "quick fixes" like sleep medications, but they'll give you more effective (and safer) results in the long run. Allow yourself at least two to four weeks to see some positive results and ten to twelve weeks for long-term improvement.

Things to Do before You Get into Bed

- **Get a comfortable bed** that allows for ease of movement and good body support. This usually means a good-quality, firm mattress that supports the spine and does not allow the body to sink in the middle of the bed. A bed board, made of 1/2- to 3/4-inch (1 to 2 cm) plywood, can be placed between the mattress and the box spring to increase the firmness.

■ **Warm your hands and feet** with gloves or socks. For painful knees, it often helps to cut the toes off warm stockings and use the remainders as sleeves over the knees.

■ **Find a comfortable sleeping position.** The best position depends on you and your condition. Sometimes small pillows placed in the right places can relieve pain and discomfort. Experiment with different positions and pillows. Also check with your health care provider for specific recommendations given your condition.

■ **Elevate the head of the bed** 4 to 6 inches (10 to 15 cm) to make breathing easier. You can prop sturdy wooden blocks under the bed legs or purchase an adjustable bed to raise your head during sleep. This is especially helpful if you have heartburn or gastric reflux. If you snore, raising your head may help alleviate the problem.

■ **Keep the room at a comfortable temperature.** This can be either warm or cool. Each of us is unique.

■ **Use a vaporizer** if you live where the air is dry. Warm, moist air often makes breathing and sleeping easier. If you prefer cool air at night, use a humidifier.

■ **Make your bedroom safe and comfortable.** Keep a lamp and telephone by your bed, within easy reach. If you use a cane, keep it by the bed where you will not trip over it. This way you can use it when you get up during the night.

■ **Keep eyeglasses by the bed** when you go to sleep. This way, if you need to get up in the middle of the night, you can easily put on your glasses and see where you are going!

Things to Avoid before Bedtime

■ **Avoid eating.** You may feel sleepy after eating a big meal, but that is not an appropriate way to help you fall asleep and get a good night's sleep. Sleep is supposed to allow your body time to rest and recover, and when it is busy digesting food, this takes valuable time and attention away from the healing process. Try to allow 10 to 12 hours between your evening and morning meal to help this healing process. If you find that going to sleep feeling hungry keeps you awake, try drinking a glass of warm milk at bedtime.

■ **Avoid using a computer, smartphone, or watching TV** for about an hour before you go to bed. The light from screens can disrupt your natural sleep rhythms.

■ **Avoid alcohol.** You may think that alcohol helps you sleep better because it makes you feel relaxed and sleepy, but in fact, alcohol disrupts your sleep cycle. Alcohol before bedtime can lead to shallow sleep and frequent awakenings throughout the night.

■ **Avoid caffeine late in the day.** Caffeine is a stimulant, and it can keep you awake. Coffee, tea, colas and other sodas, and chocolate all contain caffeine, so go easy on them after 2:00 P.M.

■ **Avoid smoking to help you sleep.** Aside from the fact that smoking itself can cause complications and a worsening of your chronic disease, falling asleep with a lit cigarette is a fire hazard. Furthermore, the nicotine contained in cigarettes is a stimulant.

- **Avoid diet pills.** Diet pills often contain stimulants, which may interfere with falling asleep and staying asleep.

- **Avoid sleeping pills.** Although the name "sleeping pills" sounds like the perfect solution for sleep problems, these remedies tend to become less effective over time. Also, many sleeping pills have a rebound effect—that is, if you stop taking them, it is more difficult to get to sleep. Thus, as they become less effective, you can have even more problems than you had when you first started taking the pills. All in all, it is best to use other approaches and to avoid using sleeping pills.

- **Avoid diuretics (water pills) before bedtime.** You may want to take them in the morning instead so that your sleep is not interrupted by frequent trips to the bathroom. Unless your doctor has recommended otherwise, don't reduce the overall amount of fluids you drink, as these are important for your health. However, you may want to limit the amount you drink right before you go to bed.

How to Develop a Routine

- **Maintain a regular rest and sleep schedule.** Try to go to bed at the same time every night and get up at the same time every morning. If you wish to take a brief nap, take one in the afternoon, but do not take a nap after dinner. Stay awake until you are ready to go to bed.

- **Reset your sleep clock when necessary.** If your sleep schedule gets off track (for example, if one day you don't get to sleep until 4:00 A.M. and then sleep until noon), you'll have to reset your internal sleep clock. To do so, try going to bed an hour earlier or later each day until you reach the hour you want to go to sleep. This may sound strange, but it seems to be the best way to reset your sleep clock.

- **Exercise at regular times each day.** Not only will the exercise help you obtain better-quality sleep, but it will also help set a regular pattern for your day. However, avoid exercising immediately before bedtime.

- **Get out in the sun every morning**, even if it is only for 15 or 20 minutes. This helps regularize your body clock and rhythms.

- **Make a habit of doing the same things every night before going to bed.** This can be anything from listening to the news to reading a chapter of a book to taking a warm bath. By developing and sticking to a "get ready for bed" routine, you will be telling your body that it's time to start winding down and relax.

- **Use your bedroom only for sleeping and sex.** If you find that you get into bed and you can't fall asleep, get out of bed and go into another room until you begin to feel sleepy again. Keep the lighting low.

What to Do When You Can't Get Back to Sleep

Many people can get to sleep without a problem but then wake up with the "middle of the night worries" and can't turn off their minds.

Then they get more worried because they cannot go back to sleep once they have awakened. Keeping your mind occupied with pleasurable or interesting thoughts will ward off the worries and help you get back to sleep. For example, try a distraction technique such as quieting your mind by counting backward from 100 by threes or by naming a flower, brand of car, or whatever interests you for every letter of the alphabet. The relaxation techniques described in Chapter 12, "Using Your Mind to Manage Symptoms," may also be helpful. If after a while you really can't sleep, get up and do something—read a book, wash your hair, play a game of solitaire (not on the computer). After 15 or 20 minutes, go back to bed.

It can also help to set a "worry time." Does a racing mind keep you awake? If it does, designate a time well before bedtime during which you write down your problems and concerns, and then make a to-do list to get them off your mind. Then you can relax and sleep well at night, knowing that you can worry again during tomorrow's worry time.

Don't worry about not getting enough sleep. If your body needs sleep, you will sleep. Also, remember that people tend to need less sleep as they get older.

Sleep Apnea and Snoring

If you fall asleep "as soon as your head hits the pillow" or fall asleep regularly in front of the TV and are tired when you wake up in the morning, even after a full night's sleep, you may have a sleep disorder. People who have the most common sleep disorder, obstructive sleep apnea, often do not know it. When they are asked about their sleep, they respond, "I sleep just fine." Sometimes the only clue is that others complain about their loud snoring. Sleep specialists believe that obstructive sleep apnea is very common and alarmingly underdiagnosed.

With sleep apnea, the soft tissue in the throat or nose relaxes during sleep and blocks the airway, requiring extreme effort to breathe. The person struggles against the blockage for up to a minute, then wakes just long enough to gasp air, and falls back to sleep to start the cycle all over again. People with sleep apnea are rarely aware that they have awakened dozens of times during the night and do not get the deep sleep needed to restore the body's energy and help with the healing process. This, in turn, leads to more symptoms such as fatigue and pain.

Sleep apnea is a serious or even life-threatening medical problem. It has been linked to heart disease and stroke and is thought to be the cause of death for many people who die in their sleep after a heart attack. Sleep experts suggest that people who are tired all the time in spite of a full night's sleep or who find that they need more sleep now than when they were younger should be evaluated for sleep apnea or other sleep disorders, especially if they (or their partner) report snoring.

Getting Professional Help for Sleep Problems

The majority of sleep problems can be solved with the techniques just mentioned, but there are times when you need professional assistance. When should you get help?

- If your insomnia persists for six months or is seriously affecting your daytime functioning (your job or your social relationships), even though you are faithfully following the self-help program described here

■ If you have great difficulty staying awake during the day, especially if your daytime sleepiness causes or comes close to causing an accident

■ If your sleep is disturbed by breathing difficulties, including loud snoring with long pauses, chest pain, heartburn, leg twitching, excessive pain, or other physical conditions

■ If your difficulty sleeping is accompanied by depression, problems with alcohol, sleeping medications, or addictive drugs

Don't put off asking for help. Some sleep problems can be dangerous. Most sleep problems can be solved. Once they're gone, you'll enjoy a better night's sleep and better health.

Depression

Most people with a chronic illness sometimes feel depressed. Depression is extremely common in people with HIV. As with pain, there are different degrees of depression. These can range from being occasionally sad or blue to serious clinical depression. Sometimes people with depression may not know they are depressed. Sometimes, people who are depressed do not want to admit it. How you handle depression makes the difference.

Depression and Bad Moods

Feeling sad sometimes is natural. "Normal" sadness is a temporary feeling, often linked to a specific event or loss. We sometimes use the word *depressed* to describe feeling sad or disappointed (e.g., "I'm really depressed about missing my friends' annual visit"). In these circumstances, we feel sad, but we can still relate to others and find joy in other areas of our lives. Sometimes depression lasts longer, as when we lose a loved one or are diagnosed with a serious illness.

If your depressed or sad feelings are severe, long-lasting, and recurrent, you may be experiencing clinical depression. It drains the pleasure out of life, leaving you feeling hopeless, helpless, and worthless. With severe depression, feelings may become numb, and even crying brings no relief. Depression affects everything: the way you think, the way you behave, the way you interact with others, and even the way your body functions.

What Causes Depression?

Depression is not caused by personal weakness, laziness, or lack of willpower. Heredity, your chronic illness, and your medications may all play a role in depression. The way you think, especially negative thoughts, can also produce and sustain a depressed mood. Negative thoughts can be automatic, recur endlessly, and are often not linked to any event or triggering cause. Certain feelings and emotions also contribute to depression, including the following:

■ **Fear, anxiety, or uncertainty about the future.** Feelings that stem from worries about the future, finances, your disease or treatment, or concerns about your family can lead to depression. By facing these issues as soon as possible, both you and your family will spend less time worrying and have more time to enjoy life. This can have a healing effect. We talk more about these issues and how to deal with them in Chapter 17, "Planning for the Future: Fears and Reality."

- **Frustration.** Frustration can have many causes. You may find yourself thinking, "I just can't do what I want," "I feel so helpless," "I used to be able to do this myself," or "Why doesn't anyone understand me?" The longer you accept these feelings, the more alone and isolated you are likely to feel.

- **Loss of control over your life.** Many things can make you feel like you are losing control. These include having to rely on medications, having to see a doctor on a regular basis, or having to count on others to help you do things you would normally do for yourself. This feeling of loss of control can make you lose faith in yourself and your abilities. Even though you may not be able to do everything yourself, you can still be in charge. You are the coach for your team.

All these factors, along with others, can contribute to an imbalance in the chemicals in your brain (neurotransmitters). This imbalance can result in changes in the way you think, feel, and act. Changing the way you think and behave can be a powerful and effective way of changing your brain chemistry, lightening depression, and improving an ordinary bad mood.

Depressed feelings can lead to such behaviors as withdrawal, isolation, drug and alcohol use, and lack of physical activity. These behaviors can cycle back to create more depressed feelings. The paradox of depression-related behavior is that the more you engage in the behavior, the more likely it is that you will drive away the people who can support and comfort you. Most of our friends and family want to help us feel better, but often they don't really know what to do to help. As their efforts to comfort and reassure us are frustrated, they may at some point throw up their hands and quit trying. Then the depressed person winds up saying, "See, nobody cares." This again reinforces the feelings of loss and loneliness.

Not all depression behavior is negative. Sometimes unrealistic cheeriness will mask what the person is really feeling, and the wise observer will recognize the brittleness or phoniness of the mood. Refusal to accept offers of help, even in the face of obvious need for it, is a frequent symptom of undiagnosed depression.

Am I Depressed?

Here is a quick test for depression: Ask yourself what you do to have fun. If you do not have a quick answer, consider the possible symptoms of depression listed here.

Consider your mood over the past two weeks. Which of the following have you experienced?

- **Little interest or pleasure in doing things.** Not enjoying life or other people may be a sign of depression. Symptoms include not wanting to talk to anyone, to go out, or to answer the phone or doorbell.

- **Feeling down, depressed, hopeless angry. or irritable.** Feeling persistently blue or irritable can be a symptom of depression.

- **Trouble falling or staying asleep or sleeping too much.** Awakening and being unable to return to sleep or sleeping too much and not wanting to get out of bed can signal a problem.

- **Feeling tired or having little energy.** Fatigue—feeling tired all the time—is often a clear-cut symptom of depression.

- **Poor appetite or overeating.** This change may range from a loss of interest in food to unusually erratic or excessive eating.

- **Feeling bad about yourself.** Have you felt that you are a failure or have let yourself or your family down? Have you had a feeling of worthlessness, a negative image of your body, or doubts about your own self-worth?

- **Trouble concentrating.** Have you found it hard to do things like reading the newspaper or watching television?

- **Lethargy or restlessness.** Have you been moving or speaking so slowly that other people may have noticed? Or the opposite: Have you been fidgety or restless and moving around a lot more than usual? Either can be a sign of depression.

- **Wishing yourself harm or worse.** Thoughts that you would be better off dead or of hurting yourself in some way are often the hallmark of severe depression.

Depressed people may also experience weight gain or loss, loss of interest in sex or intimacy, loss of interest in personal care and grooming, inability to make decisions, and more frequent accidents.

If several of these symptoms seem to apply to you, *please* seek help from your doctor, good friends, a member of the clergy, a psychologist, or a social worker. Do not wait for these feelings to pass. If you are thinking about harming yourself or others, *get help now.* Don't let a tragedy happen to you and your loved ones. *Severe depression is a biological illness, and it can be treated.*

Fortunately, the treatments for depression, including counseling, antidepressant medications, and self-help, are highly effective in decreasing the frequency, length, and severity of depression. Depression, like other symptoms, can be managed.

How to Lighten Depression and Bad Moods

The most effective treatments for depression are counseling, medications, and self-help. We discuss each of these approaches in the following material.

Counseling

Several types of psychotherapy can be highly effective to lighten depression, relieving symptoms up to 60 to 70 percent of the time. Even though it is often effective, it is important to know that counseling rarely has an immediate effect. It may be weeks (or longer) before you see improvement. Therapy does not have to last a lifetime; it can be brief, usually involving one to two sessions a week for several months. By learning new skills for ways to think and relate, psychotherapy may also help reduce the risk of recurrent depression. In addition to individual mental health therapy and counseling, there are also support groups run by counselors, some of which may be recommended by your doctor or counselor. Many people find group interactions helpful in relieving some of their depressed symptoms.

Medications for Depression

Antidepressant medications that help balance brain chemistry are highly effective. Most antidepressant medications take from several days to several weeks before they begin to work. Then they usually bring significant relief. If your doctor prescribes an antidepressant, don't be discouraged if you don't feel better immediately. Stick with it. To get the maximum benefit you may need to take certain medications for six months or more.

Like your HIV medications, side effects of antidepressant medications are usually most noticeable in the first few weeks and then lessen or go away. If you experience side effects but they are not especially severe, continue to take your medication. As your body gets used to the medication, you will begin to feel better. It is important to remember to take your antidepressant medication every day. If you stop the medication because you're feeling better (or worse), you may relapse. Antidepressant medications are not addictive, but talk with your doctor before stopping or changing the dose.

Self-Help Tools and Techniques

Self-help can also be surprisingly effective for dealing with mild depression. You can learn many successful psychotherapy techniques on your own. For mild to moderate depression or just to lift your mood, the self-help strategies discussed here can sometimes be very productive. One study showed that reading and practicing self-help advice improved depression in nearly 70 percent of patients.

The following skills and strategies can be used alone or to supplement medications and counseling:

■ **Eliminate the negative.** First let's talk about what does not help depression or bad moods. Being alone and isolating yourself, crying a lot, getting angry and yelling, blaming your failure or bad mood on others, or using alcohol or other drugs usually leaves you feeling worse. Are you taking tranquilizers, sleeping medications, narcotic/opioid painkillers, sleeping medications, or other depressants or "downers"? Medications such as Valium®, Librium®, Xanax®, Restoril®, Vicodin®, codeine, and oxycodone can intensify depression or may cause depression as a side effect. However, do not stop taking any medication before first talking with your doctor, as there may be important reasons for continuing its use or you may experience withdrawal reactions.

Do you drink alcohol to feel better? Alcohol is also a depressant or downer. There is virtually no way to escape depression unless you unload these negative influences from your brain. For most people, one or two drinks in the evening is not a problem, but if your mind is not free of alcohol during most of the day, you are having trouble with this drug. Talk this over with your doctor or call Alcoholics Anonymous.

■ **Plan for pleasure.** When you are feeling blue or depressed, the tendency is to withdraw, isolate yourself, and restrict activities. However, this may make the depression worse. Maintaining or increasing activities is one of the best antidotes for depression. Going for a walk, looking at a sunset, watching a funny movie, getting a massage, learning another language, taking a cooking class, or joining a social club can all help keep your spirits up and keep you from falling into a situation where you can get depressed.

Sometimes having fun isn't such an easy prescription. You may have to make a deliberate effort to plan pleasurable activities. Even if you don't feel like doing it, try to stick to the schedule. You may find that the nature walk, cup of tea, or half hour of listening to music will improve your mood despite your initial misgivings. Don't leave good things to chance. Make up a schedule for your free time during the week and what you'd like to do with it.

If you are feeling hardly any emotion and the world seems devoid of color, make an effort to put some sensation back into your life. Go to a bookstore and look through your favorite section. Listen or dance to some upbeat music. Exercise or ask someone to give you a massage so you can reconnect with your body. Eat some spicy food. Treat yourself to a very hot bath, or try a cold shower. Go to a garden center and smell all the flowers.

Make plans and carry them out. Look to the future. Plant some young trees. Look forward to your grandchildren's graduation from college even if your own kids are in high school. If you know that one time of the year is especially difficult, such as Christmas or a birthday, make specific plans for that period. Don't wait to see what happens. Be prepared.

■ **Take action.** Continue your daily activities. Get dressed every day, make your bed,

get out of the house, go shopping, walk your dog. Plan and cook meals. Force yourself to do these things even if you don't feel like it. Taking action to solve the problems immediately facing you provides the surest relief from a bad mood. More important than what you change or how much you change are the confidence-building feelings that come from successfully changing something—anything! Taking action is the important thing. Incorporating some simple, positive activity into your life can boost your mood. You might decide to clean or reorganize a room, for instance, or a closet or even a desk drawer. Or get a new magazine subscription or call an old friend.

Be careful not to set goals that are too difficult or take on a lot of responsibility. Break large tasks into small ones, set some priorities, and do what you can as best you can. Learn some of the proven steps for taking successful action (see Chapter 2, "Becoming an HIV Self-Manager").

When you are feeling depressed, be active—but avoid making big life decisions. For example, don't move to a new setting without first visiting for a few weeks and learning about the resources available to you in this new community. Moving can be a sign of withdrawal, and depression often intensifies when you are in a location away from friends and acquaintances. Besides, many troubles may move with you. At the same time, the support you may need to deal with your troubles may have been left behind.

- **Socialize.** Join a group. Get involved in a church or other spiritual group, a book club, a community college class, a self-help class, or art class. If you can't get out, consider a group on the Internet. (If you do this, be sure that the Internet group is moderated—that is, that someone is in charge to enforce the rules of the group.) Don't isolate yourself. Try to seek out positive, optimistic people who can lighten your heavy feelings.

- **Move your mood.** Physical activity lifts depression and negative moods. Depressed people often complain that they feel too tired to exercise. But the feelings of fatigue associated with depression are not due to physical exhaustion. Try to get at least 20 to 30 minutes a day of some type of exercise, from walking to dancing. If you can get yourself moving, you may find that you have more energy (see Chapter 13, "Physical Activity for Fun and Fitness").

- **Think positive.** Many people tend to be excessively critical of themselves, especially when they're depressed. You may find yourself thinking groundless, untrue things about yourself. Recast your automatic negative thoughts and begin to rescript the negative stories you tell yourself (see Chapter 12, "Using Your Mind to Manage Symptoms"). For example, one of your underlying beliefs may be, "Unless I do everything perfectly, I'm a failure." Perhaps this belief could be revised to, "Success is doing the best that I can in any situation." Also, when you are depressed, it's easy to forget that anything nice has happened at all. Make a list of some of the good or positive events in your life.

- **Do something for someone else.** Lending a helping hand to someone in need is one of the most effective ways to change a bad mood, but it is one of the least commonly used. Arrange to deliver food to someone who is homebound, read a story to someone who has vision problems, mentor someone newly diagnosed with HIV, or volunteer at a soup kitchen. When you're depressed, you may greet the advice of helping others with thoughts like, "I've got enough troubles of my own. I don't need anyone else's." But if you can bring yourself to help someone else, even in a small way, you'll feel better about yourself. Feeling useful is good for self-esteem, and you will be temporarily distracted from your own problems. Helping others who are needier than yourself can help you appreciate your own assets and capabilities. By comparison, your problems and difficulties may not appear as overwhelming. Sometimes helping others is the surest way to help yourself.

Don't be discouraged if it takes some time to come out of your depression and feel better. If these self-help strategies alone are not sufficient, seek help from your physician or a mental health professional. Often some "talk therapy" or the use of antidepressant medications (or both) can go a long way toward relieving depression. Seeking professional help and taking medications are not signs of weakness. They are signs of strength.

Anger

Anger is one of the most common responses to chronic illnesses such as HIV. The uncertainty and unpredictability of living with a chronic disease may threaten your independence and control. At times you may find yourself asking, "Why me?" This is a normal response to chronic illness.

You may be angry with yourself, family, friends, health care providers, God, or the world in general. For example, you may be angry at yourself for not taking better care of yourself. You may be angry at your family and friends because they don't do things the way you want. Or you might be angry at your doctors because they cannot fix your problems. Sometimes your anger may be misplaced, as when you find yourself yelling at the cat or dog.

Sometimes the health condition itself causes anger. For example, a stroke or Alzheimer's disease can affect someone's emotions, leading the person to cry inappropriately or have temper flare-ups. Some people who are depressed or have anxiety disorders express their depression or anxiety through anger.

The philosopher Aristotle (c. 384–322 B.C.E.) observed, "Anyone can get angry—that is easy—but to do this to the right person, to the right extent, at the right time, with the right motive, and in the right way, that is not for everyone, nor is it easy." The first step is recognizing or admitting that you are angry and identifying why or with whom. These are important steps to learning how to manage your anger effectively. This task also involves finding constructive ways to express your anger.

Defusing Anger

Research now suggests that people who vent their anger actually get angrier. But suppressing anger isn't the answer either. The angry feelings often smolder, only to flare up later. To better control any anger you may be feeling, remember these two things:

- You can raise your anger threshold—that is, allow fewer things to trigger your anger in the first place.
- You can choose how to react when you get angry—without either denying your feelings or giving in to the situation.

This sounds simple enough, but what gets in the way is our tendency to see anger as coming from outside ourselves—something over which we have little control. We see ourselves as helpless victims. We blame others and say, "You make me so angry!" We explode and then say, "I couldn't help it." We see friends as selfish and insensitive, bosses as snobs or bullies, friends as unappreciative. So it seems that our only choice is an outburst of hostility. But with a little practice, even a seasoned hothead can master a new repertoire of healthy and more effective responses.

Anger Management Techniques

Here are some effective tools and techniques you can use to help manage your anger.

Reason with Yourself

How you interpret and explain a situation determines whether you will feel angry or not. You can learn to defuse anger by pausing and questioning your anger-producing thoughts. If you change your thoughts, you can change your response. You can decide whether or not to get angry and then decide whether or not to act.

At the first sign of anger, count to three and ask yourself the following questions:

- **Is this really important enough to get angry about?** Maybe this incident isn't serious enough to merit the time and energy. Consider if the issue will likely make a big difference in your life. Will you remember this in a day, a week, a year?

- **Am I justified in getting angry?** You may need to gather more information to really understand the situation. Make sure that you are not jumping to conclusions or misinterpreting the intentions or actions of others.

- **Will getting angry make a difference?** More often than not, getting angry and losing your cool does not work and may even have negative consequences for you. Exploding or venting increases your angry feelings, puts a strain on your relationships, and potentially damages your health.

Cool Off

Any technique that relaxes or distracts you—such as meditating or taking a long walk—can help you put out the fire within. Slow, deep breathing is one of the quickest and simplest ways to cool off. When you notice anger building, take ten slow, relaxed breaths before responding. Sometimes withdrawing and buying some alone time can defuse the situation. Also, physical exercise provides a good natural outlet for stress and anger.

Verbalize without Blame

One important technique is to learn how to communicate your anger aloud, preferably without blaming or offending others. This can be done by learning to use "I" (rather than "you") messages to express your feelings. (Refer to Chapter 16, "Communicating with Family, Friends, and Everyone Else" for a discussion of "I" messages.) If you do choose to express your anger verbally, know that many people will not be able to help you. Many people are not very good at dealing with angry people. This is true even if the anger is justified. Therefore, you may also find it useful to seek counseling or join a support group.

Modify Your Expectations

You may benefit from modifying your expectations. You have done this throughout your life. For example, perhaps as a child you thought you could become anything—a fireman, a ballet dancer, a doctor, and so on. As you grew older, however, you reevaluated these expectations, along with your capabilities, talents, and interests. Based on this reevaluation, you modified your plans.

This same process can be used to deal with the effects of chronic illness in your life. For example, it may be unrealistic to expect that you will get "all better." However, it *is* realistic to expect that you can still do many pleasurable things. You have the ability to affect the progress of your illness by slowing your decline or preventing it from becoming worse. Changing your expectations can help you change your perspective. Instead of dwelling on the 10 percent of things you can no longer do, think about the 90 percent of things you *can* still do.

Anger is a normal response to having a chronic condition. Part of learning to manage the condition involves acknowledging this anger and finding constructive ways to deal with it.

Stress

Stress is a common problem. But what is stress? In the 1950s, the physiologist Hans Selye described stress as "the nonspecific response of the body to any demand made upon it." Others have expanded this definition to explain that the body adapts to demands, whether pleasant or unpleasant. For example, you may feel stress when you are experiencing negative events, such as the death of a loved one, or even joyful events such as marriage or a new home.

How Does the Body Respond to Stress?

Your body is used to functioning at a certain level. When there is a need to change this level, your body must adjust to meet the demand. It reacts by preparing to take some action: your heart rate increases, your blood pressure rises, your neck and shoulder muscles tense, your breathing becomes more rapid, your digestion slows, your mouth becomes dry, and you may begin sweating. These are signals of what we call stress.

Why does this happen? To move, your muscles need to be supplied with oxygen and energy. Your breathing increases in an effort to inhale as much oxygen as possible and to get rid of as much carbon dioxide as possible. Your heart rate increases to deliver the oxygen and nutrients to the muscles. To allow your body to divert even more energy to taking action, body functions that are not immediately necessary,

such as the digestion of food and the body's natural immune responses, are slowed down.

How long do these responses last? In general, they are present only until the stressful event passes. Your body then returns to its normal level of functioning. Sometimes, though, your body does not return to its former comfortable level. If the stress is present for any length of time, your body begins adapting to it. This chronic stress can contribute to the onset of some chronic conditions and can make some symptoms more difficult to manage.

Common Stressors

Regardless of the type of stressor, the changes in the body are the same. Stressors, however, are not completely independent of one another. In fact, one stressor can often lead to other stressors or even magnify the effects of existing stressors. As we saw in Figure 11.1, The Vicious Cycle of Symptoms (page 136), several stressors can also occur at the same time. For instance, shortness of breath can cause anxiety, frustration, inactivity, and loss of endurance. In the following material, we examine some of the most common sources of stress.

Physical Stressors

Physical stressors can range from something as pleasant as taking your children to the zoo to an everyday trip to the grocery store or the physical symptoms of your chronic illness. What they have in common is that all of these stressors increase your body's demand for energy. If your body is not prepared to deal with this demand, the results can range from sore muscles to fatigue to a worsening of some disease symptoms.

Mental and Emotional Stressors

Mental and emotional stressors can also be either pleasant or uncomfortable. The joys you experience from seeing a friend get married or meeting new friends may induce a similar stress response in your body as feeling frustrated or worried because of your illness. Although this fact may seem surprising, the similarity comes from the way your brain perceives the stress.

Environmental Stressors

Environmental stressors, too, can be both good and bad. They may be as varied as a sunny day, uneven sidewalks that make it difficult to walk, loud noises, bad weather, a snoring partner or spouse, or secondhand smoke. Each creates a pleasurable or apprehensive excitement that triggers the stress response.

Isn't "Good Stress" a Contradiction?

As noted earlier, some types of stress can be good, such as a job promotion, a wedding, a vacation, a new friendship, or a new baby. These stressors make you feel happy but still cause the changes in your body that we have just discussed. Another example of a good stressor is exercise.

When you exercise or do any type of physical activity, a demand is placed on the body. The heart has to work harder to deliver blood to the muscles; the lungs are working harder, and

you breathe more rapidly to keep up with your muscles' demand for oxygen. Meanwhile, your muscles are working hard to keep up with the signals from your brain, which are telling them to keep moving.

As you maintain an exercise program for several weeks, you will begin to notice a change. What once seemed virtually impossible becomes easier. Your body has adapted to this stress. There is less strain on your heart, lungs, and other muscles because they have become more efficient and you have become more fit.

The same can happen with psychological stresses. Many people become more resilient and stronger emotionally after experiencing emotional challenges and learning to adapt to them. There is an upside to learning to manage stress in healthy ways.

Recognizing When You Feel Stressed

Everyone has a certain need for stress. It helps your life run more efficiently. As long as you do not push past your body's breaking point, stress is helpful. You can tolerate more stress on some days than on others. But sometimes, if you are not aware of the different types of stress, you go beyond your breaking point and feel that your life is out of control. Often it is difficult to recognize when you are under too much stress. The following are some of the warning signs:

■ Biting your nails, pulling your hair, tapping your foot, or other repetitive habits

■ Grinding your teeth or clenching your jaw

■ Tension in your head, neck, or shoulders

■ Feeling anxious, nervous, helpless, angry, or irritable

- Frequent minor accidents
- Forgetting things you usually don't forget
- Difficulty concentrating
- Fatigue and exhaustion

Sometimes you can catch yourself when you are behaving or feeling stressed. If you do, take a few minutes to think about what it is that is making you feel tense. Take a few signal breaths and try to relax (for more on signal breathing, see Chapter 12, "Using Your Mind to Manage Symptoms"). Also, a quick body scan (also described in Chapter 12) can help you recognize stress in your body. You will find additional good ideas for coping with stress in that chapter.

Now let's examine some tools for dealing with stress.

Sorting Out Stress

Dealing effectively with stress does not need to be complicated. In fact, it can start with a simple three-step process:

1. Identify your stressors by making a list. Consider every area of your life: family, relationships, health, financial security, living environment, and so on. It may be helpful to write each stressor on a small Post-It® note.

2. **Sort your stressors.** For each stressor, ask yourself, "Is it important or unimportant?" and, "Is it changeable or unchangeable?" Then place each of your stressors in one of four categories:

   - Important and changeable
   - Important and unchangeable
   - Unimportant and changeable
   - Unimportant and unchangeable

For example, needing to quit smoking is changeable and, for most people, important. Loss of a loved one or a job is important and unchangeable. A bad season for your favorite sports team, a traffic jam, or bad weather are unchangeable and may or may not be important. What really counts is what you think about each stressor.

3. **Match your strategy to each stressor.** Different strategies work for different stressors. Here are some strategies to help you be more effective in managing each type of problem.

   - **Important and changeable stressors.** These types of stressors are best managed by taking action to change the situation and to reduce the stress associated with them. Useful decision-making and problem-solving skills include planning and goal setting (see Chapter 2, "Becoming an HIV Self-Manager"); imagery (page 180); positive thinking (page 178), effective communication (see Chapter 16, "Communicating with Family, Friends, and Everyone Else"), and seeking social support.

   - **Important and unchangeable stressors.** These stressors are often the most difficult to manage. They can make you feel helpless and hopeless. No matter what you do, you cannot make another person change, bring someone back from the dead, or delete traumatic experiences from your life. Even though you may not be able to change the situation, you may be able to use one or more of the following strategies to deal with them more constructively:

1. **Change the way you think about the problem.** For example, think how much worse it could be, focus on the positive and practice gratitude (see page 188), deny or ignore the problem, distract yourself (see page 175), or accept what you can't change.

2. **Find some part of the problem that you can reclassify as changeable.** You can't stop the hurricane, but you can take shelter and later take steps to rebuild after the storm passes.

3. **Reassess how important the problem is in light of your overall life and priorities.** Maybe your neighbor's criticism isn't so important after all.

4. **Change your emotional reactions to the situation and thereby reduce the stress.** You can't change what happened, but you can help yourself feel less distressed about it. When you feel stressed, try writing or confiding your deepest thoughts and feelings (see page 189), seeking social support, helping others, enjoying your senses, relaxing, using imagery, enjoying humor, or exercising.

   ■ **Unimportant and changeable stressors.** If the stressor is unimportant, first try just letting it go. But if you can control it with relatively little effort, go ahead and deal with it. Solving small problems helps build your skills and confidence to tackle bigger ones. Use the same strategies we described for important and changeable problems.

   ■ **Unimportant and unchangeable stressors.** The best solution for these problems is to ignore them. Starting now, you are given permission to let go of unimportant concerns. These are common hassles, and everybody has their share of them. Don't let them bother you. You can distract yourself with humor, relaxation or imagery, or focusing on more pleasurable things.

Using Problem-Solving to Deal with Stress

Whereas you can successfully manage some types of stress by modifying the situation, other types of stress can sneak up on you when you don't expect them. The approach to dealing with these types of stress also involves problem-solving.

If you know that certain situations will be stressful, develop ways to deal with them before they happen. Try to rehearse, in your mind, what you will do when the situation arises so that you will be ready. There are some situations that you no doubt recognize as stressful, such as being stuck in traffic, going on a trip, or preparing a meal. First, look at what it is about the particular situation that is stressful. Is it that you hate to be late? Are trips stressful because of uncertainty about your destination? Does meal preparation involve too many steps and demand too much energy?

Once you have determined what the problem is, begin looking for possible ways to reduce the stress. Can you leave earlier? Can you let someone else drive? Can you call someone at your destination and ask about wheelchair access, local mass transit, and other concerns? Can you prepare food in the morning? Can you take a short nap in the early afternoon before you have to cook?

After you have identified some possible solutions, select one to try the next time you are in the situation. Then evaluate the results. (This is the problem-solving approach that was discussed in Chapter 2, "Becoming an HIV Self-Manager.")

Certain chemicals you ingest can also increase stress. These include nicotine, alcohol, and caffeine. Some people smoke a cigarette, drink a glass of wine or beer, eat chocolate, or drink a cup of coffee to soothe their tension, but this may actually increase stress. Eliminating or cutting down on these stressors can help.

As noted earlier, other tools for dealing with stress include getting enough sleep, exercising, and eating well. Sometimes stress is so overwhelming that these tools are not enough. These are times when good self-managers turn to consultants such as counselors, social workers, psychologists, or psychiatrists.

In summary, stress, like every other symptom, has many causes and can therefore be managed in many different ways. It is up to you to examine the problem and try to find solutions that meet your needs and suit your lifestyle.

Itching

Itching is one of the most difficult symptoms to understand. Itching is any sensation that causes an urge to scratch. Like other symptoms, it can have many different causes. Some of these are understood by physicians. For example, when you get an insect bite or come in contact with poison ivy, your body releases histamines, which irritate nerve endings and cause itching. Or when the liver is damaged, it cannot remove bile products, and these are deposited in the skin, causing itching. Other reasons for itching are not understood. In kidney disease, itching may be severe, but the exact cause is not clear. There are also other conditions, such as psoriasis, in which the causes of itching are not easily explained. We do know that factors such as warmth, wool clothing, and stress can make itching worse. The following are some tools and techniques that may help you relieve your itching.

Countering Dryness, Irritation, and Stress

Dry skin tends to be itchy. Keeping your skin moisturized by applying moisturizing creams several times a day can help combat itching. When you choose a moisturizer, be sure to read the list of ingredients. Avoid products that contain alcohol or any other ingredient that ends in -ol, as they tend to dry the skin. In general, the greasier the product, the better it works as a moisturizer. Creams are better moisturizers than lotions, and products such as Vaseline, baby oil, olive oil, and vegetable shortening are even more effective.

When you take a bath or shower, use warm rather than hot water. In the tub, soak for not less than 10 nor more than 20 minutes. You also may want to add bath oil, baking soda, or an old remedy called "Sulzberger's household bath oil" to the water. To make this bath oil, stir two teaspoons of olive oil into a large glass of milk and add it to your bath. When you get out of the water, pat yourself dry immediately and apply your usual moisturizing cream.

During cold weather it can be especially difficult to deal with itching because indoor heating tends to dry the skin. If this is a problem for you, a humidifier might help. Also try to keep your home and office as cool as you can without being uncomfortable.

The type of clothing you wear can contribute to itching sensations. Obviously, the best rule of thumb is to wear what is comfortable. This is usually clothing made from material that is not scratchy. Most people find that natural fibers such as cotton allow the skin to "breathe" better and are the least irritating to the skin.

Anything you can do to reduce the stress in your life will also help reduce the itching. We have already discussed some of the ways to deal with stress earlier in this chapter, and some additional techniques are described in Chapter 12, "Using Your Mind to Manage Symptoms."

Medications for Itching

If your itching is caused by the release of histamines during an allergic reaction or from contact with an irritating substance, wash off the oils or offending agent, apply cold compresses, and take an antihistamine to stop the reaction. You can buy many of these products over the counter, including triprolidine (Actifed®), diphenhydramine (Benadryl®), chlorpheniramine maleate (Chlor-Trimeton®), cetirizine (Zyrtec®), loratadine (Claritin®), and fexofenadine (Allegra®).

You can also buy creams that help soothe the nerve endings, such as Bengay® and Vicks VapoRub®. Look for an anti-itch cream that contains benzocaine, lidocaine, or pramoxine. Be careful, though, because some people can have allergic reactions to these ingredients, especially benzocaine. Capsaicin creams may help itching, although they will cause a burning sensation. Steroid creams that contain cortisone can also help control some types of itching. If you are confused about what over-the-counter products to buy, ask your doctor or pharmacist.

With the exception of moisturizing creams, no cream should be used on a long-term basis without talking to your doctor. If your itching continues even after use of these over-the-counter products, you may want to talk to your doctor about trying the stronger prescription versions of these medications.

Scratching

While our natural tendency is to scratch what itches, this really does not help, especially for chronic itching. Rather, it leads to a vicious cycle. The more you scratch, the more you tend to itch. Unfortunately, it is hard to resist scratching. Instead of scratching, try rubbing, pressing, or patting the skin when you feel the need to scratch. If you are not able to break the itching/scratching cycle yourself, consult a dermatologist, who may be able to help you find alternative ways to control the itching.

Itching is a common and undoubtedly very frustrating symptom for both patients and physicians to manage. If the self-management tips described here do not seem to help, it may be time to seek the help of a physician. Often doctors can prescribe medications that can help with some specific types of itching.

Urinary Incontinence: Loss of Bladder Control

Urinary incontinence means you have trouble controlling your bladder and accidentally leak urine. If you have trouble controlling your bladder, you are not alone. Many people are coping with this problem. Although urinary incontinence can occur in both men and women, it is more common in women. In many cases, incontinence can be controlled, if not cured outright.

It is common to experience incontinence during or after pregnancy or with menopause, aging, or weight gain. Activities that put increased pressure on the bladder, such as coughing, laughing, sneezing, and physical activity, can cause urine leakage. Incontinence can be related to changes in your hormones, weakening muscles or ligaments in the pelvic area, or the use of certain medications. Infections in the bladder can also cause temporary incontinence. If you experience urinary incontinence, your first step should be to consider whether there could be an infection. For more on this, see the section on urinary infections in Chapter 10, "Evaluating Symptoms of HIV."

Urinary incontinence can affect your quality of life and lead to other health problems. Feeling embarrassed by urinary incontinence causes some people to avoid social activities or sex. Some people experience loss of confidence or depression as a result of incontinence. Leaked urine may also cause skin irritation and infections. The frequent urge to urinate can interfere with sound, restorative sleep. Slipping and falling on leaked urine when rushing to the bathroom can result in injury.

The good news is that there are many treatments that can control or even cure this condition. It may be reassuring to know that there are small things you can do at home. If none of the following solves the problem, talk to your doctor about other treatments. Don't be embarrassed. Your doctor has heard it all before.

There are three types of persistent or chronic loss of bladder control:

- **Stress incontinence** refers to small amounts of urine leaking out during exercise, coughing, laughing, sneezing, or other movements that squeeze the bladder. Kegel exercises (described below) often improve this condition.

- **Urge incontinence**, or overactive bladder, happens when the need to urinate comes on so quickly that you don't have enough time to get to the toilet.

- **Overflow incontinence** occurs when the bladder cannot empty completely.

Home Treatments for Urinary Incontinence

Small, effective changes to your lifestyle or behavior are the first treatments for urinary incontinence. For many people, the treatments we discuss in this section, such as Kegel exercises, effectively control or cure the problem.

Kegel exercises strengthen your pelvic floor muscles. This allows better control of your urine flow and prevents leaking. Learning Kegel exercises takes a bit of practice and patience. It may take a few weeks of doing Kegel exercises to feel an improvement in your symptoms. Here's how to do them:

1. First, find the muscles that stop your urine. You can do this by repeatedly stopping your urine in midstream and starting again. Focus on the muscles that you feel squeezing around your urethra (opening for the urine) and anus (opening for your bowels).

2. Practice squeezing these muscles when you are not urinating. If your stomach or buttocks move, you're not focusing on the right muscles.

3. Squeeze the muscles, hold for 3 seconds, and then relax for 3 seconds.

4. Repeat the exercise 10 to 15 times per session.

Complete at least 30 Kegel exercises every day. The wonderful thing about Kegels is that you can do them anywhere and anytime. Do them at every stop light or during all commercials while watching TV. No one will know what you are doing except you.

With urge incontinence, *retraining your bladder* may help.

■ Practice "double-voiding." Empty your bladder as much as possible, relax for a minute, and try to empty it again. This helps empty your bladder completely.

■ It sometimes helps to practice waiting a specified amount of time before urinating. This gradually retrains your bladder to require emptying less often. Train yourself to urinate on a regular schedule, about every two to four hours during the day, whether or not you feel the urge. If you now need to urinate every 30 minutes, perhaps you can start by going to the bathroom every 40 minutes and gradually work your way up to every two to four hours.

Consuming fewer beverages that stimulate the bladder and urine production, such as alcohol, coffee, tea, and other drinks that contain caffeine, can reduce your trips to the toilet.

If you carry extra weight, **losing weight** can reduce the pressure on your bladder. Studies show that a loss of just 10 percent of total body weight improves incontinence problems for many people.

Wearing absorbent pads or briefs does not cure incontinence but helps manage the condition.

Treatments and Medications for Urinary Incontinence

If changes in your lifestyle or behavior do not relieve your urinary incontinence, discuss other treatments with your doctor such as the use of medication, a pessary for women (a thin, flexible ring that can be worn inside the vagina to support the pelvic area), or, in some cases, surgery. You don't have to suffer in silence if you have urinary incontinence. Talk with your doctor.

In this chapter we have discussed some of the most common symptoms experienced by people with chronic conditions. In addition, we have described some tools that you can use to cope with your symptoms. Taking action to deal with your symptoms is necessary as you cope with HIV on a day-to-day basis. But sometimes this just doesn't seem to be enough. There are times when you may wish to escape from your surroundings and just have "your time"— a time that allows you to clear your mind and gain a fresh perspective. The following chapter, "Using Your Mind to Manage Symptoms," presents ways you can complement your physical-symptom management by using the power of your mind to help reduce and even prevent some of your symptoms.

Additional Resources

AIDS.gov: www.aids.gov/hiv-aids-basics/hiv-aids-101/signs-and-symptoms

Alzheimer's Association: www.alz.org or 24/7 Helpline, 1-800-272-3900

American Chronic Pain Association: www.theacpa.org

The Body: The Complete HIV/AIDS Resource: www.thebody.com

National Association for Continence: www.nafc.org

National Sleep Foundation: www.sleepfoundation.org

Suggested Further Reading

To learn more about the topics discussed in this chapter, we suggest that you explore the following resources:

Bourne, Edmund, and Lorna Garano. *Coping with Anxiety: 10 Simple Ways to Relieve Anxiety, Fear, and Worry.* Oakland, Calif.: New Harbinger, 2003.

Carter, Les. *The Anger Trap: Free Yourself from the Frustrations That Sabotage Your Life.* San Francisco: Jossey-Bass, 2004.

Casarjian, Robin. *Forgiveness: A Bold Choice for a Peaceful Heart.* New York: Bantam Books, 1992.

Caudill, Margaret. *Managing Pain Before It Manages You,* 4th ed. New York: Guilford Press, 2015.

Darnall, Beth. *Less Pain, Fewer Pills: Avoid the Dangers of Prescription Opioids and Gain Control over Chronic Pain.* Boulder, Colo.: Bull Publishing, 2014.

David, Martha, Elizabeth Robbins Eshelman, and Matthew McKay. *The Relaxation and*

Stress Reduction Workbook, 6th ed. Oakland, Calif.: New Harbinger, 2008.

DePaulo, J. Raymond, and Leslie Alan Horvitz. *Understanding Depression: What We Know and What You Can Do About It.* New York: Wiley, 2003.

Donoghue, Paul J., and Mary E. Siegel. *Sick and Tired of Feeling Sick and Tired: Living with Invisible Chronic Illness,* 2nd ed. New York: Norton, 2000.

Gordon, James S. *Unstuck: Your Guide to the Seven-Stage Journey Out of Depression.* New York: Penguin, 2009.

Hankins, Gary, and Carol Hankins. *Prescription for Anger,* 3rd ed. Newberg, Ore.: Barclay Press, 2000.

Hauri, Peter, and Shirley Linde. *No More Sleepless Nights.* New York: Wiley, 1996.

Jacobs, Gregg D. *Say Good Night to Insomnia.* New York: Holt, 2009.

Kabat-Zinn, Jon. *Full Catastrophe Living: Using the Wisdom of Your Body and Mind to Face Stress, Pain, and Illness.* New York: Bantam Books, 2013.

Kabat-Zinn, Jon. *Mindfulness for Beginners: Reclaiming the Present Moment—and Your Life.* Louisville, Colo.: Sounds True, 2011.

Kashdan, Todd, and Robert Biswas-Diener. *The Upside of Your Dark Side: Why Being Your Whole Self—Not Just Your "Good" Self—Drives Success and Fulfillment.* New York: Plume, 2014.

Katon, Wayne, Evette Ludman, and Gregory Simon, *The Depression Helpbook,* 2nd ed. Boulder, Colo.: Bull Publishing, 2008.

Klein, Donald F., and Paul H. Wender. *Understanding Depression: A Complete Guide to Its Diagnosis and Treatment,* 2nd ed. New York: Oxford University Press, 2005.

Kleinke, Chris L. *Coping with Life Challenges,* 2nd ed. Pacific Grove, Calif.: Brooks/Cole, 2002.

LeFort, Sandra, Lisa Webster, Kate Lorig, Halsted Holman, David Sobel, Diana Laurent, Virginia González, and Marian Minor. *Living a Healthy Life with Chronic Pain.* Boulder, Colo.: Bull Publishing, 2015.

McGonigal, Kelly. *The Upside of Stress: Why Stress Is Good for You, and How to Get Good at It.* New York: Avery, 2015.

McGonigal, Kelly. *The Willpower Instinct: How Self-Control Works, Why It Matters, and What You Can Do to Get More of It.* New York: Avery, 2013.

McKay, Matthew, Peter D. Rogers, and Judith McKay. *When Anger Hurts: Quieting the Storm Within,* 2nd ed. Oakland, Calif.: New Harbinger, 2003.

Natelson, Benjamin H. *Facing and Fighting Fatigue: A Practical Approach.* New Haven, Conn.: Yale University Press, 1998.

Sobel, David, and Robert Ornstein. *The Healthy Mind, Healthy Body Handbook* (also published under the title *The Mind and Body Health Handbook*). Los Altos, Calif.: DRx, 1996.

Stahl, Bob, and Elisha Goldstein. *A Mindfulness-Based Stress Reduction Workbook.* Oakland, Calif.: New Harbinger, 2010.

Torburn, Leslie. *Stop the Stress Habit: Change Your Perceptions and Improve Your Health.* Bloomington, Indiana: iUniverse, 2008.

Turk, Dennis, and Justin Nash. "Chronic Pain: New Ways to Cope," in *Mind/Body Medicine: How to Use Your Mind for Better Health.* New York: Consumer Reports Books, 1993.

Williams, Redford, and Virginia Williams. *Anger Kills: 17 Strategies for Controlling the Hostility That Can Harm Your Health*. New York: Random House, 1998.

Williams, Redford, and Virginia Williams. *Lifeskills: 8 Simple Ways to Build Stronger Relationships, Communicate More Clearly, and Improve Your Health*. New York: Three Rivers Press, 1998.

CHAPTER 12

Using Your Mind to Manage Symptoms

THERE IS A STRONG LINK BETWEEN thoughts, attitudes, and emotions and mental and physical health. One of our self-managers puts it this way: "It's not always mind over matter, but mind matters." Although thoughts and emotions do not directly cause chronic conditions, they can influence symptoms. Research has shown that thoughts and emotions trigger certain hormones or other chemicals that send messages throughout the body. These messages affect how the body functions; for example, thoughts and emotions can alter heart rate, blood pressure, breathing, blood sugar levels, muscle responses, immune response, concentration, the ability to get pregnant, and even the ability to fight off other illness.

All of us, at one time or another, have experienced the power of the mind and its effects on the body. Both pleasant and unpleasant thoughts and emotions can cause the body to react in different ways. Our heart rate and breathing can increase or slow down; we may experience sensations such as sweating (warm or cold), blushing, tears, and so on. Sometimes just a memory or an image can trigger these responses. For example, try this simple exercise: Imagine that you are holding a big, bright yellow

171

lemon slice. You hold it close to your nose and smell its strong citrus aroma. Now you bite into the lemon. It's juicy! The juice fills your mouth and dribbles down your chin. Imagine you begin to suck on the lemon and its tart juice. What happens? Your body responds. Your mouth puckers and starts to water. You may even smell the scent of the lemon. All of these reactions are triggered by the mind and its memory of your experience with real lemons.

This example shows the power the mind has over the body. It also inspires us to work to develop our mental abilities to help us manage our symptoms. With training and practice, we can learn to use the mind to relax the body, to reduce stress and anxiety, and to reduce the discomfort or unpleasantness caused by physical and emotional symptoms. The mind can also greatly help relieve the pain and shortness of breath associated with various diseases and may even help you depend less on some medications.

In this chapter we describe several ways in which you can begin to use your mind to manage symptoms. These are sometimes referred to as "thinking" or "cognitive" techniques because they involve the use of our thinking abilities to make changes in the body.

As you read, keep the following key principles in mind:

- **Symptoms have many causes,** which means there are multiple ways to manage most symptoms. If you understand the nature and causes of your symptoms, you will be better equipped to manage them.

- **Not all management techniques work for everyone.** It is up to you to experiment and find out what works best for you. Be flexible. This includes trying different techniques and checking the results to determine which management tool is most helpful for which symptoms and under what circumstances.

- **Learning new skills and gaining control of the situation take time.** Give yourself several weeks to practice before you decide if a new tool is working for you.

- **Don't give up too easily.** As with exercise and other new skills, using your mind to manage your health condition requires both practice and time before you notice the benefits. Even if you feel you are not accomplishing anything, don't give up. Be patient and keep on trying.

- **These techniques should not have negative effects.** If you become frightened, angry, or depressed when using one of these tools, do not continue to use it. Try another tool instead.

Relaxation Techniques

You may have heard and read about relaxation, yet still be confused as to what relaxation is, what its benefits are, and how to do it. Simply stated, relaxation involves using thinking techniques to reduce or eliminate tension from both the body and the mind. This usually results in better sleep quality and less stress, pain, and shortness of breath. Relaxation is not a cure-all, but it can be an effective part of a treatment plan.

There are different types of relaxation techniques. Each has specific guidelines and uses. Some techniques are used mostly to achieve muscle relaxation, while others are aimed at reducing anxiety and emotional stress or diverting attention, all of which aid in symptom management.

The term *relaxation* means different things to different people. We can all identify things we do that help us relax. For example, we may walk, watch TV, listen to music, knit, or garden. These methods, however, are different from most of the techniques discussed in this chapter because they include some form of physical activity or require a stimulus such as music that is outside of the mind. The relaxation *tools* we are emphasizing here require that you use your mind to help your body relax.

The goal of relaxation is to turn off the outside world so that the mind and body are at rest. This allows you to reduce the tensions that can increase the intensity or severity of symptoms.

The following guidelines can help you successfully practice relaxation:

- **Pick a quiet place and time** when you will not be disturbed for at least 15 to 20 minutes. (If this seems too long, start with five minutes. By the way, in some homes the only quiet place is the bathroom. That is just fine.)

- **Try to practice the technique twice daily** and not less than four times a week.

- **Don't expect miracles.** These techniques take practice. Sometimes it takes three to four weeks of consistent practice before you start to notice benefits.

- **Relaxation should be helpful.** At worst, you may find it boring, but if it is an unpleasant experience or makes you more nervous or anxious, consider switching to one of the other symptom management tools described in this chapter.

Relaxation Quick and Easy

Some types of relaxation are so easy, natural, and effective that people do not think of them as "relaxation techniques," especially because they can involve more physical activity than the deliberate use of the mind to elicit relaxation or refocus attention. These include some of the following:

- Take a nap or a warm, soothing bath.
- Curl up and read or listen to a good book.
- Watch a funny movie.
- Make a paper airplane and sail it across the room.
- Get a massage.
- Enjoy a glass of wine occasionally.
- Start a small garden or grow a beautiful plant indoors.
- Do some crafts such as knitting, pottery, or woodworking.
- Watch a favorite TV show.
- Read a poem or an inspirational saying.
- Go for a walk.
- Start a collection (coins, folk art, shells, or something in miniature).
- Listen to your favorite music.
- Sing.
- Crumble paper into a ball and use a wastebasket as a basketball hoop.

- Look at water (ocean waves, a lake, or a fountain).

- Watch the clouds in the sky.

- Put your head down on your desk and close your eyes for five minutes.

- Rub your hands together until they're warm, and then cup them over your closed eyes.

- Vigorously shake your hands and arms for ten seconds.

- Call up a friend or family member to chat.

- Smile and introduce yourself to someone new.

- Do something nice and unexpected for someone else.

- Play with a pet.

- Go to a vacation spot in your mind.

Relaxation Tools That Take 5 to 20 Minutes

The relaxation techniques we discuss in this section, such as signal breathing, may take a bit longer but are quite effective.

Signal Breathing

Signal breathing relies on your ability to identify the signs or "signals" in your body that indicate you are getting stressed. For example, you may feel tense muscles in different areas of your body, such as your head, jaw, neck, or shoulders. Your voice may get louder, or you may feel discomfort in your stomach. Each of us reacts differently to stress. If you pay attention to your body, you can begin to notice these changes early and use your breathing to reduce the stress before you get a head or bellyache, lose your temper, or cry.

Signal breathing is straightforward. It is like taking a "time out" from the stressful situation. To do this, first exhale or sigh to get the air out of your lungs. Then take three or four deep breaths down to your stomach. You will know you are taking deep breaths if your stomach moves more than your chest. To check that you are doing this correctly, place one hand on your chest and the other hand on your stomach. Take three or four breaths. If the hand on your stomach is moving more than the hand on your chest, you are doing it right. Don't worry if this doesn't happen for you right away. You are learning a new skill, and doing that often requires practice. With more time and practice, you will become more skilled at using this breathing technique.

Breathing techniques such as this one are not only good for reducing stress, but can also help to manage pain, anxiety, and even panic attacks. They can also be used to help you through situations or events that tend to produce stress or anxiety for you.

Body-Scan Relaxation

To relax muscles, you can learn how to scan your body and recognize where you are tense. Then you can release the tension. The first step is to become familiar with the difference between the feeling of tension and the feeling of relaxation. Body-scan relaxation allows you to compare those feelings and, with practice, spot and release tension anywhere in your body. It is best done lying down on your back, but any comfortable position can be used. You can find a body-scan script on page 176.

Relaxation Response

In the early 1970s, a physician named Herbert Benson studied what he calls the "relaxation response." According to Benson, our bodies have several natural states. One example is the "fight or flight" response experienced by people who are faced with a great danger. In times of stress the body becomes quite tense, which is followed by the body's natural tendency to relax; this is the relaxation response. As our lives become more and more hectic, our bodies tend to stay tense for longer and longer periods of time. We lose our ability to relax. Developing your relaxation response helps change this.

To elicit the response, first find a quiet place where there are few or no distractions. Find a comfortable position. You should be comfortable enough to remain in the same position for 20 minutes. Choose a pleasant word and a tranquil object or feeling. For example, repeat a word or sound (such as the word *one*) while gazing at a symbol (perhaps a flower) or concentrating on a feeling (such as peace). Adopt a passive attitude. This is of the utmost importance. Empty all thoughts and distractions from your mind. You may become aware of distracting thoughts, images, and feelings, but don't concentrate on them. Just allow them to pass on.

Follow these steps to elicit the relaxation response:

- Sit quietly in a comfortable position.

- Close your eyes.

- Relax all your muscles, beginning at your feet and progressing up to your face. Keep them relaxed.

- Breathe in through your nose. Become aware of your breathing. As you breathe out through your mouth, say the word you chose silently to yourself. Try to empty all thoughts from your mind; concentrate on the one word, symbol, or feeling you have chosen.

- Continue this for 10 to 20 minutes. You may open your eyes to check the time, but do not use an alarm. When you finish, sit quietly, at first with your eyes closed. Do not stand up for a few minutes.

- Maintain a passive attitude, and let relaxation occur at its own pace. When distracting thoughts occur, ignore them by not dwelling on them, and return to repeating the word you chose. Do not worry about whether you are successful in achieving a deep level of relaxation.

- Practice this once or twice daily.

Distraction

Our minds have trouble focusing on more than one thing at a time; therefore, we can lessen the intensity of symptoms by training our minds to focus attention on something other than our bodies and their sensations. This technique, called distraction or attention refocusing, is particularly helpful for those people who feel that their symptoms are painful or overwhelming or

Body-Scan Script

As you get into a comfortable position, allowing yourself to begin to sink comfortably into the surface below you, you may perhaps begin to allow your eyes gradually to close . . . From there, turn your attention to your breath . . . breathing in, allowing the breath gradually to go all the way down to your belly and then breathing out . . . And again, breathing in . . . and out . . . noticing the natural rhythm of your breathing . . .

Now allowing your attention to focus on your feet. Starting with your toes, notice whatever sensations are there—warmth, coolness, whatever's there . . . simply feel it. Using your mind's eye, imagine that as you breathe in, the breath goes all the way down into your toes, bringing with it new refreshing air . . . And now notice the sensations elsewhere in your feet, not judging or thinking about what you're feeling, but simply becoming aware of the experience of your feet as you allow yourself to be fully supported by the surface below you . . .

Next focus on your lower legs and knees. These muscles and joints do a lot of work for us, but often we don't give them the attention they deserve. So now breathe down into the knees, calves, and ankles, noticing whatever sensations appear . . . See if you can simply stay with the sensations . . . breathing in new fresh air, and as you exhale, releasing tension and stress and allowing the muscles to relax and soften . . .

Now move your attention to the muscles, bones, and joints of the thighs, buttocks, and hips . . . breathing down into the upper legs, noticing whatever sensations you experience. It may be warmth, coolness, a heaviness or lightness. You may become aware of the contact with the surface beneath you, or perhaps the pulsing of your blood. Whatever's there . . . what matters is that you are taking time to learn to relax . . . deeper and deeper, as you breathe . . . in . . . and out.

Move your attention now to your back and chest. Feeling the breath fill the abdomen and chest . . . Noticing whatever sensations are there . . . not judging or thinking, but simply observing what is right here right now. Allow the fresh air to nourish the muscles, bones, and joints as you breathe in, and then exhale any tension and stress.

Now focus on the neck, shoulders, arms, and hands. Inhaling down through the neck and shoulders, all the way down to the fingertips. Not trying too hard to relax, but simply becoming aware of your experience of these parts of your body in the present moment . . .

Turning now to your face and head, notice the sensations beginning at the back of your head, up along your scalp, and down into your forehead . . . Then become aware of the sensations in and around your eyes and down into your cheeks and jaw . . . Continue to allow your muscles to release and soften as you breathe in nourishing fresh air, and allow tension and stress to leave as you breathe out . . .

As you drink in fresh air, allow it to spread throughout your body, from the soles of your feet all the way up through the top of your head . . . And then exhale any remaining stress and tension . . . and now take a few moments to enjoy the stillness as you breathe in . . . and out . . . Awake, relaxed, and still . . .

Now as the body scan comes to a close, coming back into the room, bringing with you whatever sensations of relaxation . . . comfort . . . peace, whatever's there . . . knowing that you can repeat this exercise at any appropriate time and place of your choosing . . . And when you're ready, open your eyes.

▶ To order the Relaxation for Mind & Body CD, go to www.bullpub.com/catalog/relaxation-for-mind-and-body

worry that every bodily sensation might indicate a new or worsening symptom or health problem. (It is important to mention that with distraction you are not ignoring the symptoms but choosing not to dwell on them.)

Sometimes it may be difficult to put anxious thoughts out of your mind. When you try to suppress any thought, you may end up thinking more about it. For example, suppose someone asks you to try to not think about a tiger charging at you. Whatever you do, don't let the thought of a tiger enter your mind. You'll probably find it nearly impossible not to think about the tiger.

Although you can't easily stop thinking about something, you can distract yourself and redirect your attention elsewhere. For example, think about the charging tiger again. Now stand up suddenly, slam your hand on the table, and shout "*Stop!*" What happened to the tiger? Gone—at least for the moment.

Distraction works best for short activities or times when symptoms may be anticipated. For example, if you know climbing stairs will be painful or cause discomfort or that falling asleep at night is difficult, you might try one of the following distraction techniques:

■ Make plans for exactly what you will do after the unpleasant activity passes. For example, if climbing stairs is uncomfortable or painful, think about what you need to do once you get to the top. If you have trouble falling asleep, try making plans for some future event, being as detailed as possible.

■ Think of a person's name, a bird, a flower, a sports team, or whatever, for every letter of the alphabet. If you get stuck on one letter, go on to the next. (These are good distractions for pain as well as for sleep problems.)

■ Challenge yourself to count backward from 100 by threes (100, 97, 94 . . .).

■ To get through daily chores (such as sweeping, mopping, or vacuuming), imagine your floor as a map of a country or continent. Try naming all the states, provinces, or countries, moving east to west or north to south. If geography does not appeal to you, imagine your favorite store and where each of your favorite items or departments is located.

■ Try to remember words to favorite songs or the events in an old story.

■ Try the "*Stop!*" technique. If you find yourself worrying or entrapped in endlessly repeating negative thoughts, stand up suddenly, slap your hand on the table or your thigh, and shout "*Stop!*" You can practice this technique whenever your mind endlessly repeats negative thoughts. With practice, you won't have to shout out loud. Just whispering "*Stop!*" or tightening your vocal cords and moving your tongue as if saying "*Stop!*" will often work. Some people imagine a large stop sign. Others put a rubber band on their wrist and snap it hard to break the chain of negative thought. Or just pinch yourself. Do anything that redirects your attention.

■ Redirect your attention to a pleasurable experience:

   ◆ Look outside at something in nature.

   ◆ Try to identify all the sounds around you.

   ◆ Massage your hand.

   ◆ Smell a sweet or pungent odor.

There are, of course, many variations to these examples, all of which help you refocus attention away from your problem.

So far we have discussed short-term refocusing strategies that involve using only the mind for distraction. Distraction also works well for long-term projects or symptoms that tend to last longer, such as depression and some forms of chronic pain.

In these cases, the mind is focused not internally but externally on some type of activity. If you are somewhat depressed or have continuous unpleasant symptoms, find an activity that interests you and use it to distract yourself from the problem. The activity can be almost anything, from gardening to cooking to reading or going to a movie, even doing volunteer work. One of the marks of successful self-managers is that they have a variety of interests and always seems to be doing something.

Positive Thinking and Self-Talk

We all talk to ourselves all the time. For example, when waking up in the morning, we may think, "I really don't want to get out of bed. I'm tired and don't want to go to work today." Or at the end of an enjoyable evening, we think, "Gee, that was fun. I should get out more often." What we think or say to ourselves is called our self-talk. The way we talk to ourselves tends to come from how and what we think about ourselves. Our thoughts can be positive or negative, and so is our self-talk. Self-talk can be an important self-management tool when it's positive or a weapon that hurts or defeats us when it's habitually negative.

Your self-talk is learned from others and becomes a part of you as you grow up. It comes in many forms, although unfortunately for many people it is mostly negative. Negative self-statements are usually in the form of phrases that begin with something like "I just can't do . . . ," "If only I could . . . ," "If only I didn't . . . ," "I just don't have the energy . . . ," or "How could I be so stupid?" This type of negative thinking represents the doubts and fears you may have about yourself in general and about your ability to deal with your condition and its symptoms. It damages your self-esteem, attitude, and mood. Negative self-talk makes you feel bad and makes your symptoms worse.

What you say to yourself plays a major role in determining your success or failure in becoming a good self-manager. Negative thinking tends to limit abilities and actions. If you tell yourself, "I'm not very smart" or "I can't" all the time, you probably won't try to learn new skills because this just doesn't fit with what you think about yourself. Soon you can become a prisoner of your own negative beliefs. Fortunately, self-talk is not something fixed in your biological makeup, and therefore it is not completely out of your control. You can learn new, healthier ways to think about yourself so that your self-talk can work for you instead of against you. By changing the negative, self-defeating statements to positive ones, you can manage symptoms more effectively. This change, like any habit, requires practice and includes the following steps:

1. **Listen carefully to what you say to or about yourself, both out loud and silently.** If you find yourself feeling anxious,

depressed, or angry, try to identify some of the thoughts you were having just before these feelings started. Then write down all your negative self-talk statements. Pay special attention to the things you say during times that are particularly difficult for you. For example, what do you say to yourself when getting up in the morning with pain, while doing those exercises you don't really like, or at those times when you are feeling blue? Challenge these negative thoughts by asking yourself questions to identify what about the statement is really true or not true. For example, are you exaggerating the situation, generalizing, worrying too much, or assuming the worst? Are you thinking in black and white? Could there be gray? Maybe you are making an unrealistic or unfair comparison, assuming too much responsibility, taking something too personally, or expecting perfection. Are you making assumptions about what other people think about you? What do you know for a fact? Look at the evidence so that you are better able to change these negative thoughts and statements.

2. **Work on changing each negative statement to a more positive one, or find some positive statement to replace the negative one.** Write the positive statements down. For example, change negative statements such as "I don't want to get up," "I'm too tired and I hurt," "I can't do the things I like anymore, so why bother?" or "I'm good for nothing" to positive messages such as "I'm feeling pretty good today, and I'm going to do something I enjoy," "I may not be able to do everything I used to, but there are still a lot of things I can do," "People like me, and I feel good about myself," or "Other people need and depend on me; I'm worthwhile."

3. **Read and rehearse these positive statements, mentally or with another person.** It is this conscious repetition or memorization of the positive self-talk that will help you replace old, habitual negative statements.

4. **Practice these new statements in real situations.** This practice, along with time and patience, will help the new patterns of thinking become automatic.

5. **Rehearse success.** When you aren't happy with the way you handled a particular situation, try this exercise:
   ■ Write down three ways that it could have gone better.
   ■ Write down three ways it could have gone worse.
   ■ If you can't think of alternatives to the way you handled it, imagine what someone whom you greatly respect would have done. Or think about what advice you would give to someone else facing a similar situation.

Remember that mistakes aren't failures; they are good opportunities to learn. Mistakes give you the chance to rehearse other ways of handling things. This is great practice for future crises.

As you first do this, you may find it hard to change negative statements into more positive ones. A shortcut is to use either a thought stopper or a positive affirmation. A thought stopper can be anything that is meaningful to you—for example, a puppy, a polar bear, or a redwood tree. When you have a negative thought, replace it with your thought stopper. It may sound silly, but try it.

A positive affirmation is a positive phrase that you can use over and over. For example, "I am getting better every day" or "I can do this" or "God loves me." Use this to replace negative thoughts.

Imagery and Visualization Techniques

You may think that "imagination" is all in your mind. But the thoughts, words, and images that flow from your imagination can have very real affects on your body. Your brain often cannot distinguish whether you are imagining something or if it is really happening. Perhaps you've had a racing heartbeat, rapid breathing, or tension in your neck muscles while watching a movie thriller. These sensations were all produced by images and sounds on a film. During a dream, your body may respond with fear, joy, anger, or sadness—all triggered by your imagination. If you close your eyes and vividly imagine yourself by a still, quiet pool or relaxing on a warm beach, your body responds to some degree as though you were actually there. Recall the lemon exercise from the beginning of this chapter.

Guided imagery and visualization allow you to use your imagination to relieve symptoms. These techniques will help you focus your thoughts on healing images and suggestions.

Guided Imagery

This tool is like a guided daydream. It allows you to divert your attention and refocus your mind away from your symptoms by transporting you to another time and place. It has the added benefit of helping you achieve deep relaxation as you picture yourself in a peaceful environment.

In guided imagery, you focus your mind on a particular image. Imagery usually involves your sense of sight, focusing on visual images. Adding other senses—smells, tastes, and sounds—makes the guided imagery even more vivid and powerful.

Some people are highly visual and easily see images with their "mind's eye." But if your images aren't as vivid as scenes from a great movie, don't worry; it's normal for the intensity of imagery to vary. The important thing is to focus on as much detail as possible and to strengthen the images by using all your senses. Adding background music can also increase the impact of guided imagery.

With guided imagery, you are always completely in control. You're the movie director. You can project whatever thought or feeling you want onto your mental screen. If you don't like a particular image, thought, or feeling, redirect your mind to something more comfortable. You can use other images to get rid of unpleasant thoughts (for example, you might put them on a raft and watch them float away, sweep them away with a large broom, or erase them with a giant eraser), or you can open your eyes and stop the exercise.

The guided imagery scripts presented on pages 182 and 183 can help take you on this mental stroll. Here are some ways to use these scripts:

■ Read the script over several times until it is familiar. Then sit or lie down in a quiet place and try to reconstruct the scene in your mind. The script should take 15 to 20 minutes to complete.

■ Have a family member or friend read you the script slowly, pausing for about 10 seconds wherever there is a series of periods (. . .) in the script.

■ Make a recording of the script, and play it to yourself whenever convenient.

■ Use a prerecorded tape, CD, or digital audio file that has a similar guided imagery script (see examples in the "Additional Resources" section at the end of this chapter).

Visualization

Visualization is similar to guided imagery. However, this technique allows you to create your own images; this is different from guided imagery, where the images are suggested to you. Visualization is another way of using your imagination to create a picture of yourself doing the things you want to do. All of us use a form of visualization every day—when we dream, worry, read a book, or listen to a story. In all these activities the mind creates images for us to see. We also use visualization intentionally when making plans for the day, considering the possible outcomes of a decision we have to make, or rehearsing for an event or activity. Visualization can be done in different ways and can be used for longer periods of time or while you are engaged in other activities.

One way to use visualization to manage symptoms is to remember pleasant scenes from your past or create new scenes. To practice visualization, try to remember every detail of a special holiday or party that made you happy. Who was there? What happened? What did you do or talk about? Or try remembering a vacation or some other memorable and pleasant event.

Visualization can be used to plan the details of some future event or to fill in the details of a fantasy. For example, how would you spend a million dollars? What would be your ideal romantic encounter? What does your dream home or garden look like? Where would you go and what would you do on your dream vacation?

Another form of visualization involves using your mind to think of symbols that represent the discomfort or pain felt in different parts of your body. For example, a painful joint might be red or a tight chest might have a constricting band around it. After forming these images, you then try to change them. The red color might fade until there is no more color, or the constricting band will stretch and stretch until it falls off; these new images then cause the way you think of the pain or discomfort to change.

Visualization helps build confidence and skill and therefore is a useful technique to help you set and accomplish your personal goals (see Chapter 2, "Becoming an HIV Self-Manager"). After you write your weekly action plan, take a few minutes to imagine yourself taking a walk, doing your exercises, or taking your medications. You are mentally rehearsing the steps you need to take in order to achieve your goal successfully.

Imagery for Different Conditions

You have the ability to create special imagery to help (though not cure) specific symptoms or illnesses. Use any image that is strong and vivid for

Guided-Imagery Script: A Walk in the Country

You're giving yourself some time to quiet your mind and body. Allow yourself to settle comfortably, wherever you are right now. If you wish, you can close your eyes. Breathe in deeply, through your nose, expanding your abdomen and filling your lungs; and, pursing your lips, exhale through your mouth slowly and completely, allowing your body to sink heavily into the surface beneath you . . . And once again breathe in through your nose and all the way down to your abdomen, and then breathe out slowly through pursed lips—letting go of tension, letting go of anything that's on your mind right now and just allowing yourself to be present in this moment . . .

Imagine yourself walking along a peaceful old country road. The sun is gently warming your back . . . the birds are singing . . . the air is calm and fragrant . . .

With no need to hurry, you notice your walking is relaxed and easy. As you walk along in this way, taking in your surroundings, you come across an old gate. It looks inviting and you decide to take the path through the gate. The gate creaks as you open it and go through.

You find yourself in an old, overgrown garden—flowers growing where they've seeded themselves, vines climbing over a fallen tree, soft green wild grasses, shade trees.

You notice yourself breathing deeply . . . smelling the flowers . . . listening to the birds and insects . . . feeling a gentle breeze cool against your skin. All of your senses are alive and responding with pleasure to this peaceful time and place . . .

When you're ready to move on, you leisurely follow the path out behind the garden, eventually coming to a more wooded area. As you enter this area, your eyes find the trees and plant life restful. The sunlight is filtered through the leaves. The air feels mild and a little cooler . . . You savor the fragrance of trees and earth . . . and gradually become aware of the sound of a nearby stream. Pausing, you allow yourself to take in the sights and sounds, breathing in the cool and fragrant air several times . . . And with each breath, you notice how refreshed you are feeling . . .

Continuing along the path for a while, you come to the stream. It's clear and clean as it flows and tumbles over the rocks and some fallen logs. You follow the path easily along the creek for a way, and after awhile, you come out into a sunlit clearing, where you discover a small waterfall emptying into a quiet pool of water.

You find a comfortable place to sit for a while, a perfect niche where you can feel completely relaxed.

You feel good as you allow yourself to just enjoy the warmth and solitude of this peaceful place . . .

After awhile, you become aware that it is time to return. You arise and walk back down the path in a relaxed and comfortable way, through the cool and fragrant trees, out into the sun-drenched overgrown garden . . . One last smell of the flowers, and out the creaky gate.

You leave this country retreat for now and return down the road. You notice you feel calm and rested. You feel grateful and remind yourself that you can visit this special place whenever you wish to take some time to refresh yourself and renew your energy.

And now, preparing to bring this period of relaxation to a close, you may want to take a moment to picture yourself carrying this experience of calm and refreshment with you into the ordinary activities of your life . . . And when you're ready, take a nice deep breath and open your eyes.

▶ To order the Relaxation for Mind & Body CD, go to www.bullpub.com/catalog/relaxation-for-mind-and-body

Guided-Imagery Script: A Walk on the Beach

Begin by getting into a comfortable position, whether you are seated or lying down. Loosen any tight clothing to allow yourself to be as comfortable as possible. Uncross your legs and allow your hands to fall by your sides or rest in your lap, and if you are at all uncomfortable shift to a more comfortable position.

When you are ready, you may allow your eyes gradually to close and turn your attention to your breathing. Allow your belly to expand as you breathe in, bringing in fresh new air to nourish your body. And then breathing out. Notice the rhythm of your breathing—in . . . and out . . . without trying to control it in any way at all. Simply attend to the natural rhythm of your breath . . .

And now in your mind's eye, imagine yourself standing on a beautiful beach. The sky is a brilliant blue, and as some fluffy white clouds float slowly by, you drink in the beautiful colors . . . The temperature is not too hot and not too cold. The sun is shining, and you close your eyes, allowing the warmth of the sun to wash over you . . . You notice a gentle breeze caressing your face, the perfect complement to the sunshine.

Then you find yourself turn turning and looking out over the vastness of the ocean . . . you become aware of the sound of the waves gently washing up on shore . . . You notice the firmness of the wet sand beneath your feet, or If you decide to take off your shoes, you may enjoy the feeling of standing, in the cool, wet sand . . . perhaps you allow the surf to roll up and gently wash across your feet, or perhaps you stay just out of its reach. . .

In the distance you hear some seagulls calling to one another and look out to see the birds gracefully gliding through the air. And as you stand there, notice how easy it is to be here, perhaps noticing some sensations of relaxation, comfort, or peace—whatever's there . . .

Now take a walk along the shore. Turn and begin to stroll casually along the beach, enjoying the sounds of the surf, the warmth of the sun, and the gentle massage of the breeze. As you move along, taking your time, your stride becomes lighter, easier . . . you notice the scent of the ocean . . . you pause to take in the freshness of the air . . . And then you continue on your way, enjoying the peacefulness of this place.

After a time, you decide to rest a while, and find a comfortable place to sit or lie down . . . and simply allow yourself to take some time to enjoy this, your special place . . .

And now, when you feel ready to return, you stand and begin walking back down the beach in a comfortable, leisurely way, taking with you any sensations of relaxation, comfort, peace, joy—Whatever's there . . . Noticing how easy it is to be here. Continuing back until you reach the place where you began your walk . . .

And now pausing to take one last long look around. Enjoying the vibrant colors of the sky and the sea . . . The gentle sound of the waves washing up on the shore. The warmth of the sun, the cool of the breeze . . .

And as you prepare to leave this special place, taking with you any sensations of joy, relaxation, comfort, peace, whatever's there. Knowing that you may return at any appropriate time to a place of your choosing.

And now bring your awareness back into the room, focusing on your breathing . . . in and out . . . taking a few more breaths . . . and when you're ready, opening your eyes.

► To order the Relaxation for Mind & Body CD, go to www.bullpub.com/catalog/relaxation-for-mind-and-body

you—this often involves using all your senses to create the image—and one that is meaningful to you. The image does not have to be accurate for it to work. Just use your imagination and trust yourself. Here are examples of images that some people have found useful:

For a Weakened Immune System

Sluggish, sleepy white blood cells awaken, put on protective armor, and enter the fight against the virus.

White blood cells rapidly multiply like millions of seeds bursting from a single ripe seedpod.

For Infections

White blood cells with flashing red sirens arrest and imprison harmful germs.

An army equipped with powerful antibiotic missiles attacks enemy germs.

A hot flame chases germs out of your entire body.

For an Overactive Immune System (allergies, arthritis, psoriasis, etc.)

Overly alert immune cells in the fire station are reassured that the allergens have triggered a false alarm, so they turn the alarm off and go back to playing their game of poker.

The civil war ends with the warring sides agreeing not to attack their fellow citizens.

For Tension and Stress

A tight, twisted rope slowly untwists.

Wax softens and melts.

Tension swirls out of your body and down the drain.

For Pain

All of the pain is placed in a large, strong metal box that is closed, sealed tightly, and locked with a huge, strong padlock.

You grasp the TV remote control and slowly turn down the pain volume until you can barely hear it; then it disappears entirely.

The pain is washed away by a cool, calm river flowing through your entire body.

For Depression

Your troubles and feelings of sadness are attached to big colorful helium balloons and float off into a clear blue sky.

A strong, warm sun breaks through dark clouds.

You feel a sense of detachment and lightness, enabling you to float easily through your day.

For Healing of Cuts and Injuries

Plaster covers over a crack in a wall.

Cells and fibers stick together with very strong glue.

A shoe is laced up tight.

Jigsaw puzzle pieces come together.

For Arteries and Heart Disease

A miniature Roto-Rooter truck speeds through your arteries and cleans out the clogged pipes.

Water flows freely through a wide, open river.

A crew in a small boat rows in sync, easily and efficiently pulling the slender boat across the smooth water surface.

For Asthma and Lung Disease

The tiny elastic rubber bands that constrict your airways pop open.

A vacuum cleaner gently sucks the mucus from your airways.

Waves calmly rise and fall on the ocean surface.

For Diabetes

Small insulin keys unlock doors to hungry cells and allow nourishing blood sugar in.

An alarm goes off, and a sleeping pancreas gland awakens to the smell of freshly brewed coffee.

For Cancer

A shark gobbles up the cancer cells.

Tumors shrivel up like raisins in the hot sun and then evaporate completely into the air.

The faucet that controls the blood supply to the tumor is turned off, and the cancer cells starve.

Radiation or chemotherapy enters your body like healing rays of light and destroy cancer cells.

Use any of these images, or make up your own. Remember, the best ones are vivid and have meaning to you. Use your imagination for health and healing.

Prayer and Spirituality

In the medical literature, there is strong evidence of the relationship between spirituality and health. According to the American Academy of Family Physicians,* spirituality is the way we can find meaning, hope, comfort, and inner peace in our lives. Many people find spirituality through religion. Some find it through music, art, or a connection with nature. Others find it in their values and principles.

Many people are religious and share their religion with others. Others do not have a specific religion but do have spiritual beliefs. Religion and beliefs can bring a sense of meaning and purpose to life, help put things into perspective, and help us to set priorities. Our beliefs may comfort us during difficult times. Religion and beliefs can help us with acceptance and motivate us to make difficult changes. Being part of a spiritual or religious community offers a source of support when needed and the opportunity to help others.

Recent studies find that people who belong to a religious or spiritual community or who regularly engage in religious activities, such as prayer or study, have improved health. There are many types of prayer, any of which may contribute to improved health: asking for help, direction, or forgiveness; offering words of gratitude, praising, and blessing; among others. In addition, many religions have a tradition of contemplation or meditation. Prayer does not need a scientific explanation. It is probably the oldest of all self-management tools.

Although religion and spirituality cannot be "prescribed," we encourage you to explore your

---

*Adapted from the American Academy of Family Physicians: www.aafp.org/afp/2001/0101/p89.html

own beliefs. If you are religious, try practicing prayer more consistently. Also, if you are religious, consider telling your doctor and health care team. Most don't ask, so it is up to you to volunteer this information if it is important to you. Help them understand the importance of your beliefs in managing your health and life. Most hospitals have chaplains or pastoral counselors. Even if you are not in the hospital, they will probably find time to visit with you. Their advice and counsel can supplement your medical and psychological care.

Other Techniques That Use Your Mind

There are additional valuable techniques you can consider that can clear your mind, positively shift your emotional state, and reduce your tension and stress.

Mindfulness

Mindfulness involves keeping your attention in the present moment, without judging it as happy or sad, good or bad. It encourages living each moment—even painful ones—as fully and as mindfully as possible. Mindfulness is more than a relaxation technique; it is an attitude toward living. It is a way of calmly and consciously observing and accepting whatever is happening, moment to moment.

This may sound simple enough, but our restless, judging minds make it surprisingly difficult. As a restless monkey jumps from branch to branch, our mind jumps from thought to thought.

In mindfulness, you focus the mind on the present moment. The "goal" of mindfulness is simply to observe—with no intention of changing or improving anything. But people are positively changed by the practice. Observing and accepting life just as it is, with all its pleasures, pains, frustrations, disappointments, and insecurities, often enables you to become calmer, more confident, and to cope more effectively with whatever comes along.

To develop your capacity for mindfulness, sit comfortably on the floor or on a chair with your back, neck, and head straight, but not stiff. Then move through the following steps:

■ Concentrate on a single object, such as your breathing. Focus your attention on the feeling of the air as it passes in and out of your nostrils with each breath. Don't try to control your breathing by speeding it up or slowing it down. Just observe it as it is.

■ Even when you resolve to keep your attention on your breathing, your mind will quickly wander off. When this occurs, observe where your mind went: perhaps to a memory, a worry about the future, a bodily ache, or a feeling of impatience. Then gently return your attention to your breathing.

■ Use your breath as an anchor. Each time a thought or feeling arises, momentarily acknowledge it. Don't analyze it or judge it. Just observe it, and return to your breathing.

■ Let go of all thoughts of getting somewhere, or having anything special happen. Just keep stringing moments of mindfulness together, breath by breath.

- At first, practice this for just five minutes, or even one minute at a time. You may wish to gradually extend the time to 10, 20, or 30 minutes.

Because the practice of mindfulness is simply the practice of moment-to-moment awareness, you can apply it to anything: eating, showering, working, talking, running errands, or playing with your children. Mindfulness takes no extra time. Considerable research has demonstrated the benefits of mindfulness practice in relieving stress, easing pain, improving concentration, and relieving a variety of other symptoms.

Quieting Reflex

This technique was developed by a physician named Charles Stroebel. It will help you deal with short-term stress and the ways it can affect you, such as the urge to eat or smoke, succumb to road rage, or react to other annoyances. By activating what's called the sympathetic nervous system, this technique prevents you from tightening your muscles, clenching your jaw, and holding your breath.

The quieting reflex should be practiced frequently throughout the day, whenever you start to feel stressed. It can be done with your eyes opened or closed. Follow these steps:

1. *Become aware* of what is annoying you: a ringing phone, an angry comment, the urge to smoke, a worrisome thought—whatever.

2. *Repeat the phrase* "Alert mind, calm body" to yourself.

3. *Smile inwardly* with your eyes and your mouth. This stops facial muscles from making a fearful or angry expression. The inward smile is a feeling. It cannot be seen by others.

4. *Inhale slowly* to the count of three, imagining that the breath comes in through the bottom of your feet. Then exhale slowly. Feel your breath move back down your legs and out through your feet. Let your jaw, tongue, and shoulder muscles go limp.

With several months' practice, the quieting reflex becomes an automatic skill.

Nature Therapy

Many of us suffer from what has been called "nature deficit disorder," but it can be readily cured with regular doses of the outdoors. For thousands of years, exposure to natural environments has been recommended for healing. Taking a break from artificial lighting, computer and TV screens, and indoor environments is restorative. A brief walk in a park or a longer planned visit to a beautiful outdoor environment can restore the mind and body. Or bring nature indoors with plants, pets, and nature photography. Even a few minutes of playing with or stroking a pet can lower blood pressure and calm a restless mind.

Worry Time

Worrisome negative thoughts feed anxiety. Ignored problems have a way of thrusting themselves back into your consciousness. You'll find it easier to set aside worries if you make time to deal with them.

Set aside 20 to 30 minutes a day as your "worry time." Whenever a worry pops into your mind, write it down and tell yourself that you'll deal with it during worry time. Jot down the little things (Did Linda take her lunch to school?) along with the big ones (Will our children be able to find jobs?). During your scheduled worry time, don't do anything except worry, brainstorm, and write down possible solutions. For each of your worries, ask yourself the following questions:

- What is the problem?
- How likely is it that the problem will occur?
- What's the worst that could happen?
- What's the best that could happen?
- How would I cope with the problem?
- What are possible solutions?
- What is my plan of action?

Be specific. Instead of worrying about what might happen if you lose your job, ask yourself how likely it is that you will lose your job. And if you do, what will you do, with whom, and by when? Write a job search plan.

If you're anxious about getting seasick on an upcoming vacation cruise and not making it to the bathroom in time, imagine how you would manage the situation. Ask yourself if any of this is really unbearable. Remind yourself that you might feel uncomfortable or embarrassed, but you'll survive. Research ways to mitigate or avoid seasickness.

Remember, if a new worry pops up during the rest of the day, jot it down. Then distract yourself by refocusing intently on whatever you are doing. Scheduling a definite worry time cuts the amount of time spent worrying by at least a third. If you look at your list of worries later, you'll find that the vast majority of them never materialized. Or they were not nearly as bad as you had anticipated.

A Healthy Perspective

Sometimes you can relieve stress and break the cycle of negative thoughts by shifting your perspective. If you find yourself upset, ask, "How important will this be in an hour, a day, a month, or a year?" "Is this something I can change or not?" This reframing often helps to shift focus to things that are really important and need action versus the more minor annoyances that capture our attention.

Practicing Gratitude

One of the most effective ways to improve your mood and overall happiness is by focusing your attention on what's going well in your life. For what are you grateful? Psychologists have done research to demonstrate that people can increase their happiness by performing gratitude exercises. We encourage you to try these three:

- **Write a letter of thanks.** Write and then deliver a letter of gratitude to someone who has been especially kind to you but has never been properly thanked. Perhaps it's a teacher, a mentor, a friend, or a family member. Express your appreciation for the person's kindness. The letter will have more impact if you include some specific examples of what the recipient has done for you. Describe how the actions made you feel. Ideally, read your letter out loud to the person, if possible, face-to-face. Be aware of how you feel, and watch the other person's reaction.

- **Acknowledge at least three good things every day.** Each night before bed, write down at least three things that went well today. No event or feeling is too small to note. By putting your gratitude into words, you increase appreciation and memory of your blessings. Knowing that you will need to write each night changes your mental filters during the whole day. You will tend to seek out, look for, and specially note the good things that happen. If doing this daily is too much or begins to seem like a routine chore, do it once a week.

■ **Make a list of the things you take for granted.** For example, if your chronic illness has affected your lungs, you can still be grateful that your kidneys are working. Perhaps you can celebrate a day in which you don't have a headache or backache. Counting your blessings can add up to a better mood and more happiness. You can increase feelings of gratitude for positive events in your life by visualizing what your life would be like without them. By getting a taste of their absence, you should be able to appreciate their presence in your life more deeply—without actually having to lose them for real.

Listing Strengths

Make a personal inventory of your talents, skills, achievements, and qualities, big and small. Celebrate your accomplishments. When something goes wrong, consult your list of positives, and put the problem in perspective. It then becomes just one specific experience, not something that defines your whole life.

Practicing Kindness

This world is plagued by violence and suffering. When something bad happens, it's front-page news. As an antidote to this misery, despair, and cynicism, practice acts of kindness. Look for

opportunities to give without expecting anything in return. Here are some examples:

■ Hold the door open for the person behind you.

■ Give an unexpected gift of movie or concert tickets.

■ Send an anonymous gift to a friend who needs cheering up.

■ Help someone with a heavy load.

■ Tell positive stories you know of helping and kindness.

■ Cultivate an attitude of gratefulness for the kindness you have received from others.

■ Plant a tree.

■ Smile and let people cut ahead of you in line or on the freeway.

■ Pick up litter.

■ Give another driver your parking space.

Be creative. Such kindness is contagious, and it has a ripple effect. In one study, the people who were given an unexpected treat (cookies) were later more likely to help others.

Writing Away Stress

It's hard work to keep our deep negative feelings hidden. Over time, this cumulative stress undermines our body's defenses and may weaken our immunity. Confiding our feelings to others or writing them down allows us to put them into words and helps us to sort them out. Words help us understand and absorb a traumatic event and eventually put it behind us. It gives us a sense of release and control.

In his book *Opening Up*, the psychologist James Pennebaker described a series of studies that looked at the healing effects of confiding or writing. One group was asked to express their deepest thoughts and feelings about something bad that had happened to them. Another group wrote about ordinary matters such as their plans for the day. Both groups wrote for 15 to 20 minutes a day for three to five consecutive days. No one read what either group had written.

The results were surprisingly powerful. When compared with the people who wrote about ordinary events, the ones who wrote about their bad experiences reported fewer symptoms, fewer visits to the doctor, fewer days off from work, improved mood, and a more positive outlook. Their immune function was enhanced for at least six weeks after writing. This was especially true for those who expressed previously undisclosed painful feelings.

Try the "write thing" when something is bothering you: when you find yourself thinking (or dreaming) too much about an experience; when you avoid thinking about something because it is too upsetting; when there's something you would like to tell others but don't for fear of embarrassment or punishment.

Here are some guidelines for writing as a way to help you deal with any traumatic experience:

- Set a specific schedule for writing. For example, you might write 15 minutes a day for four consecutive days, or one day a week for four weeks.

- Write in a place where you won't be interrupted or distracted.

- Don't plan to share your writing—that could stop your honest expression. Save what you write or destroy it, as you wish.

- Explore your very deepest thoughts and feelings and analyze why you feel the way you do. Write about your negative feelings such as sadness, hurt, hate, anger, fear, guilt, or resentment.

- Write continuously. Don't worry about grammar, spelling, or making sense. If clarity and coherence come as you continue to write, so much the better. If you run out of things to say, just write what you have already written in different words.

- Even if you find the writing awkward at first, keep going. It gets easier. If you just cannot write, try talking into a tape recorder for 15 minutes about your deepest thoughts and feelings.

- Don't expect to feel better immediately. You may feel sad or depressed when your deepest feelings begin to surface. This usually fades within an hour or two or a day or two. The overwhelming majority of people report feelings of relief, happiness, and contentment after writing for a few consecutive days.

- Writing may help you clarify what actions you need to take, but don't use writing as a substitute for taking action or as a way of avoiding things.

Relaxation, imagery, and positive thinking can be some of the most powerful tools you can add to your self-management toolbox. They will help you manage symptoms as well as master the other skills discussed in this book.

As with exercise and other acquired skills, using your mind to manage your health condition requires both practice and time before you begin to notice the benefits. So if you feel you are not accomplishing anything, don't give up. Be patient and keep on trying.

Additional Resources

Association of Cancer Online Resources (ACOR): www.acor.org

The Body—The Complete HIV/AIDS Resource:
www.thebody.com/content/66652/stress-management-and-hiv.html

Greater Good in Action—Science-Based Practices for a Meaningful Life:
http://ggia.berkeley.edu

Greater Good Science Center: http://greatergood.berkeley.edu

Happier—Celebrate the Good Around You: www.happier.com

Happify: http://my.happify.com

Health Journeys—Resources for Mind, Body, and Spirit (guided imagery audio CDs):
www.healthjourneys.com

Mental Health America: www.liveyourlifewell.org

National Institute of Mental Health: www.nimh.nih.gov

Osher Center for Integrative Medicine (videos): www.osher.ucsf.edu/video

Regan, Catherine, and Rick Seidel. *Relaxation for Mind and Body: Pathways to Healing* [audio CD]. Boulder, Colo.: Bull, 2012.

StressStop—Stress Management Training That Works: www.stressstop.com

SuperBetter: www.superbetter.com

Weil, Andrew, and Martin Rossman. *Self-Healing with Guided Imagery* [audio CD]. Louisville, Colo.: Sounds True, 2006.

Suggested Further Reading

To learn more about the topics discussed in this chapter, we suggest that you explore the following resources:

Ben-Shahar, Tal. *Happier: Learn the Secrets to Daily Joy and Lasting Fulfillment*. New York: McGraw-Hill, 2007.

Benson, Herbert, and Eileen M. Stuart. *The Wellness Book: The Comprehensive Guide to Maintaining Health and Treating Stress-Related Illness*. New York: Fireside, 1993.

Benson, Herbert, and Miriam Z. Klipper. *The Relaxation Response*. New York: HarperCollins, 2000.

Boroson, Martin. *One Moment Meditation: Stillness for People on the Go*. New York: Winter Road Publishing, 2009.

Borysenko, Joan. *Inner Peace for Busy People: 52 Simple Strategies for Transforming Your Life*. Carlsbad, Calif.: Hay House, 2003.

Burns, David D. *The Feeling Good Handbook*, rev. ed. New York: Plume, 1999.

Caudill, Margaret. *Managing Pain Before It Manages You*. New York: Guilford Press, 2008.

Cousins, Norman. *Head First: The Biology of Hope and the Healing Power of the Human Spirit*. New York: Dutton, 1990.

Craze, Richard. *Teach Yourself Relaxation*, 3rd ed. New York: McGraw-Hill, 2009.

Davis, Martha, Elizabeth Eshelman, and Matthew McKay. *The Relaxation and Stress Reduction Workbook*, 6th ed. Oakland, Calif.: New Harbinger, 2008.

Diener, Ed, and Robert Biswas-Diener. *Happiness: Unlocking the Mysteries of Psychological Wealth*. Malden, Mass.: Blackwell, 2008.

Dossey, Larry. *Prayer Is Good Medicine*. San Francisco: HarperCollins, 1996.

Emmons, Robert A. *Thanks! How the New Science of Gratitude Can Make You Happier*. New York: Houghton Mifflin, 2007.

Emmons, Robert A. *Gratitude Works! A 21-Day Program for Creating Emotional Prosperity*. New York: Jossey-Bass, 2013.

Funk, Mary Margaret. *Tools Matter for Practicing the Spiritual Life*. New York: Continuum, 2004.

Grenville-Cleave, Bridget. *Introducing Positive Psychology: A Practical Guide*. London: Totem Books/Icon Books, 2012

Kabat-Zinn, Jon. *Coming to Our Senses: Healing Ourselves and the World Through Mindfulness*. New York: Hyperion, 2005.

Kabat-Zinn, Jon. *Wherever You Go, There You Are: Mindfulness Meditation in Everyday Life*. New York: Hyperion, 2005. Kabat-Zinn, Jon. *Full Catastrophe Living: Using the Wisdom of Your Body and Mind to Face Stress, Pain, and Illness*. New York: Bantam, 2013.

Keating, Thomas, Basil Pennington, et al. *Centering Prayer in Daily Life and Ministry*. New York: Continuum, 1998.

Keating, Thomas. *Open Mind, Open Heart: The Contemplative Dimension of the Gospel*. New York: Continuum, 2006.

Lyubomirsky, Sonja. *The How of Happiness: A New Approach to Getting the Life You Want*. New York: Penguin, 2008.

Lyubomirsky, Sonja. *The Myths of Happiness*. New York: Penguin, 2014.

McGonigal, Jane. *SuperBetter: A Revolutionary Approach to Getting Stronger, Happier, Braver, and More Resilient—Powered by the Science of Games*. New York: Penguin, 2015.

McGonigal, Kelly. *The Upside of Stress: Why Stress Is Good for You, and How to Get Good at It*. New York: Avery, 2015.

McKay, Matthew, Martha Davis, and Patrick Fanning. *Thoughts and Feelings: Taking Control of Your Moods and Your Life,* 4th ed. Oakland, Calif.: New Harbinger, 2011.

Ornstein, Robert, and David Sobel. *Healthy Pleasures*. Cambridge, Mass.: Perseus, 1989.

Peale, Norman V. *Positive Imaging: The Powerful Way to Change Your Life*. New York: Ballantine Books, 1996.

Remen, Rachel Naomi. *Kitchen Table Wisdom: Stories That Heal*. New York: Riverhead Books, 2006.

Rubin, Gretchen. *The Happiness Project*. New York: HarperCollins, 2011.

Selhub, Eva and Logan, Alan. *Your Brain on Nature: The Science of Nature's Influence on Your Health, Happiness, and Vitality*. New York: Collins, 2013.

Seligman, Martin. *Authentic Happiness: Using the New Positive Psychology to Realize Your Potential for Lasting Fulfillment*. New York: Atria, 2004.

Seligman, Martin. *Flourish: A Visionary New Understanding of Happiness and Well-Being*. New York: Free Press, 2011.

Siegel, Bernie S. and Yousaif August. *Help Me to Heal: A Practical Guidebook for Patients, Visitors, and Caregivers*. Carlsbad, Calif.: Hay House, 2003.

Siegel, Wendy Meg. *The Gratitude Habit: A Tool for Creating Positive Feelings in Your Daily Life*. Scotts Valley, Calif.: CreateSpace, 2012.

Sobel, David, and Robert Ornstein. *The Healthy Mind, Healthy Body Handbook* (also published under the title *The Mind and Body Health Handbook*). Los Altos, Calif.: DRx, 1996.

Stahl, Bob, and Elisha Goldstein. *A Mindfulness-Based Stress Reduction Workbook*. Oakland, Calif.: New Harbinger, 2010.

Wiseman, Richard. *59 Seconds: Think a Little, Change a Lot*. New York: Borzoi Books, 2009.

CHAPTER 13

Physical Activity for Fun and Fitness

REGULAR PHYSICAL ACTIVITY IS VITAL to physical and emotional health. It can also be fun and improve your fitness. Having HIV, however, can make it difficult to enjoy an active lifestyle. You may never have been really active in the first place, or you may have given up activities because of your condition or type of treatment. When you want to exercise but aren't sure what to do, physical and emotional limitations from HIV can be powerful forces to overcome. In the past, doctors even advised some people with HIV to avoid strenuous activity. Today, thanks to the research that has been conducted on people with HIV and the benefits of physical activity, we know it is safe for all people living with HIV to exercise.

Traditional medical care of chronic illness was based mainly on helping people when their illness worsened, and often involved recommendations to decrease physical activity and increase medical therapy. Unfortunately, long periods of inactivity can lead to weakness, stiffness, fatigue, poor appetite, constipation, high blood pressure, muscle loss, osteoporosis, and increased sensitivity to pain, anxiety, and depression.

muscle loss, osteoporosis, and increased sensitivity to pain, anxiety, and depression. This happens to everyone who is inactive, whether they have chronic conditions or not. No one can afford to be inactive.

For people with chronic conditions, inactivity-related problems can be caused by the illness itself or by medications, so it can be difficult to tell whether it is the illness, medication, inactivity, or a combination of the three that is responsible for these problems. Although we cannot cure HIV yet, we do know that exercise can cure inactivity and have a positive effect on a number of HIV-related problems. In this chapter we discuss the benefits of physical activity and give you pointers to help you start managing your own active lifestyle.

The Benefits of Regular Exercise

Physical activity can help you maintain a healthy weight and improve your body composition, improve your appetite, and manage your blood sugar, fats, cholesterol, and blood pressure levels. Research has shown that people with HIV-related fatty deposits (lipodystrophy) can reduce fat by exercising. (For more on this topic, see "About Distribution of Body Fat" on page 198 in this chapter.) Exercise conditions your body, helping to maintain cardiovascular and musculoskeletal fitness or restore function previously lost to disuse and illness. Exercise

Should Someone with HIV Exercise?

You may have questions about whether or not it's safe for you to exercise with HIV, and the answer is **YES**. You should follow the exact same guidelines for exercise that someone not living with HIV follows. Exercise not only promotes healthy living; it is one of the best ways to deal with many of the symptoms of HIV. In fact, exercise for people living with HIV is encouraged by all professional associations. The question is not, "Should I exercise?" but rather, "What kind of exercise program is right for me?" As you find a way to make exercise part of your life, remember the following tips:

- Check with your doctor before starting an exercise program.
- Start slowly and don't overdo it.
- When you are sick or have a fever, do not exercise.
- If you notice you are bleeding, stop exercising and (if you are at a gym or recreation center) let someone know to clean up the blood, or clean it up yourself.

Review the rest of the advice in this chapter for how to start a new exercise routine nourishes and strengthens muscles and bones, which can help increase your endurance and reduce your fatigue. Studies on HIV and exercise have shown the benefits of cardiovascular, endurance, and strengthening exercise programs, frequently combining them into a complete fitness program.

Exercise is safe for people with HIV at all ages and can have positive effects on the immune system. In general, people who are physically fit get fewer infections such as colds, and miss fewer days of work due to illness. Better fitness can also lead to better mood, coping, and quality of life. It will help you improve your health, prevent other diseases, feel better, and manage your illness better. Feeling more in control and less at the mercy of your illness is one of the biggest benefits of exercising.

If you have not exercised in a while, it is important to consult with your doctor and modify your former exercise program as needed. Symptoms such as dizziness, new numbness, vomiting, diarrhea, newly swollen joints, bleeding, or pain are reasons to stop a workout until you can speak with your doctor. (See "Advice for Exercise Problems," page 229.)

The advice in this book is not intended to take the place of specific therapeutic recommendations from your doctor or physical therapist. If an exercise plan has been prescribed for you that differs from the suggestions here, take this book to your doctor or physical therapist and ask them if this program is right for you or how you need to modify it to get the most out of the recommendations.

Developing an Active Lifestyle

One way to be more physically active is to set aside a time for a formal exercise program involving such planned activities as walking, jogging, swimming, biking, dancing, or working out with an exercise video or webcast. These kinds of formal programs are what people usually think of when they think about exercise activity. But being more physical in everyday life can also pay off. Consider taking the stairs for a floor or two instead of waiting for the elevator. Park and walk the last few blocks to work or to the store instead of circling the parking lot looking for the perfect, up-close parking space. Play with the dog. Work in the garden. Just get up and walk around the house several times a day.

These types of daily activities, if done at moderate intensity and often enough, can result in significant health benefits. Recent studies show that even small amounts of daily activity can raise fitness levels in some people, and improve health and mood—and the activities can be pleasurable, enjoyable ones! One person surveyed about activity level responded that they "*never* exercised." When asked about going dancing several times a week, they replied, "Oh, that's not exercise, that's fun." The average day is filled with excellent opportunities to be more physical and have more fun.

About Distribution of Body Fat (Lipodystrophy)

Lipodystrophy is the movement of body fat from places you typically have had it, such as your buttocks, to places you may not have had it previously, such as your chest and stomach. You can read more about lipodystrophy-related health issues in Chapter 3, "Health Problems of People with HIV," and Chapter 9, "Managing Side Effects of Medications." Although we do not understand the exact causes of lipodystrophy, we believe it is associated with the following factors:

- Use of certain HIV drugs

- Age (it is more common in older people)

- Race (it is more common in Caucasians)

- Length of HIV infection (it is more common in people who have had HIV for a long time)

- Low T-cell count

Besides changing the way your body looks and feels, lipodystrophy often goes hand in hand with high cholesterol and high insulin resistance. If this is the case for you and you develop these issues, you are more likely to have heart problems or diabetes. This means that it is important for you to discuss with your doctor any additional risks of lipodystrophy.

Although the medical community is not yet certain about how to prevent lipodystrophy, some studies suggest that exercise—especially strengthening exercise—may help to prevent or minimize it. The best current research indicates that weight training, which builds muscle, can help to change the ratio between muscle and fat, and thus combat the effects of lipodystrophy. You may want to go to a gym or recreational center whose staff is familiar with lipodystrophy. If you cannot find a fitness facility with trainers who know about this condition, follow the advice in this chapter, which is appropriate for all people with HIV.

Many health food stores, trainers, magazines, and even friends may try to get you to take supplements for lipodystrophy and other HIV-related conditions. Resist their advice at least until you have done your own research and discussed supplements with your health care team. Many supplements contain steroids or other drugs that will not help and may even harm you. Even the right drugs in the wrong dosage can be dangerous. It is important to talk with a knowledgeable health professional before trying supplements. You can find accurate, unbiased information at the excellent website www.aidsinfo.nih.gov.

Developing an Exercise Program

Although you can get lots of exercise from the activities of daily life, starting a more formal exercise program can be very helpful in achieving your health goals. Such a program usually involves setting aside a period of time, at least several times a week, to deliberately focus on increasing your fitness.

A complete, balanced exercise program can help you improve the following three aspects of fitness:

■ *Flexibility.* Flexibility refers to the ability of joints and muscles to move through a full, normal range of motion. Limited flexibility can cause pain, increase risk of injury, and make muscles less efficient. Flexibility tends to decrease with age and inactivity, but you can increase or maintain your flexibility by doing the gentle flexibility or stretching exercises described in this chapter.

■ *Strength.* Muscles need to be exercised to maintain their strength. With inactivity, they tend to weaken and shrink (atrophy). The weaker your muscles get, the less you feel like using them and the more inactive you tend to become, creating a vicious cycle. Some of the disability and lack of mobility in people with HIV is caused by decreased muscle mass and weakness. Strengthening exercises like the ones you will find in this chapter can help you maintain muscle,

reduce body fat, and bring back strength and muscle health.

■ *Endurance (Aerobic Fitness).* Our ability to sustain activity depends on certain vital capacities. The heart and lungs must work efficiently to distribute oxygen-rich blood to the muscles. The muscles must be conditioned to extract and use the oxygen. Aerobic (meaning "with oxygen") exercise builds endurance.

Aerobic exercise conditions the heart, blood vessels, and muscles. Sustained aerobic exercise uses the large muscles of your body in rhythmic, continuous activity. The most effective aerobic activities involve your whole body. Walking, jogging, swimming, dancing, and activities such as vacuuming, mowing the lawn, or raking leaves can be aerobic activities. Aerobic exercise improves cardiovascular fitness, lessens the risk of heart attack, and helps control weight. Aerobic exercise also promotes a sense of well-being—easing depression and anxiety, promoting restful sleep, and improving mood and energy levels.

Components of a Good Fitness Program

A complete fitness program combines exercises to improve each of the three important aspects of fitness: flexibility, strength, and endurance. If you haven't exercised regularly in some time or have discomfort, stiffness, shortness of breath, or weakness that interferes with your daily activities, talk with your health care providers before beginning your fitness program.

Once you are ready to begin exercising, start by choosing a number of flexibility and strengthening exercises that you are willing to do every day or every other day. After you are able to exercise comfortably for at least ten minutes at a time, you are ready to add some endurance or aerobic activities.

Physical Activity Guidelines

Many countries now have guidelines for what kinds of physical activity, and how much, people should do to be healthy. Fortunately, the guidelines are pretty much the same all over the world and apply to adults with and without chronic illness and disability.

When you read exercise guidelines, it is important to remember that *they are goals to work toward; they are not the starting point.* On average, only about 25 percent of people exercise enough to meet these guidelines. So don't think that everyone else but you is meeting the guidelines. Your goal is to gradually and safely increase your physical activity to a level that is right for you. You may be able to meet the recommended guideline level, but maybe you won't. The important point is to use the information to get you started to be more active and healthier in a way that is right for you. Start doing what you can. Even a few minutes of activity several times a day is a good beginning. The important thing is to do something that works for you, make it a habit, and gradually increase the amount of time or number of days a week that you exercise.

The following guidelines are from the U.S. Department of Health and Human Services and came out in 2008. Remember, these are a guide to where you could go, not where you must be now. Keep reading this chapter for more information that will help you get started on your exercise plan.

- Moderate aerobic (endurance) exercise for at least 150 minutes (2.5 hours) a week, or vigorous intensity activity for at least 75 minutes a week.

- Aerobic activity should be performed at least 10 minutes at a time spread out through the week.
- Moderate-intensity muscle-strengthening exercise of all major muscle groups should be done at least two days a week.
- If people cannot meet the guidelines, they should be as active as they can and avoid inactivity.

Examples of 150 Minutes a Week of Moderate Aerobic Activity

- Take a 10-minute walk at moderate intensity three times a day, five days a week.
- Take a 20-minute bike ride at moderate intensity three days a week and a 30-minute walk three days a week.
- Attend a 30-minute aerobic dance class at moderate intensity twice a week and take three 10-minute walks three days a week.
- Do gardening and yard work (digging, raking, lifting) 30 minutes a day, five days a week.

Be creative. Mix and match different activities that fit your schedule and your interests.

Examples of Muscle-Strengthening Exercise

- Twice a week do ten exercises 8 to 12 times each with enough weight or resistance that you feel slightly tired when you finish each exercise.
- Do yoga twice a week.
- Lift weights, use bands, or just work against your own body weight to do exercises for your arms, trunk, and legs.

On pages 203–213 we describe some specific exercises to build up your muscle strength.

Choose Your Goal and Make a Plan

Many people are uncertain about how to choose the right exercises and how to know what is best for them. The truth is that the best exercises are the ones that will help you do what you most want to do. Having a goal (something you want your exercise program to help you achieve) is the most important ingredient of a successful fitness program. Once you have a goal in mind, it is much easier to choose exercises that make sense for you.

If you don't see how exercise can be helpful to you personally, it is difficult to get excited about adding yet another task to your day. The steps we list here may help you get started.

1. *Choose a goal that is something you want to do* but don't do or can't do now because of physical limitations. For example, your goal might be taking a hiking trip with friends, painting your house, or having enough energy to host a family celebration.

2. *Think about why you can't or don't enjoy doing the activity now.* Maybe it is because you get tired before everybody else or you are too weak or short of breath to complete the activity.

3. *Decide what you can do to overcome the problem.* For example, you can gradually increase your endurance by walking a comfortable distance two or three times a week. Or you might practice deep breathing and strengthening exercises for your arms to help you manage your shortness of breath and upper-body weakness.

4. *Design your exercise plan.* Choose no more that 10 to 12 flexibility and strengthening exercises to start (two or three to start is fine if you are out of shape). Start by doing three to five repetitions of each, if you have not exercised for a while. As you improve, increase the number of repetitions and the number of exercises you do. To improve endurance, choose an aerobic activity you like (such as brisk walking, swimming, bicycling, or dancing). Start by doing this activity for just a few minutes at first, or for whatever period you are comfortable with now, and build up gradually. Health and fitness take time to build, but every day that you exercise makes you healthier and brings you closer to your fitness goals. That's why it is important to keep it up. Watching yourself improve even slightly week by week will build your confidence and motivation to continue.

Flexibility, Strength, and Balance Exercises

You can use flexibility exercise for many purposes: to get ready for aerobic exercise; to improve your flexibility, strength, and balance; to stretch and strengthen your back and chest for better posture and breathing; and to warm up and cool down before and after your aerobic exercise routines.

The exercises in this section are arranged in order from the head and neck down to the toes. Most of the upper-body exercises may be done

Tips for Exercising for Flexibility and Strength

- *Move slowly and gently*. Do not bounce or jerk. Such movements actually tighten and shorten muscles.

- To loosen tight muscles and limber up stiff joints, *stretch just until you feel tension*, hold for 5 to 10 seconds, and then relax.

- *Don't push your body until it hurts*. Stretching should feel good, not painful.

- *Start with no more than five repetitions of any exercise*. Take at least two weeks to increase to ten.

- Do the *same number* of repetitions for your left side as for your right.

- *Breathe naturally*. Do not hold your breath. Count out loud to make sure you are breathing easily. (If you are holding your breath, you are probably trying too hard. Reduce your intensity.)

- It is common for your muscle to "talk" to you after exercise with some slight soreness or tingling. These are signals that your body is getting stronger and more flexible! However, if you feel significantly increased symptoms or pain that lasts more than *two hours* after exercising, next time do fewer repetitions, or eliminate the exercise that seems to be causing the symptoms and try another one instead. *Don't quit exercising*.

- *All exercises should be adapted to individual needs*. If you are limited by muscle weakness or joint tightness, do the exercise as completely as you can. The benefit of doing an exercise comes from moving toward a certain position, not from being able to complete the movement perfectly the first time. In some cases you may find that after a while you can complete the movement. Other times you will continue to perform your own modified version.

either sitting or standing. Exercises done lying down can be performed on the floor or on a firm mattress. We have labeled the exercises that are particularly important for breathing and good posture "VIP" (Very Important for Posture). Exercises to improve balance by strengthening and loosening legs and ankles are marked "BB" (Better Balance). There is also a section of balance exercises that are specifically designed to help you practice balance skills.

If you see this symbol next to an exercise, this means that you can add weights (hand or ankle weights) to that exercise. When you add weights, it becomes exercise that builds your muscle strength. If you can do an exercise easily at least ten times, you can add weights. Start with 1 to 2 pounds (0.5 to 1.0 kg), and add weight gradually as you get stronger and the exercise gets easier. You can use homemade weights (e.g., cans of food, bags of beans, plastic bottles filled with water or sand) or buy small weights or dumbbells in different sizes.

You can make a routine of exercises that flow together. Arrange them so you don't have to get up and down too often. Exercise to music if you wish. An exercise CD has been designed to go with this book; see details under "Additional Resources" at the end of this chapter.

The following exercises are for both sides of the body and a full range of motion. If you are limited by muscle weakness or joint tightness, go ahead and do the exercise as completely as you can. *Remember that the benefit of doing an exercise comes from moving toward a certain position, not from being able to complete it perfectly.*

Neck Exercises

1. Heads Up (VIP)

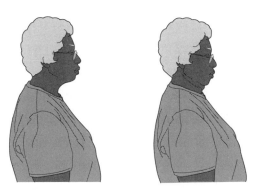

This exercise relieves jaw, neck, and upper back tension or pain and is the start of good posture. You can do it while driving, sitting at a desk, sewing, reading, or exercising.

Sit or stand straight and gently slide your chin back. Keep looking forward as your chin moves backward. You'll feel the back of your neck lengthen and straighten. To help, put your finger on your nose and draw your face straight back from your finger. (Don't worry about a little double chin—you really look much better with your neck straight once you have completed the exercise!)

Clues for Finding the Correct Position

- Ear over shoulder, not out in front
- Head balanced over neck and trunk, not in the lead
- Back of neck vertical, not leaning forward
- Bit of double chin

2. Neck Stretch

In the heads-up position (see Exercise 1, Heads Up) with your shoulders relaxed, turn slowly to look over your right shoulder. Then turn slowly to look over your left shoulder. Return your head to the centered heads-up position and then tilt your head to the right and then to the left. Move your ear toward your shoulder; do not move your shoulder up to your ear.

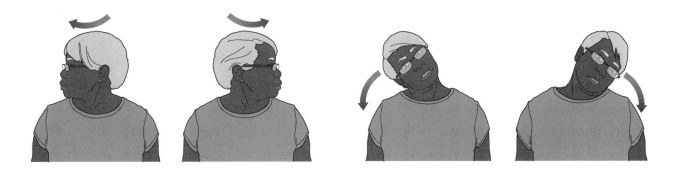

Hand and Wrist Exercises

A good place to do hand exercises is at a table that supports your forearms. Do them after washing dishes, after bathing or showering, or when taking a break from any sort of handwork. Your hands are warmer and more limber at these times.

3. Thumb Walk

Holding your wrist straight, form the letter O by lightly touching your thumb to each fingertip. After each O, straighten and spread your fingers. Use the other hand to help if needed.

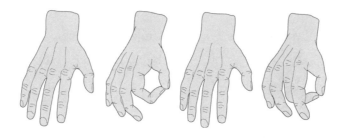

Shoulder Exercises

4. Shoulder Shape Up

This is a good exercise if the neck stretch (Exercise 2) is difficult for you.

In the heads-up position (see Exercise 1, Heads Up), slowly raise your shoulders to your ears; hold the position and then drop them. Next, raise your shoulders again to your ears and begin to slowly rotate them backward by pinching your shoulder blades together; bring your shoulders down and forward to complete a circle. Return to the heads-up position. Repeat, reversing the direction of the shoulder circles.

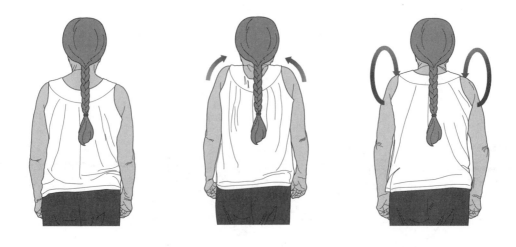

5. Good Morning (VIP)

Start with hands in gentle fists, palms down, and wrists crossed in front of you. Breathe in and stretch out your fingers while you uncross your arms and reach up for the sky. Breathe out as you stretch your arms and relax.

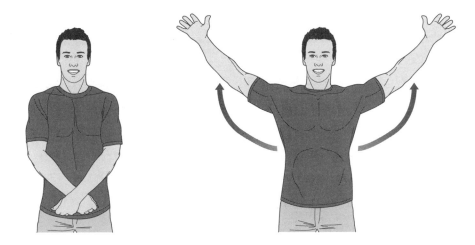

6. Wand Exercise

If one or both of your shoulders are tight or weak, you may want to give yourself a "helping hand." This shoulder exercise and the next one allow the arms to help each other.

Use a yardstick, mop handle, or cane as your wand. Place one hand on each end of your wand, and raise it as high overhead as possible. You might try this in front of a mirror. This exercise can be done standing, sitting, or lying down.

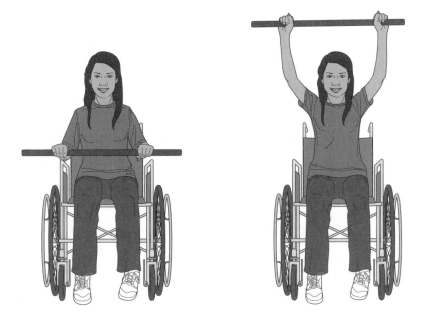

7. Pat and Reach

This double-duty exercise helps increase flexibility and strength for both shoulders.

Raise one arm up over your head, and bend your elbow to pat yourself on the back. Move your other arm down and behind your back, then bend that elbow to reach up toward the other hand. Can your fingertips touch? Relax and switch arm positions. Can you touch on that side? For most people, one side is more flexible than the other. Do not worry if you cannot touch. Many people cannot touch, but your reach will improve as you practice. If you wish, you may use a towel as if you were drying your back; this can provide you with feedback and assist in the motion.

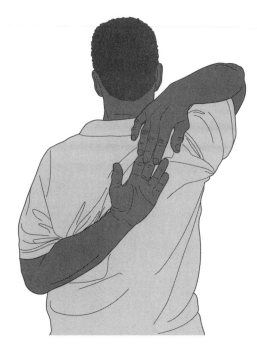

8. Shoulder Blade Pinch (VIP)

This is a good exercise to strengthen the middle and upper back and to stretch the chest. It can be especially good for individuals with breathing problems.

Sit or stand with your head in the heads-up position (see Exercise 1, Heads Up) and your shoulders relaxed. Raise your arms out to the sides with elbows bent. Pinch your shoulder blades together by moving your elbows as far back as you can. Hold briefly, and then slowly move your arms forward to touch elbows in front of your body. If this position is uncomfortable, lower your arms or rest your hands on your shoulders.

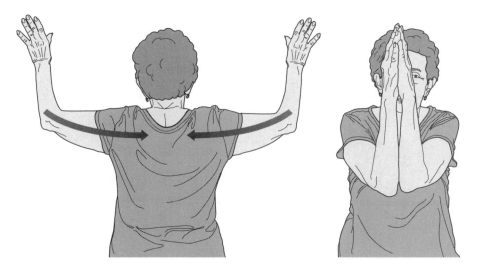

Back and Abdominal Exercises

9. Knee to Chest Stretch

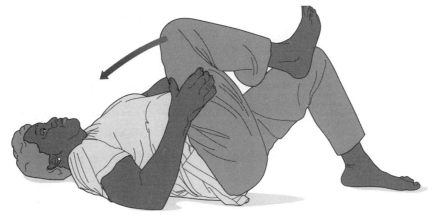

For a lower back stretch, lie on the floor with knees bent and feet flat. Bring one knee toward your chest, using your hands to help. Hold your knee near your chest for 10 seconds, and lower the leg slowly. Repeat with the other knee. You can also tuck both legs at the same time if you wish. Relax and enjoy the stretch.

10. Pelvic Tilt (VIP)

This is an excellent exercise for the lower back and can help relieve lower back pain.

Lie on your back with knees bent, feet flat. Place your hands on your abdomen. Flatten the small of your back against the floor by tightening your stomach muscles and your buttocks. When you do this exercise, you are tilting your tailbone forward and pulling your stomach back. Think about trying to pull your stomach in enough to zip a tight pair of trousers. Hold the tilt for 5 to 10 seconds. Relax. Arch your back slightly. Relax and repeat the pelvic tilt. Keep breathing. Count the seconds out loud. Once you've mastered the pelvic tilt lying down, practice it sitting, standing, and walking.

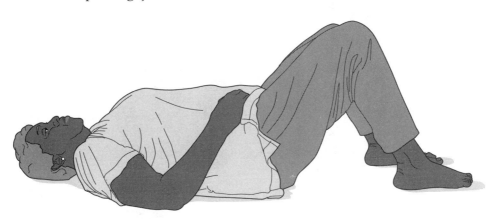

11. Back Lift (VIP)

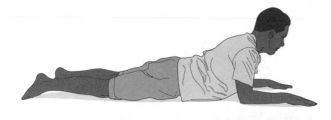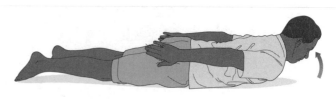

This exercise improves flexibility along your spine and helps you lift your chest for easier breathing.

Lie on your stomach, and rise up onto your forearms. Keep your back relaxed, and keep your stomach and hips down. If this is comfortable, straighten your elbows. Breathe naturally and relax for at least 10 seconds. If you have moderate to severe lower back pain, do not do this exercise unless it has been specifically prescribed for you.

To strengthen back muscles, lie on your stomach with your arms at your side or overhead. Lift your head, shoulders, and arms. Do not look up. Keep looking down with your chin tucked into that double-chin position. Count out loud as you hold for a count of 10. Relax. Alternatively, you can lift your legs, instead of your head and shoulders, off the floor.

Note that lifting both ends of your body at once is a fairly strenuous exercise. It may not be helpful for a person with back pain.

12. Low Back Rock and Roll

Lie on your back, and pull your knees up to your chest. You can keep holding on to your legs with your hands behind the thighs or stretch your arms out to your sides so they lie on the floor at shoulder level. Rest in this position for 10 seconds, and then gently roll your hips and knees to one side and then the other. Rest and relax as you roll to each side. Keep your upper back and shoulders flat on the ground.

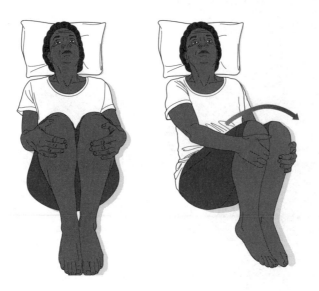

13. Curl-Up (BB)

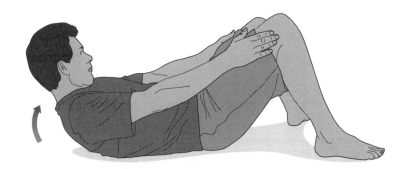

A curl-up, as shown here, is a good way to strengthen stomach muscles.

Lie on your back, knees bent, feet flat. Do the pelvic tilt (see Exercise 10, Pelvic Tilt). Slowly curl up in segments. Tuck your chin as you roll your head up and begin to lift the shoulders off the floor. Slowly uncurl back down, or hold for 10 seconds and then slowly lower. Breathe out as you curl up, and breathe in as you go back down. Do not hold your breath. If you have neck problems or if your neck hurts when you do this exercise, try the next exercise (Exercise 14, Roll-Out) instead. Never tuck your feet under a chair or have someone hold your feet!

14. Roll-Out

This is another good stomach strengthener, and it is easy on the neck. Use it instead of the curl-up (Exercise 13), or if neck pain is not a problem, do them both.

Lie on your back with knees bent and feet flat. Do the pelvic tilt (Exercise 10), and hold your lower back firmly against the floor. Slowly and carefully, move one leg away from your chest as you straighten your knee. Move your leg out until you feel your lower back start to arch. When this happens, tuck your knee back to your chest. Reset your pelvic tilt and roll your leg out again. Breathe out as your leg rolls out. Do not hold your breath. Repeat with the other leg.

You are strengthening your abdominal muscles by holding your pelvic tilt against the weight of your leg. As you get stronger, you'll be able to straighten your legs out farther and move both legs together.

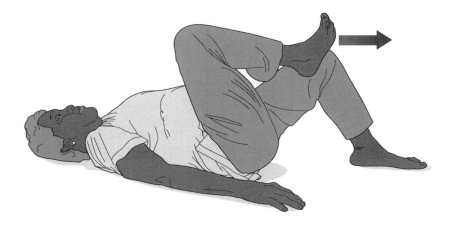

Hip and Leg Exercises

15. Straight Leg Raises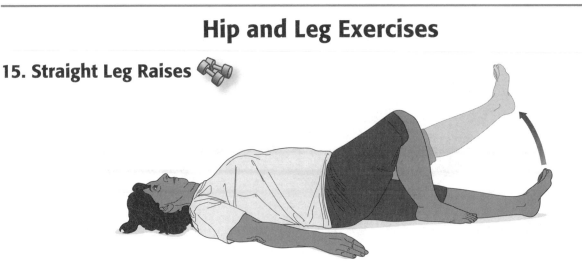

This exercise strengthens the muscles that bend the hip and straighten the knee.

Lie on your back, knees bent, feet flat. Straighten one leg. Tighten the muscle on the upper surface of that thigh, and straighten the knee as much as possible. Keeping the knee straight, raise your leg a foot or two (up to 50 cm) off the ground. Do not arch your back. Hold your leg up, and count out loud for 10 seconds. Relax. Repeat with the other leg.

16. Hip Hooray (standing only)

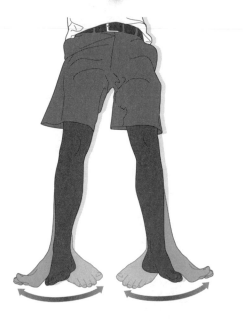
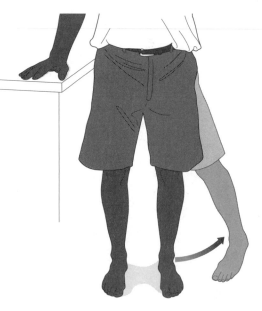

This exercise can be done standing or lying on your back. If you lie down, spread your legs as far apart as possible. Roll your legs and feet out like a duck, then in to be pigeon-toed, and then move your legs back together. If you are standing, move one leg out to your side as far as you can. Lead out with the heel and in with the toes. Hold on to a counter for support. You can make the muscles work harder while you are standing by adding a weight to your ankle.

17. Back Kick (VIP) (BB)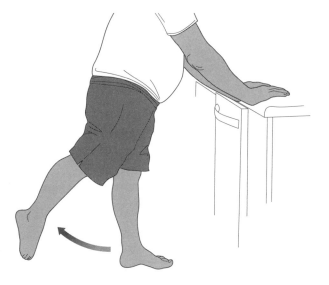

This exercise increases the backward mobility and strength of your hip. Holding on to a counter for support, move the leg up and back, knee straight. Stand tall, and do not lean forward.

18. Knee Strengthener (BB)

Strong knees are important for walking and standing comfortably. This exercise strengthens the knee.

Sitting in a chair, straighten the knee by tightening up the muscle on the upper surface of your thigh. Place your hand on your thigh and feel the muscle work. If you wish, make circles with your toes. As your knee strengthens, see if you can build up to holding your leg out for 30 seconds. Count out loud. Do not hold your breath.

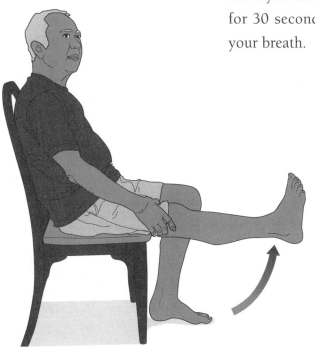

19. Power Knees

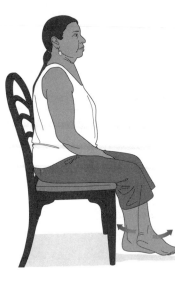

This exercise strengthens the muscles that bend and straighten your knee.

Sit in a chair and cross your legs at the ankles. Your legs can be almost straight, or you can bend your knees as much as you like. Try several positions. Push forward with your back leg, and press backward with your front leg. Exert pressure evenly so that your legs do not move. Hold and count out loud for 10 seconds. Relax. Switch leg positions. Be sure to keep breathing. Repeat.

20. Ready-Go (BB)

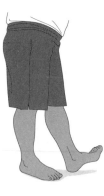

Stand with one leg slightly in front of the other with your heel on the floor as if ready to take a step with the front foot. Now tighten the muscles on the front of your thigh, making your knee firm and straight. Hold to a count of 10. Relax. Repeat with the other leg.

21. Hamstring Stretch

If you have unstable knees or "back knee" (a knee that curves backward when you stand up), do not do this exercise.

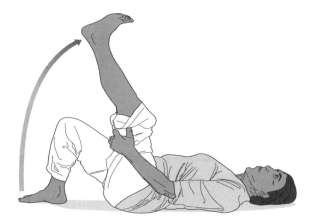

If you do have tight hamstrings, lie on your back, knees bent, feet flat. Grasp one leg at a time behind the thigh. Holding your leg out at arm's length, slowly straighten your knee. Hold your leg as straight as you can as you count to 10. You should feel a slight stretch at the back of your knee and thigh.

Be careful with this exercise. It's easy to overstretch and end up sore.

22. Achilles Stretch (BB)

This exercise helps maintain flexibility in the Achilles tendon, the large tendon at the back of your ankle. Good flexibility in this tendon helps reduce the risk of injury, calf discomfort, and heel pain. The Achilles stretch is especially helpful for cooling down after walking or cycling and for people who get cramps in the calf muscles.

Stand at a counter or with your hands against a wall. Place one foot in front of the other, toes pointing forward and heels on the ground. Lean forward, bend the knee of the forward leg, and keep the back knee straight, heel down. You will feel a good stretch in the calf (lower leg). Hold the stretch for 10 seconds. Do not bounce. Move gently. You can adjust this exercise to reach the other large calf muscle by slightly bending your back knee while you stretch the calf. Can you feel the difference?

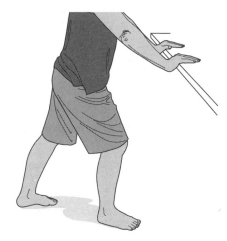

If you have trouble with standing balance or spasticity (muscle jerks), you can do a seated version of this exercise. Sit in a chair with feet flat on the floor. Keep your heel on the floor and slowly slide your foot (one foot at a time) back to bend your ankle and feel some tension on the back of your calf.

It's easy to get sore doing this exercise. If you've worn shoes with high heels for a long time, be particularly careful.

23. Tiptoes (BB)

This exercise will help strengthen your calf (lower leg) muscles and make walking, climbing stairs, and standing less tiring. It may also improve your balance.

Hold on to a counter or table for support and rise up on your tiptoes. Hold for 10 seconds. Lower yourself back down slowly. How high you go is not as important as keeping your balance and controlling your ankles. It is easier to do both legs at the same time. If your feet are too sore to do this standing, start doing it while sitting down. If this exercise makes your ankle jerk, stop doing it and talk to your therapist about other ways to strengthen your calf muscles.

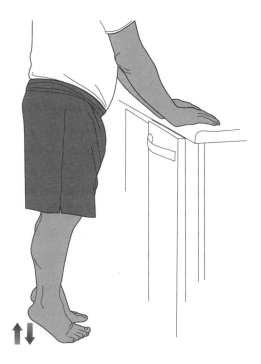

Ankle and Foot Exercises

Do these exercises sitting in a straight-backed chair with your feet bare. Have a bath towel and ten marbles next to you. These exercises are for flexibility, strength, and comfort. This is also a good time to examine your feet and toes for any signs of circulation or skin problems and to check your nails to see if they need trimming.

24. Towel Grabber

Spread a towel out in front of your chair. Place your feet on the towel, with your heels near the edge closest to you. Keep your heels down and your foot slightly raised. Scoot the towel back underneath your feet by pulling it with your toes. When you have done as much as you can, reverse the toe motion and scoot the towel out again.

25. Marble Pickup

Do this exercise one foot at a time. Place several marbles on a towel on the floor between your feet. Keep your heel down, and pivot your toes toward the marbles. Pick up a single marble with your toes, and pivot your foot to drop the marble as far as possible from where you picked it up. Repeat until all the marbles have been moved. Reverse the process and return all the marbles to the starting position. If marbles are difficult, try other objects, such as jacks, dice, or wads of paper.

26. Foot Roll

Place a rolling pin (or a large dowel or closet rod) under the arch of your foot, and roll it back and forth. It feels great and stretches the ligaments in the arch of the foot.

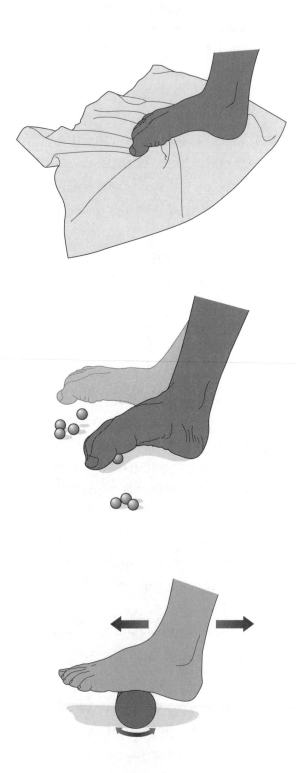

Balance Exercises

The exercises in this section are designed to let you practice balance activities in a safe and progressive way. The exercises are listed in order of difficulty. Start with the first exercises and work up to the more difficult ones as your strength and balance improve. If you feel that your balance is particularly poor, exercise with someone else nearby who can give you a supporting hand if you need one. Always practice by a counter or stable chair that you can hold on to if necessary. Signs of improving balance are being able to hold a position longer or without extra support or being able to do the exercise or hold the position with your eyes closed.

You may also be able to find some balance exercise classes in your community to help continue your progress. Tai chi is a wonderful program to help you work on balance and strength. It is low-impact and gentle on your joints. The National Institute on Aging offers a free exercise guide and video that includes other balance exercises (see "Additional Resources" at the end of this chapter), but you can use the following to get started.

27. Beginning Balance

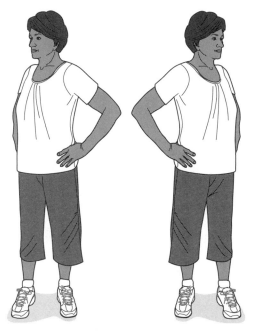

Stand quietly with your feet comfortably apart. Place your hands on your hips, and turn your head and trunk as far to the left as possible and then to the right. Repeat 5 to 10 times. To increase the difficulty, do the same thing with your eyes closed.

28. Swing and Sway

Using a counter or the back of a stable chair for support,
do each of the following 5 to 10 times:

1. Rock back on your heels and then go up on your toes.

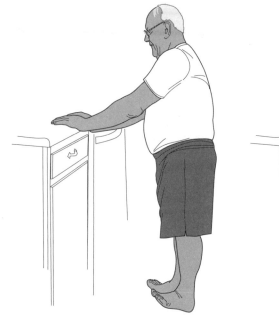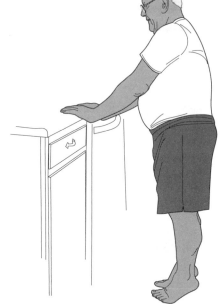

2. Do the box step (like dancing the waltz).

3. March in place, first with eyes open and then with eyes closed.

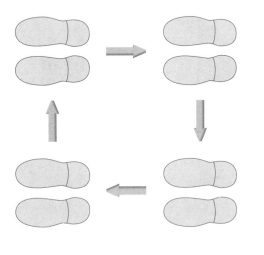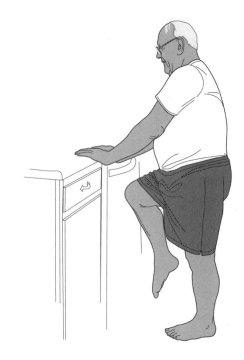

29. Base of Support

Do these exercises with someone nearby or standing close to a counter for support. The purpose of these three simple exercises is to help you improve your balance by going from a larger to a smaller base of support. Work on being able to hold each position for 10 seconds.

When you can do it with your eyes open, practice with your eyes closed.

1. Stand with feet together.

2. Stand with one foot out in front and the other back.

3. Stand heel to toe.

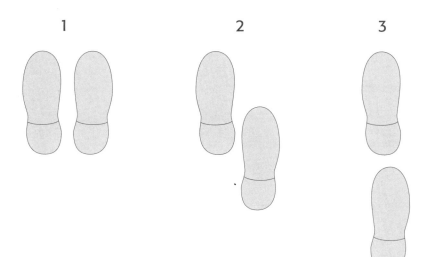

30. Toe Walk

The purpose of this exercise is to increase ankle strength and to give you practice balancing on a small base of support while moving.

Stay close to a counter for support. Rise up on your toes and walk up and back along the counter. Once you are comfortable walking on your toes without support and with your eyes open, try it with your eyes closed.

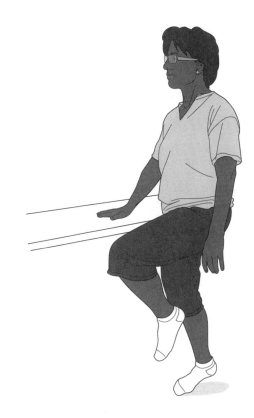

31. Heel Walk

The purpose of this exercise is to increase your lower leg strength and give you practice moving on a small base of support.

Stay close to a counter for support. Raise your toes and forefoot and walk up and back along the counter on your heels. Once you are comfortable walking on your heels without support and with your eyes open, try it with your eyes closed.

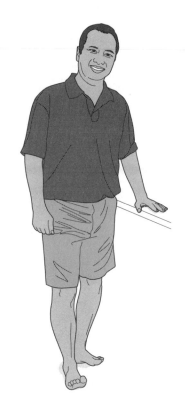

32. One-Legged Stand

Holding on to a counter or chair, lift one foot completely off the ground. Once you are balanced, lift your hand. The goal is to hold the position for 10 seconds. Once you can do this for 10 seconds without holding on, practice it with your eyes closed. Repeat with the other leg.

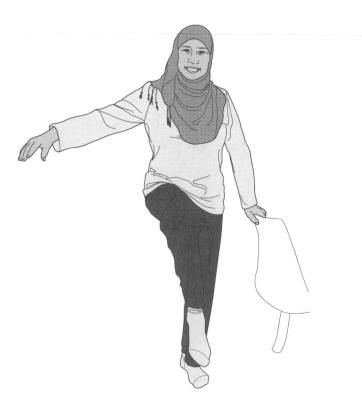

Whole Body Exercises

33. The Stretcher

This exercise is a whole-body stretch to do lying on your back. Start the motion at your ankles as explained here, or reverse the process if you want to start with your arms first.

1. Point your toes, and then pull your toes toward your nose. Relax.

2. Bend your knees. Then flatten your knees and let them relax.

3. Arch your back. Do the pelvic tilt (Exercise 10). Relax.

4. Breathe in and stretch your arms above your head. Breathe out and lower your arms. Relax.

5. Stretch your right arm above your head, and stretch your left leg by pushing away with your heel. Hold for a count of 10. Switch to the other side and repeat.

Endurance Exercise

One of the biggest problems with endurance (aerobic) exercise is that it is easy to overdo, even for people who don't have HIV. Inexperienced and misinformed exercisers think they have to work very hard for exercise to do any good. Exhaustion, very sore muscles, painful joints, and worsening shortness of breath are the consequences of starting out too hard and too fast. As a result, some people put aside their exercise programs indefinitely, thinking that exercise is just not meant for them.

There is no magic formula for determining how much exercise you need. *The most important thing to remember is that some is better than none. Every minute counts. Even a few minutes of exercise several times per week can be very beneficial.* If you start slowly and increase your efforts gradually, it is likely that you will maintain your exercise program as a lifelong habit. Generally, it is better to begin your conditioning program by *under*doing rather than *over*doing.

Fatigue, lack of cardiovascular conditioning, and poor endurance are common challenges for people with HIV. People who have had HIV for quite a while also may be at more risk for cardiovascular and bone problems. These conditions can limit the amount of exercise that can be performed, but for most people with HIV, moderate-intensity aerobic exercise can be both comfortable and safe.

You can adjust your exercise effort and work toward your goal by adjusting the three basic building blocks of an endurance exercise program: frequency, time, and intensity.

■ Frequency is how often you exercise. Most guidelines suggest doing at least some exercise most days of the week. Three to five times a week is a good choice for moderate-intensity aerobic exercise. Taking every other day off gives your body a chance to rest and recover.

- Time is the length of each exercise period. According to the guidelines, it is best if you can exercise at least 10 minutes at a time. You can add up 10-minute exercise periods all week to work toward 150 minutes. For example, three 10-minute walks a day for five days gets you to 150 minutes for the week (see "Examples of 150 Minutes a Week of Moderate Aerobic Activity" on page 200). If 10 minutes is too much at first, start with what you can do and work toward 10 minutes.

- Intensity is your exercise effort—how hard you are working. Aerobic exercise is safe and effective at a moderate intensity. When you exercise at moderate intensity, you feel warmer, you breathe more deeply and faster than usual, and your heart beats faster than normal. At the same time, if you are exercising at an appropriate intensity, you should feel that you can continue for a while. Exercise intensity is relative to your fitness. For an athlete, running a mile in 10 minutes is probably low-intensity exercise. For a person who hasn't exercised in a long time, a brisk 10-minute walk may be moderate to high intensity. For someone with severe physical limitations, a slow walk may be high intensity. The trick, of course, is to figure out what is moderate intensity for you. There are several ways to do this, which we list in the following section.

Remember, these are just rough guidelines on frequency, duration, and intensity—not a rigid prescription. Listen to your own body. Sometimes you need to tell yourself (and maybe others) that enough is enough. More exercise is not necessarily better, especially if it gives you a lot of pain or discomfort.

Intensity Guidelines

You can determine the intensity of your exercise using one of three intensity-monitoring techniques: the talk test, the perceived exertion scale, and monitoring your heart rate.

Talk Test

When exercising, talk to another person or yourself, or recite poems or music lyrics out loud. Moderate-intensity exercise allows you to speak comfortably. If you can't carry on a conversation because you are breathing too hard or are short of breath, you're working at a high intensity. Slow down to a more moderate level. The talk test is an easy and quick way to recognize your effort and regulate intensity. If you have lung disease, the talk test might not work for you. If that is the case for you, try using the perceived-exertion scale.

Perceived Exertion Scale

Another way to monitor intensity is to rate how hard you're working on a scale of perceived exertion. On the 0 to 10 scale, 0, at the low end of the scale, is lying down, doing no work at all, and 10 is equivalent to working as hard as possible—very hard work that you couldn't do for more than a few seconds. A good level for moderate aerobic exercise on the 0 to 10 scale is between 4 and 5.

Heart Rate

Unless you're taking heart-regulating medicine (such as a beta-blocker like propranolol), checking your heart rate is another way to measure

Table 13.1 Moderate-Intensity Exercise Heart Rate, by Age

Age	Exercise Pulse (beats per minute)	Exercise Pulse (15-second count)
30s	105–133	26–33
40s	99–126	25–32
50s	94–119	24–30
60s	88–112	23–28
70s	83–105	21–26
80s	77–98	19–25
90 and above	72–91	18–23

exercise intensity. The faster your heart beats, the harder you're working. (Your heart also beats fast when you are frightened or nervous, but in this case we're talking about how your heart responds to physical activity.) Endurance exercise at moderate intensity raises your heart rate to a range between 55 and 70 percent of your safe maximum heart rate. The safe maximum heart rate declines with age, so your safe exercise heart rate gets lower as you get older. You can follow the general guidelines of Table 13.1 or calculate your own exercise heart rate using the formula in the following material. Either way, you need to know how to take your pulse.

Take your pulse by placing the tips of your index and middle fingers at your wrist below the base of your thumb. Move your fingers around, but don't push down, until you feel the pulsations of blood pumping with each heartbeat. Count how many beats you feel in 15 seconds. Multiply this number by 4 to get your pulse rate. Start by taking your pulse whenever you think of it, and you'll soon learn your average resting heart rate. Most people have a resting heart rate between 60 and 100 beats per minute.

Now that you have your resting heart rate, use the following formula to calculate your exercise heart rate range:

1. Subtract your age from 220:

   Example: $220 - 60 = 160$
   You: $220 - \underline{\hspace{1cm}} = \underline{\hspace{1cm}}$

2. To find the low end of your exercise heart rate range, multiply your answer in step 1 by 0.55:

   Example: $160 \times 0.55 = 88$
   You: $\underline{\hspace{1cm}} \times 0.55 = \underline{\hspace{1cm}}$

3. To find the upper end of your moderate intensity range, multiply your answer in step 1 by 0.7:

   Example: $160 \times 0.7 = 112$
   You: $\underline{\hspace{1cm}} \times 0.7 = \underline{\hspace{1cm}}$

The exercise heart rate range for moderate intensity in our example is from 88 to 112 beats per minute. What is yours?

When checking your heart rate during exercise, you only need to count your pulse for

15 seconds, not a whole minute. To find your 15-second pulse for exercise, divide both the lower-end and upper-end numbers by 4. The person in our example should be able to count between 22 (88 ÷ 4) and 28 (112 ÷ 4) beats in 15 seconds while exercising.

The most important reason for knowing your exercise heart rate range is so that you can learn not to exercise too vigorously. After you've done your warm-up and five minutes of endurance exercise, take your pulse. If it's higher than the upper rate, don't panic. Just slow down a bit. You don't need to work so hard.

If you are taking medicine that regulates your heart rate, have trouble feeling your pulse, or think that keeping track of your heart rate is a bother, use the talk test or a perceived-exertion scale to monitor your exercise intensity.

There are many technology-based solutions for monitoring as well, such as wearable monitors and watches, phone apps, etc., that you may want to explore.

Be FIT

You can design your own endurance program by using the FIT approach. FIT stands for how often you exercise (F = Frequency), how hard you work (I = Intensity), and how long you exercise each day (T = Time). The guidelines recommend that you exercise at moderate intensity for a minimum of 150 minutes a week. You can build your exercise program by varying frequency, time, and activities. We recommend moderate-intensity exercise, so you start slowly and increase frequency and time as you work toward or even beyond 150 minutes each week. You can use different kinds or combinations of exercises. Review the programs of moderate intensity that reach 150 minutes each week on page 200 of this chapter ("Examples of 150 Minutes a Week of Moderate Aerobic Activity") and start thinking of ways you can meet your goals. For example, if you are just starting, you could begin with the following:

- Take a five-minute walk around the house three times a day, six days a week (total = 90 minutes).

- Take a water aerobics class for 40 minutes twice a week and two 10-minute walks on two other days during the week (total = 120 minutes).

- Take a low-impact aerobic class once a week (50 minutes), mow the lawn for 30 minutes, and take two 20-minute walks (total = 120 minutes).

One way to remember the guideline goal for minimum physical activity is to keep in mind that you should accumulate 30 minutes of moderate physical activity on most days of the week. This could be a combination of walking, stationary bicycling, dancing, swimming, or chores that require moderate-intensity activity.

Again, it is important to remember that 150 minutes is a goal, not necessarily your starting point. You can start small and still make progress. For example, if you begin exercising just two minutes at a time, you are likely to be able to reach the recommended 10 minutes three times a day. Almost everyone can reach the guideline goals and achieve important health benefits. If you have a setback and stop exercising for a while, restart your program by exercising for less time and less vigorously than when you stopped. It takes some time to work back up again; be patient with yourself.

Be F.I.T.

Here's a quick way to remember the three building blocks of your exercise program:

F = Frequency (how often)

I = Intensity (how hard)

T = Time (how long)

Warm Up and Cool Down

When you exercise at moderate intensity, it is important to warm up first and cool down afterward.

Warm Up

Don't exercise when your body is cold. Before building to moderate intensity, you must prepare your body to do more strenuous work. This means doing at least five minutes of a low-intensity activity to allow your muscles, heart, lungs, and circulation to gradually increase their work. If you are going for a brisk walk, warm up with five minutes of slow walking. If you are riding a stationary bike, warm up on the bike with five minutes of easy pedaling. In an aerobic exercise class, you warm up with a gentle routine before getting more vigorous. Warming up reduces the risk of injuries, soreness, and irregular heartbeat.

Cool Down

A cool-down period after moderate-intensity exercise helps your body return to its normal resting state. Repeating the five-minute warm-up activity or taking a slow walk helps your muscles gradually relax and your heart and breathing slow down. Gentle flexibility exercises during the cool-down can be relaxing, and gentle stretching after exercise helps reduce muscle soreness and stiffness.

Self Tests for Endurance

For some people, just the feelings of increased endurance and well-being are enough to indicate progress. Others may need proof that their exercise program is making a measurable difference. You can use one or both of these endurance or aerobic fitness tests. Not everyone will be able to do both tests, so pick one that works best for you. Record your results. After four weeks of exercise, repeat the test and check your improvement. Measure yourself again after four more weeks.

Distance Self-Test

■ Find a place to walk or bicycle where you can measure distance. A running track works well. On a street, measure distance with a car odometer. A stationary bicycle with an odometer provides the equivalent measurement. If you plan on swimming, you can count pool lengths.

- After a warm-up, note your starting point and either bicycle, swim, or walk as briskly as you comfortably can for five minutes. Try to move at a steady pace for the full time. At the end of five minutes, note the spot where you ended and immediately take your pulse and rate your perceived exertion from 0 to 10. Continue at a slow pace for three to five more minutes to cool down. Record the distance you covered in five minutes, your heart rate, and your perceived exertion.

- Repeat the test after several weeks of exercise. There may be a change in as little as four weeks. However, it often takes eight to twelve weeks to see improvement.

Goal: To cover more distance, lower your heart rate, or lower your perceived exertion.

Time Self-Test

- Measure a given distance to walk, bike, or swim. Estimate how far you think you can go in one to five minutes. You can pick a number of city blocks, actual distance, or lengths in a pool.

- Spend three to five minutes warming up. Start timing and start on your measured course moving steadily, briskly, and comfortably. At the finish, record how long it took you to cover your course, your heart rate, and your perceived exertion.

- Repeat after several weeks of exercise. You may see changes in as little as four weeks. However, it often takes eight to twelve weeks for a noticeable improvement.

Goal: To complete the course in less time, at a lower heart rate, or at lower perceived exertion.

What Are Your Exercise Barriers?

Fitness makes sense. Yet, when faced with the prospect of actually becoming more physically active, people can come up with many excuses, concerns, and worries. These barriers can prevent you from even taking the first step. The following are some common barriers and possible solutions.

I don't have enough time.

Everyone has the same amount of time; we just choose to use it differently. It's a matter of priorities. Some find a lot of time for television, but none to spare for fitness. It doesn't take a lot of time to become more active. Even five minutes a day is a good start, and much better than no physical activity. You may be able to combine activities, such as watching television while pedaling a stationary bicycle, or arranging "walking meetings" to discuss business or family matters.

I'm too tired.

When you're out of shape, you feel listless and tend to tire easily. Then you don't exercise because you're tired, and this becomes a vicious cycle.

You have to break out of the too-tired cycle. Regular physical activity increases your stamina and gives you more energy to do the things you like. As you get back into shape, you will recognize the difference between feeling listless or out of shape and feeling physically tired.

I'm too sick.

It may be true that you are too sick for a vigorous or strenuous exercise program, but you can still usually find some ways to be more active. Remember, it makes sense to exercise even just one minute at a time, especially if you can build up to several times a day. The enhanced physical fitness you will gain can help you better cope with your illness and prevent further problems.

I get enough exercise already.

This may be true, but for most people, their jobs and daily activities do not provide enough sustained exercise to keep them fully fit and energetic. Do you get at least 150 minutes of endurance exercise each week?

Exercise is boring.

You can make it more interesting and fun. Exercise with other people. Entertain yourself with headphones and music or listen to the radio. Vary your activities and your walking routes.

Exercise is painful.

The old saying "no pain, no gain" is simply wrong and out of date. Recent evidence shows that significant health benefits come from gentle, low-intensity, enjoyable physical activity. You may sweat or feel a bit short of breath, but if you feel more pain than before you started, something is probably wrong. More than likely

you are either exercising improperly or you're overdoing it. Talk with your physician or a fitness expert or join a supervised exercise program. You may simply need to be less vigorous or change the type of exercise that you're doing.

I'm too embarrassed.

For some, the thought of donning a skin-tight exercise outfit and walking around in public is delightful, but for others it is downright distressing. Fortunately, the options for physical activity range from exercise in the privacy of your own home to group social activities. You should be able to find something that suits you. And, no, you don't have to wear any exotic clothing to do it!

It's too cold, it's too hot, it's too dark . . .

If you are flexible and vary your type of exercise, you can generally work around the changes in weather that make certain types of exercise more difficult. Consider indoor activities such as stationary bicycling, exercising with a workout webcast or DVD at home, or working out at a gym.

I'm afraid I won't be able to do it right or be successful. I'm afraid I'll fail.

Many people don't want to start a new project because they are afraid they will fail or not be able to finish it successfully. If you feel this way about starting an exercise program, remember two things. First, whatever activities you are able to do—no matter how short or "easy"—will be much better for you than doing nothing. Be proud of what you have done, not guilty about what you haven't done. Second, new projects often seem overwhelming—until you get started and learn to enjoy each day's adventures and successes. (See "Implementing a Successful Fitness Program," page 228.)

Perhaps you have come up with some other barriers while reading this chapter. The human mind is incredibly creative. Turn that creativity to your advantage by using it to come up with even better ways to refute your excuses, and to develop positive attitudes about exercise and fitness. If you get stuck, ask others for suggestions, or try some of the self-talk suggestions in Chapter 12, "Using Your Mind to Manage Symptoms."

Finding Fitness Opportunities in Your Community

Most people who exercise regularly do so with at least one other person. Two or more people can keep each other motivated, and a whole class can build a feeling of camaraderie or even healthy competition. On the other hand, exercising alone gives you the most freedom. You may feel that there are no classes that would work for you, or no buddy with whom you can exercise. If so, start your own program; as you progress, you may find that these feelings change and you may eventually want to include others in your exercise plans.

Many communities now offer a variety of exercise classes, including special programs for people with health problems, adaptive exercises, tai chi, yoga, Pilates, Zumba, fitness trails, and others. Check with your local YMCA or YWCA, community center, department of parks and recreation, adult education program, or community college. There is a great deal of variation in the content of these programs, and in the professional experience of the exercise staff. By and large, the classes are inexpensive, and program planners are responsive to people's needs.

Health and fitness clubs usually offer aerobic studios, weight training, cardiovascular equipment, and sometimes a heated pool. For all these services they charge membership fees, which can be high. But some clubs have discounts for people with HIV. Ask about low-impact and beginners' exercise classes, both in the aerobic studio and in the pool.* Note that gyms that emphasize weight lifting exclusively generally don't have the programs or personnel to help you with a flexible, overall fitness program.

When you are choosing an exercise class or health and fitness club, look for the following qualities:

- Classes designed for *moderate- and low-intensity* exercise. You should be able to observe classes and participate in at least one class before signing up and paying.

---

*You may be wondering whether it's safe for others if you use a public pool or exercise/fitness equipment. Are you putting other people at risk for catching HIV from you? We want to be very clear here, because we don't want you avoiding exercise out of concern for others: *It is not dangerous for you to use public pools or exercise equipment or to play group sports.* No one has ever caught HIV from any kind of group sport or exercise. So just use common sense. If you're bleeding, stop your exercise and clean up after yourself. All people should do the same, whether they have HIV or not.

- Instructors with *qualifications and experience.* Knowledgeable instructors are more likely to understand special needs and be willing and able to work with you. Being knowledgeable means knowing not only about exercise but also something about working with people with HIV.

- Membership policies that allow you to pay for only a session of classes, or let you "freeze" membership at times when you can't participate. Some fitness facilities offer *different rates* depending on how many services you use.

- Facilities that are *easy to get to, park near, and enter.* Dressing/locker rooms and exercise sites should be accessible and safe, with professional staff on site.

- A pool with *"adults only"* times when children are not allowed in the lanes. Small children playing and making noise in the pool may not be good for your needs.

- Staff and other members that you feel *comfortable* being around.

Media can also be your friend when it comes to finding ways to exercise. There are many excellent webcasts (on YouTube, for instance) and DVDs for home use. They vary in intensity from very gentle chair exercises to more strenuous aerobic exercise. Ask your doctor or physical therapist for suggestions, or review the webcast or DVDs yourself. You can find some suggestions in the "Additional Resources" section at the end of this chapter.

Maintaining Your Commitment to Exercise

If you haven't exercised recently, you'll undoubtedly experience some new feelings and discomfort in the early days of your fitness program. Most of these new feelings are normal and expected, but a few may mean you should change what you're doing. See "Advice for Exercise Problems" on page 229 if you're concerned. Remember, it's normal to feel muscle tension and tenderness around joints and to be a little more tired in the evenings. Muscle or joint pain that lasts more than two hours after the exercise, or feeling tired into the next day, means that you probably did too much too fast. *Don't stop;* just exercise less vigorously or for a shorter time the next day.

When you do aerobic exercise, it's natural to feel your heart beat faster, your breathing speed up, and your body get warmer. However, irregular or very rapid heartbeats, excessive shortness of breath, or dizziness are not what you want. If this happens to you, stop exercising and discontinue your program until you check with your doctor.

If you have symptoms such as fatigue, shortness of breath, or physical discomfort, it can be difficult at first to figure out whether these are caused by the illness, medication, exercise, or some combination of these. Talking to other people with HIV about their experiences with starting an exercise program may help. Once you are able to sort out some of these sensations, you'll be able to exercise with confidence.

Expect setbacks. During the first year of an exercise program, people average two to three

Implementing a Successful Fitness Program

- Keep your exercise goal in mind.

- Choose exercises you want to do. Combine activities that move you toward your goal and are recommended by your health care providers.

- Choose the time and place to exercise. Tell your partner, family, and friends your plan.

- Make an action plan for yourself. Decide how long you'll stick with these particular exercises. Six to eight weeks is a reasonable time commitment for a new program.

- Keep an exercise diary or calendar, leaving space to write down your exercises, how long you do them, your heart rate or perceived exertion score, and your feelings before and after exercise. Put your diary where you can see it, and fill it out after every exercise activity.

- Do some self-tests to keep track of your progress. Distance and time self-tests appear on pages 223–224. Record the date and results. You may also use your exercise diary for this purpose.

- Start your program. Remember to begin gradually and proceed slowly, especially if you haven't exercised in a while.

- Repeat self-tests at regular intervals, record the results, and check the changes.

- Revise your program. At the end of six to eight weeks, decide what you liked, what worked, and what made exercising difficult. Modify your program and make another action plan for the next few weeks. You may decide to change some of the exercises, the place or time that you exercise, or your exercise partners.

- Reward yourself for a job well done. Many people who start an exercise program find that the rewards come with improved fitness and endurance. Being able to enjoy outings, a refreshing walk, or trips to a store, the library, a concert, or a museum are great rewards to look forward to.

interruptions in their exercise schedule, often because of minor injuries or illnesses unrelated to their exercise. You may find yourself sidelined or derailed temporarily. Don't be discouraged. Try a different activity or simply rest. When you are feeling better, resume your program, but begin at a lower, more gentle level. *As a rule of thumb, it will take you the same amount of time to get back into shape as you were out.* For instance, if you missed three weeks, it may take

at least three weeks to get back to your previous level. Go slowly. Be kind to yourself. You're in this for the long haul.

Think of your head as the coach and your body as the team. For success, all parts of your team need attention. Be a good coach. *Encourage and praise yourself.* Design "plays" you feel your team can execute successfully. Choose places that are safe and hospitable. A good coach knows his or her team, sets good goals, and

Advice for Exercise Problems

Problem	Advice*
Irregular or very rapid heartbeat	Stop exercising. Check your pulse. Are the beats regular or irregular? How fast is your heartbeat? Make a note of this information, and discuss it with your doctor before exercising again
Pain, tightness, or pressure in your chest, jaw, arms, neck, or back	Stop exercising and sit or lie down. If the pain, tightness, or pressure lasts more than 15 minutes, call 911 or go to an emergency department AT ONCE! Don't wait. Check with your doctor about these symptoms before exercising again
Unusual, extreme shortness of breath, persisting 10 minutes after you exercise	Notify your doctor and get clearance before exercising again.
Light-headedness, dizziness, fainting, cold sweat, or confusion	Lie down with your feet up, or sit down and put your head between your legs. If it happens more than once, check with your doctor before exercising again.
Excessive tiredness after exercise, especially if you're still tired 24 hours after you exercise	Don't exercise so vigorously next time. If the excessive tiredness persists, check with your doctor.

*Your physician knows you and your medical condition, so they may give you different or more specific advice than is listed here. Follow that advice.

helps the team succeed. A good coach is loyal. A good coach does not belittle, nag, or make anyone feel guilty. Be a good coach.

Besides a good coach, everyone needs an enthusiastic cheerleader or two. Of course, you can be your own cheerleader, but being both coach and cheerleader is a lot to do. A successful exerciser usually has at least one family member or close friend who actively supports his or her exercise program. Your cheerleader can exercise with you, help you get chores done so you have time to exercise, praise your accomplishments, or just take your exercise time into consideration when making plans. Sometimes cheerleaders pop up by themselves, but don't be bashful about asking for a hand.

With exercise experience, you develop a sense of control in your life. You learn how to alternate your activities to fit your day-to-day needs. You know when to do less and when to do more. You know that a change in symptoms or a period of inactivity are usually only temporary and don't have to be devastating. You know you have the tools to get back on track again.

Give your exercise plan a chance to succeed. Set reasonable goals and enjoy your success. Stay motivated. When it comes to your personal fitness program, sticking with it and doing it your way make you a definite winner.

Exercise Resources

- Adult education classes
- Hospitals, health care clinics, and HIV case management organizations
- Community colleges

- Parks and recreation programs
- Health and fitness clubs
- YMCA, YWCA

Additional Resources

Physical Activity Guidelines

    Australia: www.health.gov.au/internet/main/publishing.nsf/content /health-pubhlth-strateg-phys-act-guidelines

    Canada: www.phac-aspc.gc.ca/hp-ps/hl-mvs/pa-ap

    United States: http://health.gov/paguidelines

AIDS Info: www.aidsinfo.nih.gov

American Heart Association Recommendations for Physical Activity in Adults: www.heart.org/HEARTORG/GettingHealthy/PhysicalActivity/FitnessBasics/American-Heart-Association-Recommendations-for-Physical-Activity-in-Adults_UCM_307976_Article.jsp

BeFIT: www.youtube.com/user/BeFit

Centers for Disease Control and Prevention, Physical Activity: www.cdc.gov/physicalactivity

Dance Workout for Beginners: www.youtube.com/watch?v=LRqMnMdMv3s

Everybody Walk—The Movement to Get America Walking: http://everybodywalk.org

Fitness Blender: www.youtube.com/user/FitnessBlender

Low Impact Cardio Workout for Beginners (women): www.youtube.com/watch?v=bSZj19AUU5I

Low Impact Workout for Beginners (men): www.youtube.com/watch?v=QiuJ3ZFAiBg

Medline Plus, Exercise and Physical Fitness: www.nlm.nih.gov/medlineplus/exerciseandphysicalfitness.html

My Fabulous Disease (gym workout specific to HIV): www.youtube.com/watch?v=oBvqXrnqha8

National Center on Health, Physical Activity and Disability: www.nchpad.org

National Institute on Aging, *Exercise and Physical Activity: Your Everyday Guide from the National Institute on Aging:* www.nia.nih.gov/health/publication/exercise-physical-activity/introduction

STEADI (Stopping Elderly Accidents, Deaths, and Injuries) Older Adult Fall Prevention: www.cdc.gov/steadi/patient.html

Suggested Further Reading

To learn more about the topics discussed in this chapter, we suggest that you explore the following resources:

Cooper, Kenneth H. *Overcoming Hypertension.* New York: Bantam Books, 2012.

Dahm, Diane, and Jay Smith, eds. *Mayo Clinic Fitness for Everybody.* Rochester, Minn.: Mayo Clinic Health Information, 2005.

Fortmann, Stephen P., and Prudence E. Breitrose. *The Blood Pressure Book: How to Get It Down and Keep It Down,* 3rd ed. Boulder, Colo.: Bull Publishing, 2006.

Huey, Lynda, and Robert Forster. *The Complete Waterpower Workout Book: Programs for Fitness, Injury Prevention, and Healing.* New York: Random House, 1993.

Karpay, Ellen. *The Everything Total Fitness Book.* Avon, Mass.: Adams Media, 2000.

Knopf, Karl. *Make the Pool Your Gym: No-Impact Water Workouts for Getting Fit, Building Strength, and Rehabbing from Injury.* Berkeley, Calif.: Ulysses Press, 2012.

Moffat, Marilyn, and Steve Vickery. *Book of Body Maintenance and Repair.* New York: Henry Holt, 1999.

Nelson, Miriam E, Alice H. Lichtenstein, and Lawrence Lindner. *Strong Women, Strong Hearts: Proven Strategies to Prevent and Reverse Heart Disease Now.* New York: Putnam, 2005.

Nelson, Miriam E., and Sarah Wernick. *Strong Women Stay Young,* rev. ed. New York: Bantam Books, 2005.

O'Brien, K., et al. "Aerobic Exercise Interventions for Adults Living with HIV/AIDS." *Cochrane Database of Systematic Reviews,* no. 8 (August 2010): CD001796, www.ncbi.nlm.nih.gov/pubmed/20687068

Stewart, Gordon W. *Active Living: The Miracle Medicine for a Long and Healthy Life.* Champaign, Ill.: Human Kinetics, 1995.

Van Fulpen, Charles D. *Guide to Contented Hearts: Cardiac Risk Management.* Kalamazoo, Mich.: Contented Hearts, Inc., 1995.

Vedral, Joyce L. *Bone Building Body Shaping Workout: Strength, Health, Beauty in Just 16 Minutes a Day.* New York: Fireside, 1998.

White, Martha. *Water Exercise: 78 Safe and Effective Exercises for Fitness and Therapy.* Champaign, Ill.: Human Kinetics, 1995.

Special thanks to Bonnie Bruce, DrPH, RD, and Yvonne Mullan, MSc, RD, for their help with this chapter.

CHAPTER **14**

Healthy Eating

HEALTHY EATING IS ONE OF THE BEST **personal investments** you can make in your life. It is a central factor that influences your health, and an important tool for managing your HIV. Eating healthy means that most of the time you make good and healthful food choices. It does not mean being rigid or perfect. No matter what the media or your friends say, there is no one best way of eating that fits everyone; there is no perfect food, nor a perfect diet. Healthy eating can mean finding new or different ways to prepare your meals to make them tasty and appealing. If you have certain health conditions such as HIV, it may mean that you have to be choosier. Eating well does not usually mean you can never again enjoy the foods you like most.

Unfortunately, thanks to the Internet, books, magazines, television, friends, and relatives, you can get overloaded with information about what you should and should not eat. The whole eating thing gets very confusing. In this chapter we give you basic science-based nutrition and dietary information. We do not tell you what to eat or how to eat. That is your decision. We do tell you what is known about nutrition for adults and some ways to help you apply that information to your specific likes and needs.

We hope this chapter will help you start making changes and begin eating healthier. In the next chapter, we give more specific information for individuals with the most common long-term health conditions.

Why Is Healthy Eating So Important?

The human body is a very complex and marvelous machine, somewhat like an automobile. Autos need the proper mix of fuel to run right. Without it, they may run rough and may even stop working. The human body is similar. It needs the proper mix of good food (fuel) to keep it running well. It does not run right on the wrong fuel or on empty.

Healthy eating cuts across every part of your life. It is linked to your body and your mind's well-being, including how your body responds to some illnesses.

When you give your body the right fuel and nourishment, here's what happens:

- You have more energy and feel less tired.

- You increase your chances of potentially preventing, slowing, or lessening further problems such as unpleasant side effects of medication, weight loss, high blood sugar, and high cholesterol that can result from health conditions such as HIV, heart disease, diabetes, and cancer.

- You feed your brain, which can help you handle life's challenges as well as emotional ups and downs, improving your quality of life.

What Is Healthy Eating?

At the heart of healthy eating are the choices you make over the long run. Healthy eating includes being flexible and allowing yourself to occasionally enjoy small amounts of foods that may not be so healthy. Being too strict or rigid and not allowing yourself ever to have a treat will likely cause your best efforts to fail.

For some people, healthy eating means having to be somewhat choosy about foods. For example, people with HIV may need to eat larger portions or increase the number of meals and snacks in a day to fuel the body's immune system so it can fight infection. In contrast, people with diabetes need to watch their carbohydrate intake to manage their blood sugar levels. They do best each day by deciding which carbohydrate foods, such as fruit, breads, beans, cereals, and rice, they will eat. Others, who have heart disease or are at risk for heart disease, find that watching the amount and kinds of fat they eat helps control blood cholesterol levels. Those with high blood pressure find that they may be able to lower their blood pressure by eating lots of fruits, vegetables, and low-fat dairy foods.

Some people with high blood pressure have to cut back on salt. People trying to lose or gain weight need to pay attention to how many calories they consume.

We have come a long way since meat and potatoes were thought of as the backbone of a great diet. Today we know that vegetables, fruits, whole grains, low-fat milk and low-fat milk products, lean meats, poultry, and fish are at the core of a healthy diet. There is still a place for meat and potatoes; it is just not the central place at every meal.

The real issue for most people is not the healthy foods we choose but the less healthy ones. One-third of the diet of most North Americans is made up of foods that are high in added sugars, solid fats (butter, stick margarine, shortening, and beef, pork, and chicken fats), and sodium (salt). North Americans also eat a lot of food that is made from white flour and other refined grains. Added sugars, fats, and sodium contribute to high blood pressure, diabetes, and obesity.

Trade-offs are a big part of healthy eating. This means learning how food affects you and then deciding when you can treat yourself and when you should pass. For instance, it may be important for you to have a very special meal on your birthday. If so, then you can make healthier choices when you are out for a casual weekday lunch. Trading off is a skill that can help you stay on the path of healthy eating. As you get better at this, you will find making trade-offs gets easier and even becomes part of your everyday decision making.

A good starting place for eating more healthily is to eat more plant foods: whole grains, fruits, vegetables, cooked dry beans and peas, lentils, nuts, and seeds. This does not mean giving up meats and other foods high in sugar, fat, or sodium but rather eating them in smaller amounts or less often. Many current dietary guidelines recommend eating moderate amounts of lean meats, poultry, and eggs. The key is to maintain the proper balance in the kinds of foods you eat and how much you eat. (We'll have more to say about this a little later in this chapter.)

This all sounds simple, but every day we are faced with hundreds of food choices. It is often easier and quicker to grab something less healthful than to think about what healthy food you will eat, much less prepare. So how do we put together meals that are tasty and enjoyable yet healthful? In this chapter we try to make it as simple as possible.

Key Principles of Healthy Eating

■ **Choose foods as nature originally made them.** This means the less processed your food the better. *Processed* describes foods that have been changed from their original state by having ingredients added (often sugar, salt, or fat) or removed (often fiber or nutrients) to make them tastier—for example, whole grains made into white flour for bakery products, or animal foods made into luncheon or deli meats. Food choices that are less processed include a grilled chicken breast instead of fried breaded chicken nuggets, a baked potato (with skin) rather than French fries, and whole-grain bread and pasta and brown rice instead of refined grains such as white bread and white rice.

- **Get your nutrients from food, not supplements.** For most people, vitamin, mineral, and other dietary supplements cannot completely take the place of food. Unprocessed foods contain nutrients and other healthy compounds (such as fiber) in the right combinations and amounts to help the body do its work properly. When manufacturers remove nutrients from food, the foods may not fuel the body the way they should. They may even have harmful side effects.

  For instance, consider beta carotene, an important source of vitamin A, found in plant foods such as carrots and winter squash. When consumed as part of these foods, it helps vision and enhances immune system functioning. However, artificial beta carotene supplements have been shown to increase some cancer risks in some people. This same risk does not happen when beta carotene is eaten as it is naturally found in food.

  Another reason to get your nutrition from foods as close as possible to how nature made them is that these choices may contain as yet unknown healthy compounds. When you take a supplement such as a vitamin pill, you could be missing out on many other helpful substances that are naturally packaged with the food from which the vitamin was removed.

  In many countries, including the United States, diet and nutrition supplements do not have to follow government rules for quality or effectiveness. Unlike over-the-counter medications, with supplements there is no guarantee that you are getting what you pay for or that you are not getting harmful substances.

  Can dietary supplements ever play a role in healthy eating? Yes, sometimes people cannot get enough of one or more of the nutrients they need. For example, people with HIV and older people need larger amounts of calcium or vitamin D to help prevent or slow osteoporosis. Although people can get enough calcium from milk and milk products such as yogurt or cheese, getting the amount needed can be a challenge at times, so calcium supplements can be a good idea. If you are thinking of taking a supplement, talk to your health care professional or a registered dietitian first.

- **Eat a wide variety of colorful and minimally processed foods.** The more variety in your foods, the better; the more colors on your plate, the better; and the less processed your food, the better. By following these three simple rules, your body will probably get all the good things it needs. This means your plate should contain minimally processed meat, fish, or poultry and a lot of colorful fruits and vegetables—think blue and purple for blueberries and grapes; yellow and orange for pineapple, oranges, and carrots; red for tomatoes, strawberries, and watermelon; and green for spinach and green beans—along with the white and warm brown tones from mushrooms, onions, cauliflower, and whole grains such as brown rice.

■ **Eat foods high in phytochemicals.** Phytochemicals are compounds that are found only in plant foods—fruits, vegetables, whole grains, nuts, and seeds (*phyto* means "plant"). There are hundreds of health-promoting and disease-fighting phytochemicals. These include compounds that give fruits and vegetables their bright colors. Whenever a food is refined or processed, as when whole wheat is made into white flour, phytochemicals are lost. The more often you choose foods that are not refined and as close as possible to how nature made them, the better.

■ **Eat regularly.** A gas-fueled vehicle will not run without the gas, and a fire eventually burns out without more wood. Your body is much the same. It needs refueling regularly to work at its best. Eating something, even a little bit, at regular intervals helps keep your "fire" burning.

Eating at regular times during the day, preferably at evenly spaced intervals, helps maintain and balance your blood sugar level. Blood sugar is a key player in supplying the body, especially the brain, with energy. Usually, the brain can only use blood sugar for energy. If you do not eat regularly your blood sugar drops, and depending on how low it gets, low blood sugar (hypoglycemia) can cause weakness, sweating, shaking, mood changes (irritability, anxiety, or anger, for example), nausea, headaches, or poor coordination. Low blood sugar can be dangerous for many people.

Eating regularly helps you get the nutrients you need, and helps your body use those nutrients. Of course, not skipping meals or not letting too many hours go between meals also helps keep you from getting overly hungry. Being overly hungry often leads to overeating. This can in turn lead to such problems as indigestion, heartburn, and weight gain.

Finally, eating regularly does not mean that you must stick to the same routine every day. Nor does it mean that you must follow the "normal" pattern of eating three meals a day. Allow yourself room for give and take. If you have certain health conditions, such as HIV or cancer, you may find that sometimes several small meals throughout the day works well while at other times, fewer, bigger meals work best. For people with diabetes, spacing meals regularly and balancing what you eat is important, but this could mean several small meals a day, three meals mixed with a snack, or just three meals, based on what is best for you.

■ **Eat what your body needs (not more or less).** This is easy to say but more difficult to put into action. How much you should eat depends on things like the following:

♦ Your age (we need fewer calories as we get older)

♦ Your body size and shape (in general, if you are taller or have more muscle, you can eat more)

♦ Your health needs (some conditions like HIV affect how your body uses calories)

♦ Your activity level (the more you move or exercise, the more calories you can eat)

A Note About Breakfast

Breakfast is just that: "breaking the fast." It refuels your body after going without eating for many hours and may help you resist the urge to eat extra snacks or overeat during the rest of the day.

We know that you may not want to eat breakfast, not only because you don't have the time or aren't hungry but maybe because you do not like the usual breakfast foods. The good news is that there are no set rules about what or when you should eat in the morning. Breakfast can be small and include anything—fruit, beans, rice, bread, broccoli, even leftovers. The important thing is to kick-start your body each day by refueling it.

Tips to Help You Manage How Much You Eat

- **Stop eating when you first begin to feel full.** This helps you control the amount you eat and helps prevent overeating. Pay attention to your body so you can learn what being full feels like. Like all new skills, it takes some practice. If it is hard to stop eating when you begin to feel full, remove your plate or get up from the table if you can.

- **Eat slowly.** Eating slowly gives you more enjoyment and helps prevent overeating. Make your meals last at least 15 to 20 minutes. It takes this much time for the brain to catch up and tell your stomach that it is getting full. If you finish quickly, wait at least 15 minutes before getting another portion or eating dessert. If you find this difficult to do, follow the tips in Chapter 15, "Eating for Specific Long-Term Conditions," pages 267–268.

- **Pay attention to what you eat.** If you are not aware of what you are doing, it is easy to eat an entire bag of chips or cookies or eat too much of any bite-sized pieces of food without knowing it. This can happen easily when you are with friends, using the computer, or watching television. In these situations, try portioning out what you want to eat or keeping food out of reach or out of sight.

- **Know a serving size when you see one.** To do this, you need to know a little about what a serving size or portion looks like. A half-cup (125 mL) portion is about the size of a tennis ball or a closed fist. A three-ounce (84 g) portion of cooked meat, fish, or poultry is about the size of a deck of playing cards or the palm of your hand. The end of your thumb to the first joint is about one teaspoon (5 mL); three times that is a tablespoon (15 mL). (Tip: Using a measuring cup and measuring spoons is a great way to see what a serving size looks like.)

- **Watch out for supersizing and portion inflation.** In recent years, serving sizes at restaurants and in packaged foods have literally "beefed up." The typical adult cheeseburger used to have about 330 calories; now it has a whopping 590 calories. Twenty years ago, an average cookie was about 1½ inches (3.8 cm) wide and had 55 calories; now it is 3½ inches (8.9 cm) wide and has 275 calories—*five times* the calories! Soda typically came in 6½-ounce (195 mL) bottles with 85 calories; today it's 20 ounces (600 mL) to a bottle, with 250 calories. When eating away from home, select appetizers or first courses over main entrées, or order a child's meal. This will help you eat fewer calories. Over a year, it takes only an extra 100 calories a day to put on 10 pounds (4 kg). This is like eating only an extra third of a bagel a day. There are many published ranges of recommended serving sizes for different foods. Table 14.2, "Food Guide for Healthy Meal Planning," on pages 252–259, lists some common serving sizes for a variety of foods, along with information on selected nutrients.

- **Select single-size portions when practical.** Foods that come prepackaged as single servings can help you see what a suggested serving should look like. If the recommended serving size seems too small compared to what you would usually eat, start slowly by cutting how much you now eat by just a small amount at a time. For example, if you usually eat one cup of rice, try eating a half cup instead. Especially when first starting to make changes, measure out your portions—and do this frequently over time. It is amazing just how easily a half cup of rice can "grow" to a one-cup serving.

- **Choose a smaller plate.** Sometimes a smaller plate will make the portions seem larger.

- **Make your food attractive.** We really do eat with our eyes! Compare the mouth-watering appeal of a plate with white fish, white rice, and white cauliflower with one of golden brown chicken, grilled sweet potato, and bright green spinach. Which of these two meals sounds more appetizing?

A Map for Healthy Eating

A map helps you along your path and gets you to where you are going. The U.S. Department of Agriculture's "Map for Healthy Eating" in Figure 14.1 illustrates what a healthy meal should look like. Put your meal together so that one-fourth of the plate is covered with colorful fruit, one-fourth with vegetables, one-fourth with a protein source (lean meat, fish, or poultry, or better yet, plant foods such as tofu, cooked dry beans, or lentils), and the remaining one-fourth with grains (preferably at least half from whole grains) or other starches such as potatoes, rice, yams, or winter squash. Finish off your plate with calcium-rich foods. These could be milk or foods made from milk (preferably fat-free or low-fat), such as cheese, yogurt, frozen yogurt, puddings, or calcium-fortified soy foods such as soy milk. Of course, your food choices and amounts depend on what you like and need. If you would like more information about this way of eating, check out the USDA's ChooseMyPlate website at www.choosemyplate.gov.

For people with diabetes, the American Diabetes Association recommends a similar plate, "Create Your Plate." You can find it in Chapter 15 on page 263 and in the "Food and Fitness" section of their website at www.diabetes.org.

Just using this map as a guideline is not always enough; calories and portion sizes are important too. Plate sizes are now larger, making it is easier to get more calories than you want or need. Table 14.1 on pages 246–247 can help you plan. It gives you examples of recommended daily portions from different food groups. Note that these amounts are general recommendations and may be different if you have special dietary needs. If you have questions, check with your doctor or a registered dietitian.

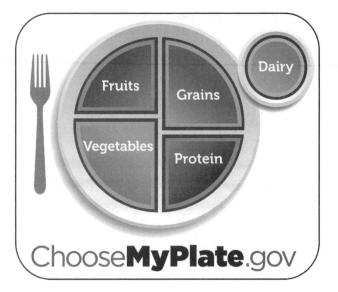

Figure 14.1 **ChooseMyPlate: A Map for Healthy Eating**

Note, too, that when you go to the Internet, you will find many people who say they are nutrition experts, but they may not be. If you want a real expert, look for a registered dietitian (RD). These health professionals are specially trained and are the best sources for diet and nutrition advice and information.

Nutrients: What the Body Needs

Earlier we talked about the need to get nutrients from food. In the following sections, we talk about carbohydrates, fats, protein, a few vitamins and minerals, and water. Although it is technically not a nutrient, we also talk about fiber.

Table 14.1 on pages 246–247 shows the number of recommended servings for adults, along with examples of serving sizes. These recommendations are for people who do less than 30 minutes of moderate exercise a day and eat 1,000 to 3,000 calories. If you have a special health problem or condition, such as HIV and/or diabetes,

you may need to change how much you eat of certain foods. Even so, you can still follow the Map for Healthy Eating. We discuss some special dietary issues for different health conditions in the next chapter.

Carbohydrates: Your Body's Chief Energy Source

With few exceptions, carbohydrates are the go-to fuel for the brain, central nervous system, and red blood cells. Carbohydrates largely determine your blood glucose (sugar) level—more so

Tips for Choosing Healthier Carbohydrates and Increasing Fiber

- Fill at least half of your plate with a variety of vegetables and whole fruits.

- At least half of the grains you eat should be whole grains (brown rice, whole-grain breads and rolls, whole-grain pasta and tortillas).

- Choose foods that list whole wheat or a whole grain (such as oats) as the first ingredient on the food label.

- Choose dried beans and peas, lentils, or whole-grain pasta instead of meat for your main course or as a side dish at least a few times a week.

- Choose whole fruit rather than fruit juice. Whole fruit contains fiber, takes longer to eat, fills you up better than juice, and can help keep you from overeating.

- Choose higher-fiber breakfast cereals such as shredded wheat, Grape-Nuts, or raisin bran.

- Eat higher-fiber crackers, such as whole-rye or multigrain crackers and whole-grain flatbread.

- Snack on whole-grain crackers or breads, whole fruit, or nonfat yogurt rather than sweets, pastries, or chips.

- When you add fiber to your diet, do it gradually over a period of a few weeks. Drink plenty of water to process the fiber and prevent constipation.

than protein or fat. But carbohydrates also do a great deal more. They provide you with basic materials to help make other vital parts for the body. Nearly every part of your body, from your toenails to the top of your head, including hormones, fats, cholesterol, and even some vitamins and proteins, probably used some part of a carbohydrate in its construction.

Carbohydrates are found mostly in plant foods. Milk and yogurt are about the only animal foods with more than minimal amounts of carbohydrate. Foods with carbohydrates can be categorized by whether they are high in sugar or high in starch. Foods that are high in sugar usually break down faster, get into your blood faster, and give you energy faster than high-starch foods. Sugary carbohydrates are found in fruit and juice, milk, yogurt, table sugar, honey, jellies, syrups, and sugar-sweetened drinks. There are other sugars (maltose and dextrose among them) that are both found naturally in foods and are added to processed foods.

Starchy carbohydrates are found in vegetables such as corn, green peas, potatoes, winter squash, dried beans and peas, lentils, and grains such as rice. Pasta, tortillas, and bread are also high in starchy carbohydrates. The amount of carbohydrate in whole grains, brown rice, and whole wheat bread is similar to that in refined grains, such as white bread and white rice. The big difference between them is that processing removes nutrients, phytochemicals, and fiber so the refined grains have less of the things that are good for you.

Many minimally processed plant foods also contain fiber. Although fiber is essentially not

The Nutrition Facts Label: "What's in That Package of Food?"

Food labels inform you about what is in the packaged foods you eat. The Nutrition Facts panel and the ingredients list are two important sources of information. Together they tell you what a food contains, which can help you make better choices. Reading and understanding the information on food labels isn't as daunting as it may seem. The following guidelines focus on the serving size, calories, total fat, trans fat, cholesterol, sodium, and total carbohydrates.

Serving Size

Look at the serving size information first. All the other information on the label is based on the serving size. If you will be having a single serving, then interpreting the Nutrition Facts panel is a straightforward process. But the serving size on the package may not be the amount you usually eat. If you would usually have less or more than the stated serving size, you need to adjust all the amounts listed in the Nutrition Facts. For example, if a serving size is one half a cup of cooked rice and you eat one cup, which is two servings, you need to double all the values. Most serving sizes are stated in cups, ounces, or pieces of the food. Beware: many packages that appear to be a single serving size contain more than one serving.

Calories

Total calories are given for the stated serving size, so if you eat more or less than one serving, you again will have to do a little arithmetic. There is also a listing for the number for calories from fat, although it doesn't tell you the kind of fat. You can calculate the percentage of fat calories in a food. This is important if you are interested in how much fat you are eating. Divide the calories from fat by the calories in the serving size and then multiply by 100. For the label

Nutrition Facts

Serving Size	1 cup (228g)
Servings Per Container	2

Amount Per Serving

Calories 250   Calories from Fat 110

% Daily Value*

Total Fat 12g	18%
Saturated Fat 3g	15%
Trans Fat 3g	
Cholesterol 30mg	10%
Sodium 470mg	20%
Potassium 700mg	20%
Total Carbohydrate 31g	10%
Dietary Fiber 0g	0%
Sugars 5g	
Protein 5g	

Vitamin A	4%
Vitamin C	2%
Calcium	20%
Iron	4%

*Percent Daily Values are based on a 2,000 calorie diet. Your daily values may be higher or lower depending on your calorie needs.

	Calories:	2000	2500
Total fat	Less than	65 g	80 g
Sat fat	Less than	20 g	25 g
Cholesterol	Less than	300 mg	300 mg
Sodium	Less than	2,400 mg	2,400 mg
Total Carbohydrate		300 g	375 g
Dietary Fiber		25 g	30 g

Figure 14.2

in Figure 13.2, divide the 110 fat calories by the 250 in the serving and you get 0.44. Then multiply by 100 to get 44 percent.

Total Fat, Cholesterol, and Sodium

The total fat number includes good fat (polyunsaturated and monounsaturated), bad fat (saturated), and trans fat in grams (a unit of weight). If you are more comfortable thinking in terms of calories, you can change grams to calories by multiplying by 9. For the label in Figure 14.2 multiply the 12 g (total fat) by 9 to get 108 calories. This is the same number of calories shown in the calories from fat line. The amount of calories in all the fats should add up (or at least be close) to the calories for total fat.

Remember our warning about deadly trans fats! Due to the way food companies are allowed to do the arithmetic, any food with up to 1/2 (0.5) g per serving of trans fat can be listed as having no trans fat, but you still may be getting some. If the ingredients list has the words *partially hydrogenated* or *hydrogenated*, the product contains trans fat (even if the amount of trans fats per serving is 0 g).

So when you eat anything that lists *partially hydrogenated* or *hydrogenated* fat on the ingredients label, trans fats could add up, especially if you have more than one serving.

The cholesterol line tells you the amount of cholesterol by serving size. Because cholesterol is found only in animal foods, this line may be missing or show 0 g for foods not made with animal products. If you are watching the amount of cholesterol you eat, you need to be especially careful because even if a food does not have any cholesterol, it may contain bad or trans fat, particularly if it is a processed food. Trans fats cause your body to make cholesterol and can raise your cholesterol level more than cholesterol from food.

To tell if the fat, cholesterol, or sodium is high or low, look at the "% Daily Value" or "% DV" column. Any value of 20 percent or more is high. If you want to eat less fat, cholesterol, or salt, or you plan to eat more than one serving, look for values of 5 percent or less. In this example the food has cholesterol and trans fat, and is high is sodium. Also note that there are two portions per container. Note that percent values are not available for trans fats and protein, as there are no recommended Daily Values for them. If you want to learn more about these recommended Daily Values, go to the MyPlate website (www.choosemyplate.gov).

Total Carbohydrate, Dietary Fiber, and Sugars

This section breaks out values for dietary fiber and sugars. It is important for people who want to monitor their carbohydrates or get more fiber in their diet. (Most of us should be eating more fiber.) Note that there is no Daily Value percent for sugar. However, for many people with diabetes, it's the total amount of carbohydrate that matters, not the specific kind. A general guideline is to keep this amount between 45 and 60 g per meal, assuming three meals a day.

Ingredients List

Always check a package's ingredients list. It will show you what is in the food you will be eating. Ingredients are listed in order *by weight.* If you see sugar listed first, then the food contains more sugar than anything else. And remember: when you see the words *partially hydrogenated* or *hydrogenated*, the product contains trans fats (even if the amount for trans fats is 0 g).

absorbed into the body and does not have calories, it helps you in important ways. Fiber is found naturally in whole and minimally processed plant foods with "skins, seeds, and strings." For example, whole grains, dried beans, peas, lentils, fruits, vegetables, nuts, and seeds all have some fiber. Animal-based foods and refined and processed foods (white flour, bread, many baked and snack foods) have little or no fiber unless it was added by the manufacturer during processing.

Different types of fiber help your body in different ways. Wheat bran, some fruits and vegetables, and whole grains act as "nature's broom"; they keep your digestive system moving and help prevent constipation. The fiber in oat bran, barley, nuts, seeds, beans, apples, citrus fruits, carrots, and psyllium seed can help regulate your blood sugar because they help slow the amount of time it takes for sugar to get into the bloodstream. They can also help lower blood cholesterol. High fiber diets are also thought to help reduce the risk of rectal and colon cancers.

Oils and Solid Fats: The Good, the Bad, and the Deadly

Most people think that all fat is bad for them. But you need some fat for survival and for your body to work properly. The body needs about one tablespoon (15 mL) of fat a day. Although all fats have the same number of calories per portion size, some fats are more healthful than others (we call these good fats), and some fats are harmful when we eat too much (bad fats).

Good fats (also called unsaturated fats) are by and large oils that are usually liquid at room temperature. These fats help keep your cells healthy, and some can help reduce blood cholesterol. Good fats include soybean, safflower, corn, peanut, sunflower, canola, and olive oils. Nuts, seeds, and olives (and their oils), as well as avocados, are also rich in good fats.

There is another group of good fats, the omega-3s, which can be helpful for some people in reducing the risk of heart disease and may help with rheumatoid arthritis symptoms. These fats are found in fatty fish such as salmon, mackerel, trout, and tuna. Other sources of omega-3s include wheat germ, flaxseed, and walnuts, although the body may not be able to use omega-3s from plants as well as it does the omega-3s from fish.

The bad fats (also called saturated fats) are usually solid at room temperature (think shortening, butter, lard, and bacon grease). They can increase blood cholesterol and the risk of heart disease. Most bad fats are found in animal foods such as butter, beef fat (tallow, suet), chicken fat, and pork fat (lard). Other foods high in bad fats include stick margarines, red meat, regular ground meat, processed meats (sausage, bacon, luncheon and deli meats), poultry skin, whole- and low-fat milk and cheeses including cream cheese and sour cream. Palm kernel oil, coconut oil, and cocoa butter are also considered bad fats because they are high in saturated fat.

The fats classified as "deadly" are the trans fats. They can increase blood cholesterol and risk of heart disease even more than the bad fats. Trans fats are found in many processed foods, including pastries, cakes, cookies, crackers, icing, margarine, and most microwave popcorn. These fats are listed on food labels as "partially hydrogenated" or "hydrogenated" oils. Be warned! Food companies can legally claim "no"

Tips for Choosing Good Fats and Healthier Fats

The following tips can help you eat less bad fat and more good fat. Be sure that if you decide to choose more good fats, you are eating less bad fat. You do not want to increase the total amount of fat you eat.

When Choosing Foods

- Eat cooked portions of meat, fish, and poultry that are two to three ounces (56 to 84 g). This amount is about the size of a deck of cards or the palm of your hand.

- Eat more fish rich in omega-3s (salmon, tuna, and mackerel).

- Choose leaner cuts of meat (round, sirloin, or flank).

- Choose low-fat or fat-free milk and dairy foods (cheese, sour cream, cottage cheese, yogurt, and ice cream).

When Preparing Foods

- Use a nonstick pan without oil or a pan with small amounts of cooking oil spray.

- When cooking and baking, use oil (such as olive or canola oil) and soft (tub) margarines instead of shortening, lard, butter, or stick margarine.

- Broil, barbecue, or grill meats.

- Avoid frying or deep-frying foods.

- Do not eat the skin on poultry.

- Trim off all the fat you can see from meat before cooking it.

- Skim the fat from stews and soups during cooking. (If you refrigerate them overnight, solid fat collects on the surface and lifts off easily.)

- Use less butter, margarine, gravies, meat-based and cream sauces, spreads, and creamy salad dressings.

or "0" trans fats on the label even when the food has up to half a gram (0.5 g) per serving. The best advice is to eat as little trans fats as possible.

There are no specific daily recommendations for how much fat you should eat. Most people get more than enough in their regular diet. The best recommendation is to eat very little bad and deadly fats and to instead choose foods with the good fats, without increasing the total amount of fat you eat.

There is one more thing you should know about fat. All fats contain twice the calories per teaspoon as protein or carbohydrate. Calories

from fat add up quickly. For instance, one teaspoon (5 mL) of sugar has about 20 calories, but the same amount of oil or solid fat has about 35 calories. When we eat more calories than we need—no matter where they come from—the extra calories get stored as body fat, which leads to weight gain.

Protein: Muscle Builder and More

Protein is vital for hundreds of biological processes that keep you alive and healthy. Protein is part of your red blood cells, your muscles, and the enzymes and hormones that help regulate

Table 14.1 **Daily Recommended Amounts, with Examples for Healthy Meal Planning**

These recommendations are for average adults (19 years and older) who exercise less than 30 minutes daily and eat 1,000 to 3,000 calories. They are based on the United States Dietary Guidelines. (For Canada's guidelines, please see www.healthcanada.gc.ca/foodguide.)

   If you have a special condition, you may need to modify portion sizes of certain foods but should still aim for an overall balance.

Household Measure Equivalencies

Imperial (United States)	Metric (Canada)
1 teaspoon (tsp)	5 milliliters (mL)
1 tablespoon (Tbsp)	15 mL
1/4 cup	60 mL
1/3 cup	75 mL
1/2 cup	125 mL
2/3 cup	150 mL

Imperial (United States)	Metric (Canada)
3/4 cup	175 mL
1 cup	250 mL
1 ounce (oz)	28 grams (g)
1 fluid ounce (oz)	30 mL
1 inch	2.54 centimeters (cm)

Recommended Daily Amount			
Protein-Rich Foods	**Women**	**Men**	**Examples**
Animal (meat, fish, poultry) and plant sources (beans, nuts, seeds)	5–5½ ounces (140–154 g)	5½–6½ ounces (154–182 g)	**What counts as a 1-ounce (28 g) serving:** _Contains Little to No Carbohydrate_ 1 ounce (28 g) cooked lean meat, poultry, or fish 1 egg 1 tablespoon (15 mL) nut butter (peanut, almond, soy, etc.) About 2 tablespoons (1 ounce, 30 mL, or 30 g) nuts (12 almonds, 7 walnut halves) _Contains Carbohydrates_ 1/2 cup (125 mL) cooked dry beans, peas, or lentils 1/2 cup (125 mL) baked or refried beans 1 ounce (28 g) cooked tempeh 2 tablespoons (30 mL) hummus 1/2 cup (125 mL) roasted soybeans 4-ounce (112 g) falafel patty
Milk, cheese (except cream cheese), yogurt, milk-based desserts (Choose fat-free or low-fat most of the time)	3 cups (750 mL)	3 cups (750 mL)	**What counts as a 1-cup (250 mL) serving:** _Contains Little to No Carbohydrate_ 1½ ounces (42 g) cheese 1/3 cup (75 mL) shredded cheese 2 cups (500 mL) cottage cheese _Contains Carbohydrates_ 1 cup (250 mL) milk, yogurt, or kefir 1 cup (250 mL) pudding or frozen yogurt 1½ ounces (42 g) ice cream 2 ounces (56 g) processed cheese or cottage cheese

Recommended Daily Amount			
Grains	**Women**	**Men**	**Examples**
Grains (At least half should be whole grains)	5–6 ounces (140–168 g)	6–8 ounces (168–224 g)	**What counts as a 1-ounce (28 g) serving:** 1-ounce (28 g) slice of bread 1/2 English muffin 1 cup (250 mL) ready-to-eat flaked cereal 1/2 cup (125 mL) cooked rice, cooked pasta, or cooked cereal 6-inch flour or corn tortilla
Vegetables and Fruits	**Women**	**Men**	**Examples**
Vegetables	2–2½ cups (500–625 mL)	2½–3 cups (625–750 mL)	**What counts as a 1-cup (250 mL) serving:** *Low in Starch* 1 cup (250 mL) cooked vegetables (greens, broccoli family, green beans) or vegetable juice 2 cups (500 mL) raw leafy greens 12 medium baby carrots *High in Starch* 1 cup (250 mL) cooked sweet potato, white potato, or winter squash 1 cup (250 mL) cooked dry beans, peas, or lentils 1 cup (8 ounces) (250 mL or 224 g) tofu 1 cup (250 mL) corn or green peas
Fruit	1½–2 cups (375–500 mL)	2 cups (500 mL)	**What counts as a 1-cup (250 mL) serving:** 1 cup (250 mL) fruit 1 cup (250 mL) 100% juice 1/2 cup (125 mL) dried fruit 1 banana (8–9 inches) (20–23 cms) 8 large strawberries
Fats	**Women**	**Men**	**Examples**
Oils and Solid Fats	5–6 teaspoons (25–30 mL)	6–7 teaspoons (30–35 mL)	**What counts as a 1-teaspoon (5 mL) serving:** About 1 teaspoon (5 mL) salad or cooking oil, margarine, mayonnaise, or salad dressing 1 teaspoon (5 mL) butter or margarine

your body. It helps your immune system fight infection and builds and repairs damaged tissues. Protein can also give you some energy. But like fat, protein is not as good a source of energy for the body as is carbohydrate.

There are two types of proteins. Complete proteins have all the right parts in the right amounts. Your body uses them just as they are. Complete proteins are found in animal foods—meat, fish, poultry, eggs, milk, and other dairy products—as well as in soy foods such as soybeans, tofu, and tempeh. Incomplete proteins are low in one or more parts. Incomplete proteins are found in plant foods such as grains, dried beans and peas, lentils, nuts, and seeds. Most fruits and vegetables contain minimal protein if they contain any at all. For your body to be able to use incomplete proteins best, eat them with at least one other incomplete protein or along with a complete protein.

Over centuries, people have learned to survive by eating protein combinations. Two of the most plentiful and commonly eaten incomplete protein pairs are beans and rice and peanut butter and bread. Unfortunately, many people get most of their protein from meat, which tends to be high in the bad fats. The best way to get protein is mainly from plant foods along with small amounts of lean meat, poultry, or fish. Although nearly all plant proteins are incomplete proteins, they are at the heart of eating healthy. By eating a small amount of an animal protein (such as chicken) with a plant food such as lentils or black beans, you get all the benefits of a complete protein. In addition, some plant foods, such as nuts and seeds, are sources of the good fats, and many plants foods are good sources of fiber. Plant foods have no cholesterol and little or no trans fats.

The good news is that most people eat more than enough protein. Unless you have been told by your health care provider that you have a medical condition and you need to increase your protein consumption, there is no need to be concerned.

Vitamins and Minerals

Vitamins help regulate the body's inner workings. Minerals are part of many cells and cause important reactions to happen in the body. Vitamins and minerals are essential for survival and health, and most of us get all the vitamins and minerals we need from healthy eating. But three minerals—sodium, potassium, and calcium—stand out. They are related to current health problems because many of us eat either too much or too little of these nutrients.

Sodium

For some people, too much sodium can raise blood pressure. This can lead to heart disease, stroke, and kidney failure. Cutting back on sodium can help lower blood pressure, and it can help prevent high blood pressure.

It is easy to get enough sodium to meet the body's needs, but most people get way too much. People need only about 500 milligrams a day (in terms of table salt, this is less than a fifth of a teaspoon, or 1 mL). Yet most people eat 8 to 12 times that much. Adults should limit sodium intake to 2,300 mg a day, which is about the amount in 1 teaspoon (5 mL) of table salt. People who have high blood pressure, kidney disease, or diabetes, are African American, or who are middle-aged (about 40 years) or older should not have more than 1,500 mg of sodium a day.

You get sodium from most foods you eat—from trace amounts in some plant foods to higher amounts in some animal foods. But the real culprits are processed foods, which typically contain a lot of added sodium.

Eating less sodium takes some getting used to, but over time you will learn to enjoy the natural flavors of food. Here are some tips to help you keep your sodium intake in check:

■ Always taste your food before salting it. Most times you'll find it tastes good as is.

■ Don't add salt to food when cooking; season instead with spices, herbs, pepper, garlic, onion, or lemon.

■ Use fresh or frozen minimally processed poultry, fish, and lean meat, instead of canned, breaded, or prepared packaged food.

■ Choose foods labeled "low sodium" or those with 140 mg or less per serving. (Check out the Nutrition Facts label on page 242 for more on how to read these labels.)

■ Save high-sodium food for special occasions. Serve bacon, luncheon or deli meats, frozen dinners, packaged mixes, salted nuts, salad dressings, and high-sodium canned soups as part of celebrations, not as everyday fare.

■ In restaurants, ask that your food not be salted during preparation.

Potassium

This mineral helps regulate the heartbeat, among other important jobs in the body. In contrast to sodium, which raises blood pressure, potassium can help lower blood pressure. When you follow the Map for Healthy Eating (page 240), it is easy to get enough potassium. Good sources include vegetables such as broccoli, peas, lima beans, tomatoes, potatoes, sweet potatoes, and winter squash; fruits, including citrus fruits, cantaloupe, bananas, kiwifruit, prunes, and apricots; and nuts. Meat and poultry, some fish (salmon, cod, flounder, and sardines), milk, buttermilk, and yogurt also contain some potassium.

Calcium

You probably know that calcium helps build bones, but did you know that it is needed for blood clotting and helps you maintain a healthy blood pressure? It may also help protect against colon cancer, kidney stones, and breast cancer.

Unfortunately, most people, especially women and young children, do not get enough calcium. Most women under 60 should get the amount of calcium found in three cups (750 mL) of milk every day. Other good sources of calcium are yogurt and kefir (a beverage similar to yogurt); calcium-fortified soy, rice, and almond milks and orange juice; seaweed; and leafy greens (bok choy, kale, Brussels sprouts, broccoli, kohlrabi, collards, and some others). Unfortunately, our bodies cannot easily access the calcium in spinach, Swiss chard, and rhubarb even though they are green and leafy plants.

Most fruits are low in calcium, except for dried figs (there's not much in fig cookies, though) and the tropical cherimoya (custard apple).

Water

Water is the most important nutrient. Like the air you breathe, you cannot live without it. More than half of your body is made up of water, and each cell is bathed in it. Water helps keep your kidneys working, helps prevent constipation, and can help you eat less by making you feel full. It also helps prevent some medication side effects.

Although most people can last weeks without food, people cannot typically live longer than a week or so without water. Most adults lose about 10 cups (2500 mL) of water a day. However, we usually have no problem getting the six to eight glasses each day many experts recommend. This is especially true when you consider that most liquids and foods we consume contain some water. Remember, you get water from what you drink as well as the food you eat. Even the driest cracker has a tiny bit of water.

To see if you are drinking enough, check your urine. If it is light colored, you are fine.

When you start to get thirsty, you need more water. Milk, juice, and many fruits and vegetables are good sources of water. Coffee, tea, and other drinks with caffeine, as well as alcohol, however, can act like a mild diuretic which may cause you to lose water. Do not depend only on these drinks for your water.

If you have kidney disease or congestive heart failure or are taking special medications, your needs for water may be different. Talk to a registered dietitian or your health care provider. People with HIV or other conditions that suppress the immune system may prefer to use bottled water. This can be distilled water, spring water filtered to two microns, or carbonated soda water. If you want to use tap water and have a very low CD4 T-cell count, you may want to boil it for at least five minutes to kill any possible germs before drinking or making ice cubes with it. Also, if you drink bottled juices, choose those that are pasteurized to avoid bacteria that can make you sick. A person living with HIV should never drink water directly from lakes or rivers because of the risk of waterborne infection.

After reading this chapter, you may feel that we have taken all the fun out of food and made eating a big hassle. Luckily, however, it doesn't have to be that way. If you choose to make some of the changes suggested here, consider what you are doing as something positive and wonderful for yourself, not as punishment. As a self-manager, it's up to you to find the changes that are best for you. And if you experience setbacks, identify the problems and work at resolving them. You can do it! With some thought, planning, and practice, mealtime can be one of the best parts of your day. By making healthy choices and taking safety precautions, you will enjoy your food more and feel more in control of your health!

Additional Resources

Academy of Nutrition and Dietetics: www.eatright.org

American Cancer Society: www.cancer.org/healthy/eathealthygetactive/index

American Diabetes Association: www.diabetes.org/food-and-fitness

American Heart Association: www.heart.org/nutrition

Center for Science in the Public Interest, Nutrition Action Health Letter:
www.cspinet.org/nah/index.htm

Environmental Nutrition: The Newsletter of Food, Nutrition, and Health:
www.environmentalnutrition.com

Harvard School of Public Health: www.hsph.harvard.edu/nutritionsource

International Food Information Council Foundation: www.ific.org

Mayo Clinic, "Nutrition and Healthy Eating":
www.mayoclinic.com/health/nutrition-and-healthy-eating/MY00431

Tufts University Health and Nutrition Letter: www.healthletter.tufts.edu

University of California, Berkeley, Wellness Letter: www.wellnessletter.com

U.S. Department of Agriculture, ChooseMyPlate: www.choosemyplate.gov

U.S. Department of Agriculture, Food and Nutrition Information Center: http://fnic.nal.usda.gov

U.S. Department of Health and Human Services, "Heart Healthy Home Cooking, African
American Style": www.nhlbi.nih.gov/files/docs/public/heart/cooking.pdf

Suggested Further Reading

To learn more about the topics discussed in this chapter, we suggest that you explore the following resources:

Duyff, Roberta Larson. *American Dietetic Association's Complete Food and Nutrition Guide*, 4th ed. Hoboken, N.J.: John Wiley & Sons, 2012.

Warshaw, Hope. *Eat Out, Eat Well: The Guide to Eating Healthy in Any Restaurant.* Alexandria, Va.: American Diabetes Association, 2015.

Woodruff, Sandra, and Leah Gilbert-Henderson. *Soft Foods for Easier Eating Cookbook: Easy-to-Follow Recipes for People Who Have Chewing and Swallowing Problems.* Garden City Park, N.Y.: Square One, 2010.

Table 14.2 Food Guide for Healthy Meal Planning

Nutritional values are based on data from the U.S. Department of Agriculture and the American Diabetes Association.

Abbreviations:
g = grams, mg = milligrams, oz = ounce, c = cup, Tbsp = tablespoon, tsp = teaspoon
mL = milliliters, cm = centimeters

PROTEIN FOODS

Protein Sources with Little or No Carbohydrate

Serving Size: 3–4 oz (84–112 g), cooked, NOT breaded, fried, or cooked with added fat unless noted. This portion is the size of the palm of your hand and 1/2 to 1 inch (1.0–2.5 cm) thick.
Per Serving: approx. 21–28 g protein; fat and calories vary

Beef, Pork, Lamb, Veal, Poultry, and Fish	
Lean *(up to 9 g fat, 135–180 calories per serving)*	Beef (fat trimmed) from the round, sirloin, and flank, tenderloin sirloin, ground round
	Pork, fresh, cured, boiled ham, Canadian bacon, tenderloin, center loin chop
	Lamb and veal, rib roast, chop, leg
	Chicken and turkey, white or dark meat, no skin
	Duck and goose, drained of fat, no skin
	Game, buffalo, ostrich, rabbit, venison
	Fish (fresh or frozen), catfish, cod, flounder, haddock, halibut, orange roughy, salmon, tilapia
	Fish (canned), tuna, in water or oil, drained; herring, uncreamed or smoked, 6–8 sardines
	Shellfish, clams, crab, lobster, scallops, shrimp, imitation shellfish
	Oysters (fresh or frozen), 18 medium
	Processed meats (luncheon meat, deli meat), turkey ham, kielbasa, pastrami, chipped beef, shaved meats
Medium-fat *(12–21 g fat, 150–300 calories per serving)*	Ground beef, meatloaf, corned beef, short ribs, prime rib, tongue
	Pork, shoulder roast, Boston butt (picnic), cutlets
	Lamb, rib roast and chops, roasts, ground
	Veal, cutlet
	Chicken, turkey, with skin, fried, ground
	Pheasant, dove, wild duck, wild goose
	Fish, all fried
High-fat *(24 g or more fat, 300–400 calories per serving)*	Pork, spareribs, ground
	Sausage, pork, bratwurst, chorizo, Italian, Polish, smoked, summer
	Processed meats, luncheon meat and deli meats, bologna, salami
	Bacon, 6 slices

Protein Sources with Little or No Carbohydrate (*continued*)

Organ Meats *Serving Size: 2–3 oz (56–84 g)* *Per Serving: 14–21 g protein; fat and calories vary; high in cholesterol*	Kidney (1–3 g fat, 70–105 calories) Liver, heart (6–9 g fat, 55–100 calories)
Eggs *Per Serving: 7 g protein*	Whole egg, 1 large, cooked (5 g fat, 75 calories) Egg whites, 2 large, cooked (0–1 g fat, 35 calories) Egg substitute, plain, 1/4 c (60 mL) (1 g fat, about 50 calories)
Cheese *Per Serving: 7 g protein; fat and calories vary*	
Fat-free and low-fat *(0–1 g fat, 35 calories)*	Fresh (Mexican) and nonfat cheese, 1 oz (28 g) Cottage cheese, fat-free, 1/4 c (2 oz) (60 mL or 56 g)
Medium-fat *(4–7 g fat, 75 calories)*	Feta, skim-milk mozzarella, string cheese, reduced-fat and processed cheese spreads, 1–2 oz (28–56 g) Ricotta, 1/4 c (2 oz) (60 mL or 56 g) Grated parmesan, 2 Tbsp (1 oz or 30 mL)
High-fat *(8 g fat, 100+ calories)*	All regular full-fat cheese: American, blue, Brie, Swiss, cheddar, Monterey jack, provolone, whole-milk mozzarella, goat, queso fresco, 1–2 oz (28–56 g)
Nuts and Seeds* *Per Serving: Little to no carbohydrate; fat and calories vary* *(These foods contain good fats—see page 244.)	Almonds, cashews, mixed nuts, 6 nuts Peanuts, 10 nuts Pecans, walnuts, 4 halves Tahini (sesame paste), 1 Tbsp (15 mL) Pumpkin seeds, sunflower seeds, 1 Tbsp (15 mL) Nut butters (peanut, almond, etc.), 2 Tbsp (30 mL) (8 g fat)

continues ▶

PROTEIN FOODS (*continued*)

Protein Foods with Carbohydrate

Milk *Serving Size: 1 c (250 mL)* *Per Serving: 8 g protein,* *12 g carbohydrate; fat and* *calories vary*	Nonfat, fresh or evaporated 1%, nonfat or low-fat buttermilk (0–3 g fat, 100 calories) Low-fat (2%) sweet acidophilus (5 g fat, 120 calories) Whole, fresh or evaporated cow milk, goat milk, buttermilk (8 g fat, 160 calories)
Yogurt *Per Serving: 8 g protein,* *12 g carbohydrate; fat and* *calories vary*	Nonfat, plain, or flavored with artificial sweetener, 2/3 c (5 oz) (150 mL) (0–3 g fat, 90–100 calories) Low-fat, sugar-sweetened, with fruit, 2/3 c (5 oz) (150 mL) (5 g fat, 120 calories) Plain whole milk, kefir, 3/4 c (6 oz) (175 mL) (8 g fat, 150 calories) Nonfat fruit-flavored, sweetened with sugar, 1 c (8 oz) (250 mL) (3 g carbohydrate, 0–3 g fat, 100–150 calories) Nonfat or low-fat fruit-flavored, sweetened with sugar substitute, 1 c (8 oz) (250 mL) (0–3 g fat, 90–130 calories)
Plant Protein Sources *Per Serving: as noted*	Soy milk, regular, 1 c (250 mL) (2–3 g carbohydrate, 8 g protein, 4 g fat, 100 calories) Dried beans and peas, lentils, cooked, 1/2 c (125 mL) (15 g carbohydrate, 7 g protein, 0–1 g fat, 80 calories) Edamame (soybeans), 1/2 c (125 mL) (8 g carbohydrate, 7 g protein, 0–1 g fat, approx. 60 calories) Hummus (garbanzo bean spread), 1/3 c (75 mL) (15 g carbohydrate, 7 g protein, approx. 8 g fat, 100 calories) Refried beans, canned, 1/2 c (125 mL) (15 g carbohydrate, 7 g protein, 0–3 g fat, approx. 100 calories) Tofu, regular, 1/2 c (4 oz) (125 mL) (3 g carbohydrate, 8 g protein, 5 g fat, 75 calories)

CARBOHYDRATE FOODS

Per Serving: 15 g carbohydrate, 3 g protein, 0–1 g fat, 80 calories

Tip: Choose whole grains as often as you can.

Breads and Grains	
Breads, Rolls, Muffins, and Tortillas *Good source of fiber	Bagel, large, 1/4 Bread, white, whole grain,* rye, pumpernickel, 1 slice Buns, hot dog or hamburger, 1/2 English muffin, plain, 1/2 Pancake, 4 inches (10 cm) across, 1 Pita bread, 6 inches (15 cm) across, 1/2 Roll, regular, 1/2 Tortilla, corn or flour, 6 inches (15 cm) across, 1 Waffle, 4½ inches (11 cm) square, reduced-fat, 1
Cereals *Good source of fiber	Bran flakes, spoon-size shredded wheat,* 1/2 c (125 mL) Granola,* low-fat or regular, Grape-Nuts* 1/4 c (60 mL) Oats,* cooked, 1/2 c (125 mL) Puffed cereal, unfrosted, 1½ c (375 mL)
Grains *Good source of fiber	Bulgur wheat,* grits, cooked, tabbouleh, prepared, 1/2 c (125 mL) Pasta, barley, couscous, quinoa, cooked, 1/3 c (75 mL) Rice, white, or brown,* cooked, 1/3 c (75 mL) Wheat germ,* dry, 3 Tbsp (45 mL) Wild rice,* cooked, 1/2 c (125 mL)
Crackers and Snacks	Graham crackers, 2½ inches (6 cm) square, 3 Matzo, 3/4 oz (21 g) Melba toast, 2 x 4 inches (5 cm x 10 cm), 4 Pretzels, 3/4 oz (21 g) Rice cakes, 4 inches (5 cm) across, 2 Saltines, 6 Whole-wheat crackers, no fat added, 3–4 oz (84–112 g), 2–5

continues ▶

CARBOHYDRATE FOODS (*continued*)

Low-Starch Vegetables

Per Serving: approx. 5 g carbohydrate, 2 g protein, no fat, 25 calories
Serving Size: 1/2 c (125 mL) cooked or vegetable juice, 1 c (250 mL) raw fresh, frozen, or canned (frozen or canned may be high in sodium)

Amaranth	Cucumber	Rutabaga
Artichoke	Eggplant (aubergine)	Salad greens
Asparagus	Garlic	Snap peas
Bamboo shoots	Green beans	Spinach
Bean sprouts	Green onion, scallions	Summer squash (yellow squash, zucchini)
Beets	Greens (collard, kale, mustard, turnip)	Sweet peppers
Broccoli		
Brussels sprouts	Jicama	Tomatoes (raw, canned, sauce)
Cabbage, Chinese cabbage	Kohlrabi	Turnips
Carrots	Mushrooms	Vegetable juice (usually high in sodium)
Cauliflower	Nopales (cactus)	
Celery	Okra	Watercress
Chayote (vegetable pear)	Onions	
Chicory	Pea pods	
Chilies, spicy	Radishes	

Starchy Vegetables

Per Serving: 15 g carbohydrate, 0–3 g protein, 0–1 g fat, 80 calories

Corn, 1/2 c (125 mL) or 1/2 large cob	Succotash (lima beans and corn), 1/2 c (125 mL)
Mixed vegetables with corn, peas, or pasta, 1 c (250 mL)	Winter squash (acorn, butternut, pumpkin), 1 c (250 mL)
Parsnips, 1/2 c (125 mL)	Yam, sweet potato, 1/2 c (125 mL)
Plantain, ripe, 1/3 c (75 mL)	Yautia, yuca (cassava), 1/2 c (125 mL)
Potato, baked or boiled, large, with skin, 1	

CARBOHYDRATE FOODS (*continued*)

Fruit

Per Serving: 15 g carbohydrate, no protein, 0–1 g fat, approx. 80 calories

Fresh

Apple, small, 2 inches (5 cm), 1

Apricots, 4

Banana, extra small, 1 (4 oz) (112 g)

Berries (strawberries, blueberries, raspberries) 3/4–1 c (175–250 mL)

Cherries, 1/2 c (125 mL) (approx. 12)

Coconut, fresh (shredded), 1/2 c (125 mL)

Dates, 3

Figs, large, 2

Fruit cocktail, 1/2 c (125 mL)

Grapefruit, small, 1/2

Grapes, small, 1/2 c (125 mL)

Guava, medium, 2

Kiwifruit, large, 1

Lemon, lime, large, 1

Mango, cubed, 1/2 c (125 mL)

Melon (honeydew, cantaloupe), 1/4 (60 mL)

Orange, small, 1

Papaya, small, cubed, 1 c (250 mL)

Peach, nectarine, 1

Pear, 1/2

Persimmon, medium, 1

Pineapple, cubed, 3/4 c (175 mL)

Plum, small, 2

Tangerine, small, 2

Watermelon, cubed, 1/2 c (125 mL)

Canned

Unsweetened, 1/4–1/2 c (60–125 mL)

In sugar syrup, 1/4 c (60 mL)

Dried

Apricots, 8 halves

Figs, 2

Prunes, 3

Raisins, 1 Tbsp (15 mL)

Tamarind, 1/2 c (125 mL)

Fruit Drinks

(If the label doesn't say 100% juice, it usually contains added sugar)

Unsweetened

Apple, grapefruit, orange, pineapple, 1/2 c (125 mL)

Apricot nectar, 1/2 c (125 mL)

Grape, prune, juice blends, 1/3 c (75 mL)

Sweetened

Carbonated juice drinks, 1/2 c (125 mL)

Cranberry cocktail, 1/3 c (75 mL)

continues ▶

OILS AND SOLID FATS

Per Serving: little or no carbohydrate, 5 g fat, 45 calories
Tip: Choose good fats as often as you can.

Good fats

Unsaturated fats, see page 244

Avocado, medium, 1/4

Margarine (soft), reduced-fat, 1 tsp (5 mL)

Mayonnaise, reduced-fat, 1 Tbsp (15 mL)

Mayonnaise, regular, 1 tsp (5 mL)

Olives, all types, large, 5

Salad and cooking oils (corn, olive, safflower, soybean, etc.), 1 tsp (5 mL)

Salad dressing, 1 Tbsp (15 mL)

Bad fats

Saturated fats, see pages 244

Bacon fat, 1 tsp (5 mL)

Butter, reduced-fat, 1 Tbsp (15 mL)

Butter, regular, 1 tsp (5 mL)

Cream, half-and-half, whipped, 2 Tbsp (30 mL)

Cream, liquid nondairy creamer, 1 Tbsp (15 mL)

Cream cheese, 1 Tbsp (15 mL)

Margarine (stick), regular, made with hydrogenated fat, 1 tsp (5 mL)

Shortening, lard, 1 tsp (5 mL)

Sour cream, regular, 1 Tbsp (15 mL)

ADDITIONAL FOODS AND DRINKS

Extras

Tip: These foods are high in fat or sugar or both; they're best saved for special occasions.

Cake with frosting, 1 small slice or 2-inch (5 cm) square

Cookies, small, 2

Danish, small, 1

Flan, with milk, 1/2 c (125 mL)

Fruit tart or pie, 1 slice

Honey, 1 Tbsp (15 mL)

Ice cream (regular), 1/2 c (125 mL)

Jam or jelly (low-sugar or light), 2 Tbsp (30 mL)

Jam or jelly (regular), 1 Tbsp (15 mL)

Juice bar (frozen, 100% juice), 1

Pudding, 1/2 c (125 mL)

Sherbet, sorbet, 1/2 c (125 mL)

Syrup (regular), 1 Tbsp (15 mL)

Syrup (sugar-free), 2 Tbsp (30 mL)

Alcoholic Beverages

Per Serving: no protein or fat; carbohydrate and calories vary

Beer, lite or nonalcoholic, 12 oz (360 mL) (approx. 5 g carbohydrate, 60–120 calories)

Beer, regular, 12 oz (360 mL) (approx. 13 g carbohydrate, about 160 calories)

Distilled spirits, 80 proof, 1½ oz (45 mL) (0 g carbohydrate, 80–110 calories)

Liqueurs, 1½ oz (45 mL) (approx. 20 g carbohydrate, 125 calories)

Mixed drinks (margarita, mojito, gin and tonic, etc.), 1 drink (approx. 12 g carbohydrate, 150–250 calories)

Wine, red, white, dry, sparkling, 4 oz (120 mL) (1–2 g carbohydrate, 80 calories)

Wine, sweet or dessert, 4 oz (120 mL) (approx. 14 g carbohydrate, 120 calories)

ADDITIONAL FOODS AND DRINKS (*continued*)

Free Foods

Per Serving: up to 5 g carbohydrate, up to 20 calories; enjoy moderate servings as often as you like

Atol (cornmeal drink), 1 c (250 mL)	Herbs, spices
Bouillon, broth, consommé	Horchata (rice drink)
Candy, hard (sugar-free)	Hot pepper sauces
Chewing gum (sugar-free)	Soft drinks (sugar-free)
Club soda, mineral water	Soy sauce*
Coffee or tea, unsweetened or with sugar substitute, no milk, cream, or whitener	Worcestershire sauce*
Gelatin (sugar-free or unflavored)	*Use low sodium versions to reduce salt intake.

Sugar substitutes

Approved by the U.S. Food and Drug Administration

Equal (aspartame)	Sweet One (acesulfame K)
Splenda (sucralose)	Sweet-10 (saccharin)
Sprinkle Sweet (saccharin)	Sweet'N Low (saccharin)
Sugar Twin (saccharin)	

CHAPTER 15

Eating for Specific Long-Term Conditions

*T*HE PREVIOUS CHAPTER PROVIDED GENERAL INFORMATION on healthy eating that will work for most people. However, people with specific long-term conditions often have different considerations and needs. In this chapter, we present some information and guidelines for selected long-term health problems that can affect people with HIV. We also address common challenges for people who need to gain or lose weight, or who just need to eat better in general, as well as specific eating challenges for people with HIV.

If you have specific concerns about what to eat, talk to your doctor or a registered dietitian. These professionals can tell you what's best for you as well as help you fit our recommendations to your unique health needs.

HIV

Healthy eating is important for all people with HIV. If you do not have any symptoms, then following the suggestions offered in this chapter and the previous chapter will help you stay healthy. If you are having symptoms, then you may need to make some changes. For example, you may need to increase the amount of protein and calories you eat to maintain your lean body mass (muscles). Some tips for doing this are provided on page 269. You may also need extra vitamins and minerals, more than you get from foods, to help repair and heal damaged cells. To find out whether or not you should take vitamins and mineral supplements, which ones, and what dose, talk with your HIV health care provider.

If you are taking medications for HIV, you may be experiencing side effects that interfere with your body's ability to eat, absorb, and use needed nutrients. Some of these side effects include nausea, vomiting, diarrhea, loss of appetite, and mouth and swallowing problems.

The tips on pages 276–279, "Managing Specific Eating Challenges with HIV," may be useful for managing some of these problems. There is also information in Chapter 8, "Managing Medications for HIV," that may help.

If you have a low CD4 T-cell count (200 or less), make sure that you do not eat raw or undercooked eggs, poultry, beef, pork, or seafood. You also want to avoid unpasteurized fruit juices and dairy products. A good way to ensure your meat is cooked is to use a food thermometer, and make sure that you cook your meat until the internal temperature is between 145°F (63°C) for whole cuts of beef and pork and 165°F (74°C) for poultry. No matter what your CD4 T-cell count, make sure to wash your hands, utensils, and cutting boards with soap and hot water after each use. Also, before traveling abroad, talk with your doctor about additional steps you may want to take to protect yourself from water- or food-borne illnesses. See "Food Safety and Preparation Tips," page 279–282, for more on this topic.

Diabetes

People living with HIV have an increased risk for diabetes, so it is important to understand what diabetes is so you can take steps to prevent it. When a person eats a meal, the body breaks down the carbohydrates into glucose (sugar), the basic fuel for the body's cells, which is then absorbed into the bloodstream. (Protein and fat usually contribute little to the body's blood sugar.) The hormone

insulin takes the glucose into the cells. In people with diabetes, cells do not absorb or use glucose very well. Glucose builds up in their bloodstreams, which can lead to other health problems. Managing blood sugar levels is one of the prime goals in diabetes care and involves many different things, including taking medication, exercising, and keeping a careful eye on your diet.

In years past, people with diabetes were told that they could not eat sweets and that they could only eat certain types of carbohydrates. As the medical community learned more about the disease, recommendations changed. Doctors now know that people with diabetes do not have to avoid any specific food. However, they do need to watch what and how much they eat. These things will vary from person to person.

The American Diabetes Association (ADA) recommends that you "Create Your Plate" to plan meals (Figure 15.1). To create your plate, first look at your plate and divide it in half. Then take one of those halves and divide it in half again. You should have three sections on the plate now.

■ Half of the plate should be non-starchy vegetables, such as spinach or other greens, carrots, lettuce, cabbage, bok choy, broccoli, green beans, tomatoes, cauliflower, salsa, cucumber, okra, peppers, mushrooms, beets, or turnips.

■ One small section (a quarter of the plate) should be starchy food, such as whole-grain breads, whole-grain cereal, rice, pasta, tortillas, dal, oatmeal hominy, grits, cooked beans and peas, potatoes, corn, lima beans, green peas, sweet potatoes, fat-free popcorn, low-fat crackers, or pretzels.

■ The other small section should be meat or meat substitute, such as chicken or turkey (without the skin), fish, lean cuts of beef or pork, eggs, low-fat cheese, or tofu.

Add to that one eight-ounce (240 mL) glass of non- or low-fat milk, or six ounces (175 mL) of light yogurt, and a small piece of fruit or 1/2 cup (125 mL) of fruit salad

Here are some general points about healthy eating for people with diabetes:

■ Follow either the ADA's Create Your Plate or the USDA's Map for Healthy Eating (page 240) recommendations. People with diabetes are at higher risk for heart disease and other chronic health conditions. Following these guidelines is especially important to help prevent future problems.

■ Start each day with something to eat. Eating something in the morning is truly "breaking the fast." It helps fuel the body after a long night of resting and not having any food; it gives you energy to start the day's activities.

■ Space your meals and snacks at regular intervals throughout the day, and don't skip meals. Spacing your meals at usual times gives your body the chance to produce and use its insulin. It also gives your medication time to work and helps you keep up your energy level. The number of meals you eat and the time between your meals will

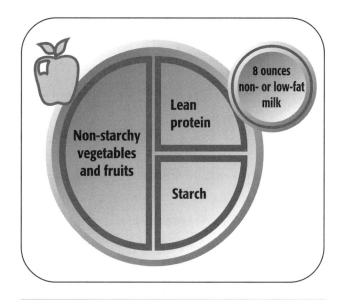

Figure 15.1 **"Create Your Plate" from the American Diabetes Association (ADA)**

vary depending on your personal health and lifestyle. Many people eat three meals a day, while others may prefer or need to eat smaller meals more frequently.

- Eat the same amount of food at each meal. This helps you maintain an even energy flow and blood sugar level throughout the day. Skipping meals or alternating large meals and small meals can throw off your energy level. It can also lead to overeating or making less healthy food choices. Eating poorly or overeating can cause swings in your blood sugar and results in symptoms such as irritability, mood swings, shakiness, difficulty sleeping, and pain or difficulties breathing due to stomach bloating, heartburn, or indigestion.

It is important that you learn to manage the carbohydrates you eat. Nearly all carbohydrates break down into glucose, so they have the greatest effect on your blood sugar of all the nutrients you eat. Too much carbohydrate causes blood sugar to increase; too little makes your blood sugar low. General guidelines suggest eating between 45 and 60 grams of carbohydrates per meal, but this amount may vary widely from person to person.

For most people with diabetes, there is no such thing as a bad carbohydrate or one that is off limits. What matters most is the total amount of carbohydrates, not the specific kind, although some people may feel that certain foods affect them in particularly negative or positive ways. Review the material on pages 240–241 and 244 about carbohydrates.

Because it increases the risk of heart disease and stroke, it is very important to eat fewer bad fats. Replace bad fats with good fats such as olive and canola oils, but just be sure not to add to your total fat intake. In addition, eat more plant foods and fewer animal foods. Review the material on saturated and trans fats on page 244. Get less sodium by eating fewer processed and prepared foods, and use the saltshaker sparingly, if at all. If you are carrying extra weight, losing some weight can help lower your blood sugar. Even a small loss of 5 to 10 pounds (2–4 kg) can make a big difference in your blood sugar level. (See the tips for healthier eating in the boxes on pages 241, and find tips for choosing healthy fats on page 245).

Heart Disease and Stroke

Healthy eating for people with heart disease or those who have had a stroke usually involves keeping arteries from hardening or getting clogged. To accomplish this, it is important to watch the amount and kind of fat you eat. Get most of the fat you eat from the good (unsaturated) fats and very little from the bad (saturated) fats. Eat little to no trans fat. (Review the material on saturated and trans fats on page 244.) Also, increasing the amount of fiber you eat—especially from oats, barley, dried beans and peas, lentils, apples, citrus fruits, carrots, and psyllium seed—can be helpful in managing high blood cholesterol, a major risk factor for heart disease. As we discussed on pages 248–249, eating less salt and sodium can help prevent or control high blood pressure. Limit the daily total amount of sodium you get to less than 1 teaspoon (15 mL) of table salt (about 1,500 mg). Use herbs, spices, lemon, and vinegar for flavor instead of salt. The tips on page 241 and 245 also provide suggestions for ways to make healthy fat choices and increase fiber in your eating plan.

Lung Disease

People with lung disease, especially emphysema, sometimes need to increase the amount of protein they eat. This helps increase energy, strength, and the ability to fight lung infections. When you have little or no appetite and it is hard for you to eat enough food, try eating higher-calorie foods—fruit nectars instead of juice, dried fruit instead of fresh fruit, sweet potato instead of white potato—or try nibbling on a small handful of nuts over the course of the day. Our discussion of the common challenges of gaining weight on pages 269–271 gives some tips to help you increase the amount of healthy foods you eat.

Osteoporosis

Osteoporosis makes your bones brittle and easily broken. It has been called a silent disease because it is often not obvious and its first symptom can be a bone fracture, especially in the spine, hip, or wrist. Even if it is not discovered early, it is never too late to help slow its progress. You can help by getting enough calcium and vitamin D, regularly doing muscle-strengthening and weight-bearing exercise (such as walking; see Chapter 13, "Physical Activity for Fun and Fitness"), and following your health care professional's recommendations, such as taking prescribed medications for bone loss.

Osteoporosis is technically not a calcium deficiency disease, so after bone has been lost, getting more calcium will not fix it. But getting vitamin D along with enough calcium can help the body absorb the calcium. Everybody needs some calcium every day. The best sources are milk and foods made from milk. But some people avoid milk products because they don't like them, do not eat animal products, or have problems digesting milk sugar (lactose intolerance). You can get enough calcium from your diet even if you have problems with milk sugar. Many people can enjoy milk products if they take them in small amounts or eat other foods at the same time, such as cereal with milk; if they use lactase tablets to help digest the lactose; or if they can eat foods such as kefir or yogurt. As we noted on page 247, there are also some fruits and vegetables that are high in calcium as well as foods with added calcium, such as soy milk, juices, cereals, and pasta. If you think you may not be getting enough calcium, talk to your doctor or a registered dietitian about your diet and whether calcium supplements are required to meet your calcium needs.

Eating and Your Thoughts

Do you eat when you're bored, down in the dumps or sad, or feeling lonely? Many people find comfort in food, or they eat just as something to do when they need to take their minds off something or have nothing else to do. Some eat when they are feeling angry, anxious, or depressed. At these times, it is easy to lose track of what and how much you eat. These are also the times when celery sticks, apples, or popcorn just won't do and you may crave less healthy options. Here are some ways to help control these urges:

- Keep a food-mood diary. Every day, list what, how much, and when you eat. Note how you are feeling when you have the urge to eat. Try to spot patterns so you can anticipate when you may want to eat without really being hungry.

- If you catch yourself feeling bored and are thinking about eating, ask yourself, "Am I really hungry?" If the answer is no, make yourself do something else for two to three minutes—go for a short walk around the house or around the block, work on a jigsaw puzzle, or play a computer game.

- Keep your mind and hands busy with a favorite hobby or activity.

- Write down action plans for the times when stressful or other situations make you think about food when you are not hungry. Sometimes it is easier to refer to the written word than to remember what you said you would do.

Common Challenges to Making Healthier Food Choices

Remember, healthy eating means enjoying a moderate amount of a wide variety of minimally processed foods in the proper amounts for your body while allowing for occasional treats. Eating this way can help you maintain your health, help prevent future health problems, and help you manage your disease symptoms as best as possible. Eating healthy may mean making some changes to what you are now doing. Healthy eating is equally important whether you want to lose weight and keep it off, maintain your weight, or gain weight (see pages 269–275). The following material will help you address some of the more common challenges we all face when trying to eat well.

"Healthy food doesn't taste the same as food I am used to. When I eat, I want something with substance, like meat and potatoes or a piece of apple pie! The healthy stuff just doesn't fill me up!"

Making healthier food choices does not mean that you can never have something you want or crave. It means trading off to fit in favorites while making the better choices most of the time. And healthy food can be delicious and satisfying! There are many excellent cookbooks with healthy recipes, as well as Internet sites with good, healthful recipe ideas.

"I know certain foods are good for me, but I just don't like them."

If you don't like a certain food, try substituting another food from the same food group. Maybe you don't care for winter squash as a source of potassium, but you might like sweet or regular potatoes with the skin on instead. If you don't like an entire food group, you may need to consult a registered dietitian to find foods from other groups that can give you similar nutrients.

"I don't like vegetables."

Try raw vegetables with tasty and healthy dips or sauces to add flavor. Grated or frozen vegetables can be added to soups, stews, or meat loaf. Try vegetable casseroles, such as vegetable lasagna. If vegetables still don't appeal to you, increase the amount of fruits you eat.

"I can't or don't like to drink milk."

Instead of drinking glasses of milk, add milk (or dry milk powder) to foods such as soups, meat loaf, or casseroles. You can also choose low-fat pudding, yogurt, cottage cheese, or ice cream in place of milk. Try yogurt in a salad dressing or in a vegetable or fruit dip. Melt some cheese on vegetables, potatoes, beans, tortillas, sandwiches, or pizza, or incorporate it into a dip. To get some of the same nutrients that are in milk without eating cheese or yogurt, try broccoli, greens (such as kale or collard or beet greens), tofu, beans, canned salmon, or corn tortillas. If milk or milk products make you feel bloated and cause diarrhea or gas, see the discussion of dairy products and lactose intolerance on page 265.

"I love to cook and I don't want to cook boring healthy food!"

If you love to cook, you are in luck. Take a new cooking class, begin watching one on television or YouTube, check out a new cookbook on healthy cooking from the library, or find an Internet site or smartphone app with healthy recipes. If you have odds and ends, even leftovers, in your kitchen, do a computer search to see what recipes you can find. Play around with ways to modify your favorite recipes, making them lower in fat, sugar, and sodium.

"I've never really been a cook, and I'm not sure I want to start now."

Keep it simple. Keep your freezer stocked with prepared meals, precut vegetables, and other convenience foods. Try easy-to-prepare meals such as a sandwich with vegetables on whole-wheat bread, egg or egg whites and whole-wheat toast, high-fiber cereal and low-fat milk, or pasta with fresh tomatoes. Check the Internet or go to the library or a bookstore and look through some cookbooks to get ideas for quick meals. When you do cook, make larger amounts and freeze portions to reheat later.

"I'm living alone now, and I'm not used to cooking for one. I find myself overeating so that food isn't wasted."

This can be a problem, particularly when the situation is new. You may be overeating or eating a "second dinner" to fill in time. Maybe you are one of those people who will eat for as long as food is in front of you. Whatever the reason, here are some ways to help you deal with the extra food:

■ Don't eat "family style" by putting serving dishes on the table. Put as much as you feel you can comfortably eat on a small plate, and bring only that plate to the table.

■ As soon as you have finished eating, or even right after you have served your portion, immediately put leftovers in the refrigerator or freezer. This will also give you leftovers for the next day or whenever you don't feel like fixing a meal.

- Ask others over for dinner once in a while, so that you can share food and other people's company. Plan a potluck supper with neighbors, relatives, or members of your house of worship, clubs, or other groups.

"I love to eat out, so how do I know if I'm eating well?"

Whether it is because you don't have time, you hate to cook, or you just don't have the energy to shop for groceries or fix meals, eating out may suit your needs. This is not necessarily bad if you know how to make the best choices possible. Here are some tips on eating out:

- Select restaurants that have a variety of menu items prepared in healthy ways (for example, grilled or steamed dishes in addition to or instead of fried foods).

- Ask what is in a dish and how it is prepared, especially if you are eating in a restaurant where the dishes are new to you.

- Before you go out, decide what type of food you will eat and how much. Many restaurants post their menus on the Internet or at the front of the restaurant.

- Order small plates or appetizers instead of main courses.

- When you are with a group, order first so that you aren't tempted to change your mind after hearing what others have selected.

- Ask if you can split an entrée with a dining companion, or order a half portion. You can also plan to eat only half of what you are

served and take the rest home for another meal. Ask to have the take-home container brought to you with your food, and box half of it up before you start eating.

- Choose menu items that are low in fat, sodium, and sugar, or ask if they can be prepared that way.

- Whenever possible, order broiled, barbecued, baked, grilled, or steamed dishes rather than food that has been breaded, fried, sautéed, creamed, or covered in cheese.

- Ask for your vegetables steamed or raw without butter, sauces, or dips.

- Ask that no bread be served, or eat bread without butter. You can also ask that no butter or dipping oil be served with your bread.

- Request salad with dressing on the side, and dip your fork into the dressing before spearing each mouthful.

- For dessert, select fruit, nonfat yogurt, sorbet, or sherbet.

- Share dessert with at least one other person.

"I snack while I am doing other things—watching TV, working on the computer, or reading."

If this is a problem for you, plan ahead by keeping a list of healthier snacks to grab. Here are some examples:

- Rather than snacking on crackers, chips, and cookies, munch on fresh fruit, raw vegetables, or fat-free or plain popcorn.

- Measure out your snack in a single-portion size so you won't be tempted to eat more.

- Designate specific places at home and work as "eating areas," and don't eat anywhere else.

Common Challenges to Gaining Weight

Sometimes long-term health problems like HIV make it difficult to gain weight or keep it on. This could be because your condition or its treatment makes it hard for you to eat because you aren't hungry, you are sad or depressed, your body is unable to use the food it gets, or it burns up calories faster than you can replace them.

When you aren't hungry or have trouble eating, few foods sound appealing. This is when it is more important to eat anything rather than worry about whether the foods you choose are "healthful." You need to eat for energy and strength and to support the body's nutrition needs, and that overrides being sure that what you eat is healthy. During those times, feel comfortable about eating whatever you can; it will probably only be temporary and then you can return to healthier eating.

If you experience continual or extreme weight loss or have trouble keeping weight on, you're not alone. Let's look at some common challenges and some ideas for dealing with them.

"I don't know how to add calories to my current diet."

Here are some ways to increase the calories and nutrients you eat without increasing the amount of food you need to eat:

■ Because fat gives us many more calories than carbohydrate or protein, choose foods that are higher in fat, but try to stick with foods that contain good fats (see pages 244–245). For example, snack on calorie-rich but healthy foods such as avocados, nuts, seeds, or nut butter.

■ Eat dried fruit or drink nectars instead of fresh fruit or regular juice.

■ Choose sweet potatoes instead of white potatoes.

■ Use whole milk instead of lower-fat dairy products, and use whole milk instead of broth or water in soups and sauces.

■ Try a liquid supplement drink with or between meals.

■ Drink high-calorie beverages such as shakes, malts, fruit whips, and eggnogs.

■ Top salads, soups, and casseroles with shredded cheese, nuts, dried fruits, or seeds.

"Food doesn't taste as good as before."

Many things can affect how food tastes. Mouth infections such as thrush, surgery, certain medications, being on oxygen, and even the common cold can make food taste off, bad, or funny. When this happens, you tend to eat less. Many people automatically add extra salt to their food to try to make it taste better. Unfortunately, this can cause you to retain water or feel bloated, which can increase blood pressure.

The following are some ways to make foods taste better:

■ Rinse your mouth with a mixture of one teaspoon (5 mL) of hydrogen peroxide or baking soda in a glass of warm distilled water before eating. Swish the mixture around in your mouth, but do not swallow. Also, if oral or esophageal thrush is a problem for you, remember to take your antifungal medication to prevent it.

- Use flavored toothpaste on a soft-bristled toothbrush to clean your teeth and tongue before and after you eat.

- Try drinking orange, cranberry, or pineapple juice; lemonade; or another tart drink to mask the bad taste.

- Marinate meat, poultry, fish, or tofu in vinegar or low-sodium salad dressing or soy sauce to make it more flavorful.

- Use herbs (basil, oregano, tarragon) and spices (cinnamon, cumin, curry, ginger, nutmeg) when you cook, or sprinkle them on top of finished dishes.

- Squirt fresh lemon juice on foods.

- Use a small amount of vinegar in or on top of hot or cold foods. There are dozens of different kinds, from balsamic to berry- and fruit-flavored varieties; experiment with new flavors.

- Add healthy ingredients to the foods you usually eat (carrots or barley to soup, for example, or dried fruits and nuts to salads) to give them more texture and make them tastier.

- Eat cold foods such as low-fat sherbet, fruit ice, frozen yogurt, and ice cream to cleanse your palate and numb the taste buds.

- Chew your food slowly and well. This will allow the food to remain in your mouth longer and release more flavor.

If the lack of taste is keeping you from eating enough, you may need to add more calories to your meals or snacks. Tips for doing this are given on page 269.

"It takes so long to prepare meals. By the time I'm done, I'm too tired to eat."

This is common, especially when you do not have much energy. This situation calls for planning to help make sure that you do eat. Here are some hints to help:

- When you do have some energy, cook enough for two, three, or even more servings or meals, especially if it is something you really like.

- Do a meal exchange with friends or family, and freeze what you get in single-serving sizes for times when you are too tired to cook.

- Break your food preparation into steps, resting in between.

- Ask for help, especially for big holiday meals or family gatherings.

"Sometimes eating causes discomfort."

"I'm afraid I'll become short of breath while I'm eating."

People who experience shortness of breath or who find it difficult and physically uncomfortable to eat meals tend to eat less. For some, eating a large meal causes stomach problems such as indigestion, discomfort, or nausea. Indigestion, along with a full stomach, reduces the space your breathing muscles have to expand and contract. This can aggravate breathing problems.

If these are challenges you sometimes face, try the following:

- Eat four to six small meals a day, rather than the usual three large meals. You will be using less energy for each meal.

- Avoid foods that produce gas or make you feel bloated. Many foods can produce gas, although foods affect people differently. Among the more common foods that can cause discomfort are cabbage, broccoli, Brussels sprouts, onions, beans, and certain fruits, including bananas, apples, melons, and avocados.

- Eat slowly, take small bites, and chew your food well. Pause occasionally during a meal. Eating quickly to avoid an episode of shortness of breath can actually cause shortness of breath. Slowing down and breathing evenly reduces the amount of air you swallow while eating.

- Choose food that is easy to eat, such as yogurt or pudding, or easy to drink, such as a smoothie or fruit nectar. Also, consider asking your doctor, nurse, or registered dietitian to recommend a nutritional supplement drink.

- Avoid filling up on liquids before you eat. Drink small amounts when you eat, and sip fluids between your eating times.

- Do a relaxation exercise about half an hour before mealtime, or take time out for a few deep breaths during the meal.

"I can't eat very much in one sitting."

"I get full too fast."

There is no rule that says we must eat only three meals a day. In fact, many people, especially those with HIV, find that four to six smaller meals work better. If you choose to eat more frequently, include no-fuss, high-calorie snacks such as smoothies, muffins and other baked products, and protein or meal bars as part of these extra meals. If you still can't finish a whole meal, eat the portion of your meal that is highest in protein and calories first.

"I just don't have much of an appetite."

Check with your doctor or a registered dietitian to see if the following tips are appropriate for you.

- Eat smaller meals several times a day.

- Keep high-calorie, high-protein snacks on hand, such as nuts or dried fruit, and eat a few pieces each time you walk past the bowl. Or snack on crackers with cheese or peanut butter.

- Eat the highest-calorie foods first, saving lower-calorie foods for later (for example, eat buttered bread before cooked spinach).

- Add extra whole milk or milk powder to sauces, gravies, cereals, soups, and casseroles.

- Add melted cheese to vegetables and other dishes.

- Use butter, margarine, or sour cream as toppings.

- Consider keeping snacks at your bedside so that you can sit up and eat something if you wake in the middle of the night, or pack them with you when you go out.

- Do light exercise before you eat to help stimulate your appetite.

- Ask your doctor about medications or natural remedies that stimulate appetite. If you have HIV, it is important to eat enough calories and nutrients to avoid weight loss.

Common Challenges to Losing Weight and Keeping It Off

While most people tend to relate HIV with weight loss and wasting, it is common for people with HIV to be overweight. If you are physically inactive (sit for more than four hours a day), do not sleep well, have low thyroid function, low testosterone blood levels, or take HIV medications that slow your metabolism and increase your insulin resistance, you may gain weight even when eating healthy. Studies show that eating fewer calories and being physically active are both important for successful weight loss. Just eating less is usually not enough. Being active not only helps you burn calories, but it also helps you build muscle (which burns more calories than fat) and gives you more strength and zip. You will be able to move and breathe better, and your energy level will increase. You will find more information about exercise and tips for choosing activities that suit your needs and lifestyle in Chapter 13, "Physical Activity for Fun and Fitness." Review the following pointers as well as the "Tips to Help You Manage How Much You Eat" on pages 238–239 when you are trying to lose weight.

- **Set small, gradual weight loss goals.** Break the total amount of weight you want to lose into small, reachable goals. Think in terms of, say, 1 to 2 pounds (1/2 to 1 kg) a week or 5 to 7 pounds (about 2–3 kg) a month instead of looking at the total number, especially if you have a lot of weight you would like to lose. For most people, aiming to lose 1 to 2 pounds (1/2 to 1 kg) a week is realistic and doable. When you set small goals rather than large ones—say 5 pounds (about 2 kg) instead of 20 pounds (9 kg)—your goals become more possible and practical.

- **Identify the exact specific steps you will take to lose your weight.** For example, walking 20 minutes a day five days a week, not eating between meals, and eating more slowly.

- **Keep on top of what is happening.** Keep track of your weight. Studies have shown that people who lose weight and keep it off are most successful when they weigh themselves daily.

- **Think long-term.** Instead of "I really need to lose 10 pounds (about 5 kg) right away," tell yourself, "Losing this weight gradually will help me keep it off for good."

Now with these basic principles in mind, let's look at some common challenges and ideas for dealing with them.

"I need to lose 10 pounds (about 5 kg) in the next two weeks. I want to look good for a special event."

Sound familiar? Almost everyone who has tried to lose weight wants it off fast. There are hundreds of weight loss diets promising fast and easy ways to lose weight. However, these promises are false. There is no "magic bullet." If it sounds too good to be true, it probably is.

During the first few days of almost any weight loss plan, your body loses mostly water, along with some muscle. This can amount to 5 or even 10 pounds (about 2–5 kg). Because of this, fad and fast-weight-loss diets can say they are successful. But the pounds (or kg) come right back on just as soon as you return to your old ways. Also, when you use fad diets, you may experience light-headedness, headaches, constipation, fatigue, and poor sleep, because such diets are often badly imbalanced in the kinds and amounts of foods allowed. Fat loss, what you really want, typically comes about after a few weeks of eating fewer calories than your body needs.

Rather than wasting time with fad diets, do it right. Set small, realistic goals; do action planning; and use positive thinking and self-talk. (These activities are discussed in greater detail in Chapter 2, "Becoming an HIV Self-Manager," and Chapter 12, "Using Your Mind to Manage Symptoms.") The weight didn't go on overnight. It won't go away overnight.

"I just can't seem to lose those last few pounds (kilos)."

Almost everyone reaches a time where weight loss stops (a plateau) despite continued hard work. This is frustrating and often makes us want to give up. Plateaus are often temporary. They can mean that your body now needs fewer calories and has adapted to its lower calorie intake and higher activity level. While your first impulse may be to cut your calories even further, this could actually make your body burn fewer calories, making more weight loss even harder.

This is a good time to ask yourself how much of a difference those last one, two, or even five pounds (1/2, 1, or even 2 kg) really makes. If you are feeling good and doing well with your blood sugar or cholesterol or other health issues, chances are you may not need to lose more weight. If you are relatively healthy,

staying active, and eating a healthy diet, it is usually not bad to carry a few extra pounds. Also, if you have begun to exercise, you may have replaced some of your body fat with muscle, which weighs more than fat—this type of weight gain is good. However, if you decide that those pounds (kilos) must go, try the following tactics:

- Instead of focusing on weight loss, for at least a few weeks focus on staying at the same weight and not gaining any weight; then go back to your weight loss plan.

- Increase your physical activity. Your body may have adjusted to your lower weight and therefore needs fewer calories, so you may need to exercise more to burn more calories. Adding more exercise could help kick-start your body into burning more calories. (You can find tips for safely increasing your exercise in Chapter 13, "Physical Activity for Fun and Fitness.")

- Keep thinking positive. Remind yourself of how much you have achieved. (Here's a tip: write positive comments on sticky notes and post them where you will see them.)

"I always feel so deprived of the foods I love when I try to lose weight."

You are a special person. This means that the changes you decide to make have to meet your special likes, dislikes, and needs. Unfortunately, our brains can get channeled into what we don't want to do or should not be doing instead of being supportive or encouraging, especially when it comes to losing weight.

You think using both pictures and words. This calls for teaching yourself how to see things in a better light and telling your brain to stop thinking about certain things, and to replace those thoughts with positive ones that work for you (more on positive thinking can be found in Chapter 12, "Using Your Mind to Manage Symptoms"). Here are a few examples:

- Replace thoughts that include the words *never*, *always*, and *avoid*. Instead, tell yourself that you can enjoy things occasionally, "but a healthier choice is better for me most of the time."

- Tell yourself that you are retraining your taste buds and that making healthier choices can help you manage your weight and feel better.

"I eat too fast or I finish eating before everyone else and find myself reaching for seconds."

If you are finishing meals in just a few minutes or before everyone else at the table, you are most likely eating too fast. You may be doing this for a number of reasons. You may be letting yourself get too hungry because too much time passes between meals or snacks and then you wolf food down when you finally do get to eat. You may be hurried, anxious, or stressed when you sit down to eat. Slowing down your eating pace can help you eat less and enjoy your food more. Here are some tips for cutting down your eating speed:

- Do not skip meals; avoid becoming overly hungry.

- Make it a game not to be the first person at the table to be finished eating.

- After eating something, if you find yourself saying, "I think that was good—I better have more to make sure," that usually means you aren't paying attention to what you eat. Work on thinking about what you are eating and how you are enjoying it. Practice this without things at the table that divert your attention, such as friends, computer games, your cell phone, or television.

- Take small bites, chew slowly, and be sure to swallow each bite before taking another. Chewing your food well also helps you enjoy your food more and feel better after the meal by lessening heartburn or other digestive upsets.

- Try a relaxation technique about a half hour before you eat. Several methods are discussed in Chapter 12 "Using Your Mind to Manage Symptoms."

"I can't do it on my own."

Losing weight is challenging, and sometimes you just need some outside support and guidance. For help, you can contact any of the following resources:

- A registered dietitian through your health plan, local hospital, or the Academy of Nutrition and Dietetics website, www.eatright.org. This site also provides ratings for many of the smartphone apps offering diet and nutrition information.

- A support group such as Weight Watchers or Take Off Pounds Sensibly (TOPS), where you can meet other people who are trying to lose or maintain a healthy weight. Weight Watchers also has an app for your smartphone.

- A weight loss program offered by your local health department, hospital, health plan, community school, recreational center or YMCA, or employer.

"I've been on a lot of diets before and lost a lot of weight. But I've always gained it back, and then some. It's so frustrating and I just don't understand why this happens!"

This happens to many people. In fact, it is the downside of quick-weight-loss diets, because they typically involve drastic changes. They do not focus on lifelong changes in eating habits, exercise, and lifestyle. Typically, after you have gotten tired of the diet or have reached your goal weight, you return to your old ways, and the weight comes back on. Sometimes you even gain back more weight than you lost.

The key to maintaining a healthy weight is to develop healthy eating and exercise habits that you enjoy, that fit into your lifestyle, and that are part of a lifestyle that you can stick with. We have already given you many tips earlier in this chapter. Here are two more:

- Set a personal weight gain "alarm"—say, a specific number of pounds (kilos) gained (perhaps 3 pounds, or 1–2 kg). If you hit this mark, go back on your regular program. The sooner you start, the faster the newly added pounds will come off.

- Monitor your activity level. Once you have lost some weight, exercise three to five times a week to improve your chances of keeping the weight off. Research suggests that to maintain weight loss, some people should be exercising nearly an hour a day—but no need to fear, this includes normal activities during the day as well as planned physical exercise. Also remember that increasing activity does not just mean exercising longer. It can mean going faster or doing something that is harder to do, such as walking uphill or

swimming with paddles. Your body gets efficient and good at doing the things you have been doing for a while and starts to burn fewer calories when you do them. Changing your exercise routine can prevent this from happening (and keep you from getting bored). Also, for some people, using a journal or an app to record your physical activity and what you eat each day can also be helpful. It keeps you mindful of your habits.

"I do OK keeping weight off for a short time. Then something happens beyond my control, and I stop caring about what I eat. Before I know it, I've slipped back into my old eating habits."

Everyone is going to slip at one time or another; no one is perfect. If it is only a little slip, don't worry about it. Just continue as if nothing happened and get back on your plan. If the slip is bigger, try to figure out why. Is there something that is taking a lot of your attention now? If so, weight management may need to take a backseat for a while. That's okay. The sooner you realize this, the better; just set a date when you will restart your weight management program. You may even want to join a support group and stay with it for at least four to six months. If so, look for a weight loss support group that:

- emphasizes healthy eating.

- emphasizes lifelong changes in eating habits and lifestyle patterns.

- gives support in the form of ongoing meetings or other long-term follow-up.

- does not make miraculous claims or guarantees. (Remember, if something sounds too good to be true, it probably is.)

- does not rely on special meals or supplements.

Managing Specific Eating Challenges with HIV

There are a number of special challenges that are of particular importance for many people with HIV. Let's look at some positive proven suggestions for addressing these issues.

"When I eat, I feel like I'm going to throw up."

An infection or a medication side effect can cause nausea, making foods unappealing. The following suggestions may help:

- Eat smaller, snack-sized meals throughout the day. Nausea is often worse when the stomach is empty

- Drink high-calorie fluids one hour after eating, not during meals.

- Avoid spicy and fatty foods and caffeine. These can irritate the stomach and intestines.

- Eat cold, blander-tasting foods such as ice cream, frozen yogurt, gelatin, pudding or custard, cottage cheese and fruit, juice, cold cereal, or a sandwich. These may be easier to take.

- Try salty or dry foods, such as bread or crackers. These may help calm your stomach.

- Rest between meals, but do not lie down completely flat. Elevate your upper body or sit up for at least two hours after eating.

- If the smell of food bothers you, ask someone else to cook; make sure the cooking area is well ventilated so that food smells don't linger.

- Avoid eating your favorite foods when you feel sick so that you don't start to associate them with nausea and begin to dislike them.

- Drink a cup of herbal tea (chamomile or peppermint) with honey or a piece of fresh ginger, or chew on a small piece of fresh ginger to help settle your stomach.

- If your medication causes nausea, talk to your doctor or a pharmacist about timing your doses so that you take them when eating or right after you eat.

- Ask your doctor about taking taking medication for nausea. If one medication doesn't work, ask for a different one. Take the medication as directed—typically one half hour before meals.

"Diarrhea is a problem for me."

Diarrhea can be caused by many things, including medications, stress, infections, or severe weight loss. Whatever the cause, diarrhea means that your body is not getting the fluids and nutrients it needs from the foods you eat. For this reason, it is critical that you pay attention to your fluid intake to prevent dehydration.

The following tips can help you deal with or lessen your diarrhea:

- Drink high-calorie fluids (at least eight glasses per day), such as juices, clear carbonated beverages, broth, and fruit or sports drinks. Water should not be the only fluid you drink, because it lacks the calories and nutrients your body must replace. Avoid drinks that have caffeine or alcohol; these stimulate the intestines and can cause further dehydration. Drink fluids at room temperature; very hot or cold fluids may stimulate the intestines and make diarrhea worse.

■ Potassium is a vital mineral that is lost when you have diarrhea; this can lead to muscle cramping and fatigue. Replace lost potassium by eating bananas, raisins, sports drinks, fruit juices (especially orange juice and nectars), vegetable juices, mashed potatoes, or canned fruits without seeds or skins.

■ Even if you do not feel like eating much, try not to skip meals. You may be able to tolerate plain white rice, noodles, mashed potatoes, crackers, white toast, eggs, hot cereal, applesauce or other canned fruits without seeds or skins, bananas, gelatin, ice cream, sherbet, or broth-type soups.

■ Avoid greasy or fatty foods with large amounts of butter, margarine, or oils, and foods that are fried.

■ Avoid high-fiber foods as well as ones with skins or seeds; these can be irritating and hard to digest. Avoid raw fruits and vegetables and whole-grain breads or cereals. Low-fiber foods, such as cooked vegetables, canned fruits without skins or seeds, ripe bananas, white rice, and white bread are good choices.

■ Avoid milk and milk products for a while. Drink low-fat milk and eat lean meats if you can tolerate them. Dairy aids containing lactase can help you digest and absorb the milk sugar that sometimes causes problems such as bloating and diarrhea. Stick to plain boiled, baked, or broiled meats, and stay away from fried, spicy foods and spicy sauces.

■ Cramps often accompany diarrhea and can be a sign of gas or air in your intestines. Avoid carbonated beverages that can worsen this problem. Also avoid foods that cause gas, such as raw apples, beans, cabbage, broccoli, cauliflower, onions, green peppers, and beer.

■ Try a tablespoon of Metamucil or other fiber product mixed with juice to help make the stool bulky.

■ Ask your doctor about antidiarrheal medications if your diarrhea increases in frequency or lasts more than a week. Unchecked diarrhea can cause further problems, such as dehydration and potassium loss that must be prevented or corrected.

"What if I am constipated?"

Constipation is often the result of not drinking enough fluids, not eating enough food or fiber, and/or not being physically active. Constipation may also develop as a side effect of certain medications, especially narcotic-based pain medications. In addition to drinking enough fluids, try these suggestions:

■ Eat foods high in insoluble fiber, such as whole-grain breads and cereals, fresh fruits and vegetables, cooked beans and chickpeas, nuts, and seeds.

■ Add small amounts of bran to food or liquids to increase fiber.

■ Include some aerobic exercise in your daily schedule.

■ Ask your doctor about medications to relieve constipation.

"I have trouble digesting fat."

If you need to gain weight, fats are an excellent source of calories, but they can be hard to digest. Fat intolerance—difficulty digesting and absorbing fats—can be a problem for people with HIV. If you experience discomfort after eating foods high in fat, you may need to reduce the amount of fat you eat. It is not a good idea to completely eliminate fat unless you are having prolonged and severe diarrhea. If fat intolerance becomes a chronic problem, avoid all fat-rich foods, such as the ones listed in Table 14.2, "Food Guide for Healthy Meal Planning," on pages 252–259.

If your problem digesting fat is severe, choose nonfat foods that have extra calories and protein. Also, there are some products with a special, easily digestible form of fat that may help keep your calorie intake and weight at appropriate levels.

Some people, particularly people taking ART medications, have lipodystrophy (fatty deposits on their bodies) and high blood cholesterol. If this is true for you, you need to avoid the bad (saturated and trans) fats to lower your blood cholesterol.

"I don't feel well when I eat dairy products."

If you notice that milk, cheese, and ice cream cause cramping, gas, bloating, or diarrhea, you may have lactose intolerance. This means your body has trouble digesting lactose, a type of sugar found in milk and milk products. If your reactions subside with time, you can start eating these dairy foods again. After all, they are good protein and calcium sources.

The following suggestions can help you avoid the more troublesome dairy products and find ones you are able to tolerate:

- Avoid foods containing milk, such as pudding, custard, ice cream, cream soups, cream pies, gravies, and sauces. In place of milk, try nondairy products like enriched soy, rice, almond, or other milk substitutes.

- Buy milk and milk products that contain an enzyme called lactase to help you digest lactose. These items are found in the dairy section of your supermarket. Check the labels carefully.

- Some dairy products contain less lactose and therefore may be easier to tolerate. These include buttermilk, cottage cheese, sour cream, aged cheeses, sherbet, and yogurt.

- Look for kosher foods labeled pareve or parve; they are milk-free.

- Take lactase pills or drops before eating foods with large amounts of lactose. You can buy these over the counter at any drugstore and at many grocery stores.

"My dry mouth and mouth sores make it hard to eat anything."

Your mouth may feel dry as a side effect of some medications or from not drinking enough fluids. Also, infections in your mouth and throat can cause sores that make it painful to eat or swallow. See the information about ways to make foods taste better on pages 269–270. The following tips may also help:

- Avoid smoking and drinking alcohol; these irritate the mouth and throat.

- Choose soft foods that are smooth in consistency and easy to swallow. Blend or puree foods to make swallowing easier. Eat casseroles and stews, or add butter, gravy, sauce, or salad dressing to moisten food. Add liquids to foods or dunk them in soup, milk, juice, or hot chocolate. This makes them less irritating to your mouth and throat.

- Avoid spicy foods, foods with a high acid content (such as orange juice or tomatoes), and carbonated sodas. These can make mouth sores burn. Cold foods, such as ice pops, ice cream, sherbet, frozen yogurt, and thick milk shakes, can numb your mouth and are easy to swallow.

- If you find that you gag easily, avoid sticky foods, such as peanut butter, and slippery foods like gelatin.

- Use a straw for drinking fluids and a cup or glass for eating soup. Tilt your head back to make swallowing easier.

- Try eating soft, bland foods, such as pudding, custard, eggs, canned fruits, cottage cheese, yogurt, bananas, and creamed cereals.

- Avoid foods that require a lot of chewing or are tough and fibrous.

- Suck on sugar-free or sour hard candy and on Popsicles or ice, or chew sugarless gum to stimulate salivation.

- Rinse your mouth frequently and drink lots of fluids to help with dryness. If dryness continues to be a problem even when you moisten your foods, ask your doctor or dentist to prescribe artificial saliva for you.

- Sleep with a humidifier in your room, and keep fluids by your bedside to sip on during the night if you are thirsty.

Food Safety and Preparation Tips

Just as eating well is important, so is protecting yourself from bacteria, viruses, and parasites that can cause food poisoning. People with HIV are more likely than people with strong immune systems to acquire food-borne illnesses that can be hard to treat.

Food poisoning can cause nausea, vomiting, and diarrhea, all of which make you miserable and interfere with your eating. This, in turn, leads to weight loss, further weakens your immune system, and hastens the progression of disease. Although for most people, food poisoning can be treated with rest and plenty of fluids, this is not always true for people with HIV. You may experience more serious and prolonged symptoms that are difficult to treat, which can require a doctor's care.

Because most food contamination results from the improper handling of food, you can protect yourself by following some basic safety guidelines when buying, preparing, serving, and storing foods. The guidelines listed below are also important to keep in mind when eating away from home or traveling abroad.

Precautions When Shopping for Food

- Read food labels carefully. Avoid products that contain raw or undercooked meat and dairy products. Avoid all dairy products that are not pasteurized.

- Check the use-by dates on food packages. Don't buy or use packaged food whose "best if used by . . ." or expiration date has passed.

- Don't buy food with damaged packaging or food that has been handled, stored, or displayed improperly.

- Put packaged meat, poultry, or fish into a plastic bag before placing it in your shopping cart.

- When grocery shopping, select cold and frozen foods last, and ask that cold foods be packed in the same bag.

- Carry a cooler in your car to store the cold and frozen foods if the trip home takes longer than 30 minutes.

- Check your refrigerator regularly and throw away foods whose expiration date has passed.

Proper Food Storage

- Storing foods properly is the key to food safety. Be sure to refrigerate or freeze foods that require cold storage as soon as possible after buying them. The temperature in your refrigerator should be 40°F (–4°C) or lower, and the freezer temperature should be 0°F (–18°C) or lower. Use a refrigerator thermometer to make sure temperatures are in the proper range. See "Lifespan of Refrigerated Products," page 281.

- Label your stored foods with the date of purchase, and follow the recommended storage times for each type of food. Foods that contain harmful bacteria do not always look or smell spoiled. When in doubt, throw it out.

- Always thaw frozen foods in the refrigerator or microwave. Do not allow drippings from defrosting foods (especially meat, poultry, or fish) to touch other foods in the refrigerator. Place them in a separate container on the bottom shelf of the refrigerator to thaw.

- Put leftover prepared foods containing meat, eggs, or milk products in the refrigerator or freezer immediately. Store portions in small containers for easy use later.

- Cover food tightly with plastic wrap or store in airtight containers.

- Don't eat leftovers that have been in the refrigerator for more than two days.

Food Preparation and Cooking

- Always begin by washing your hands with soapy water. Remember to wash your hands again after handling any raw foods and before handling cooked food.

- Use only cutting boards that can be sanitized in the dishwasher for meat, poultry, or fish, or soak the board for ten minutes in a solution of one to two tablespoons of bleach per gallon of warm water.

- Clean all utensils and chipped china or crockery in the dishwasher, or wash them in hot, soapy water (at least 140°F, or 60°C) and rinse them well.

- Clean utensils, countertops, shelves, refrigerator, and freezer with a bleach and warm water solution as an additional safety step.

- Keep towels and sponges clean. Replace sponges often, and use different sponges for washing dishes and for other types of cleaning. Put wet sponges in the microwave oven and heat for two minutes to sanitize.

Lifespan of Refrigerated Products

Stored at 35° to 40°F (1°C to 4°C) Food Product	Use Within
Raw beefsteak and roasts, raw pork chops, raw lamb chops and roasts, cooked ham, lunch meat	3–5 days
Ground beef, turkey, pork, or lamb; sausage	1–2 days
Hot dogs	1 week
Raw chicken or turkey, giblets, fish	1–2 days
Leftover cooked meat and meat dishes; soups and stews	3–4 days
Leftover gravy and meat broth	1–2 days
Leftover cooked poultry and poultry dishes	3–4 days
Leftover cooked poultry covered with broth or gravy; leftover chicken nuggets, patties, or fried chicken	1–2 days
Fresh eggs in the shell	3 weeks
Raw egg yolks or whites (out of the shell)	2–4 days
Hard-cooked eggs	1 week

Meat, poultry, and fish

■ Never eat raw meat, poultry, or fish of any kind. Even steak tartare, carpaccio, raw oysters, raw shrimp, sashimi, or sushi topped with raw fish can cause serious infections.

■ Cook meats and poultry to 165°F (74°C) or higher. Use a meat thermometer to check the temperature.

■ Cook all meats completely. Red meat should be well-done, and poultry should be cooked until the juices are clear.

■ Reheat all leftovers thoroughly before eating, to 165°F (74°C) or higher.

■ When barbecuing, precook meats partially before putting them on the grill to make sure that the inside reaches the proper temperature.

■ Eat meats and meat dishes while they are hot, and store leftovers in the refrigerator immediately. Don't let leftovers sit out at room temperature for more than two hours, or one hour if room temperature is over 90°F (32°C).

Eggs

■ Check at the store to make sure you don't buy eggs with cracked shells. Refrigerate eggs as soon as you get home. Never let eggs or dishes prepared with eggs sit out at room temperature.

■ Don't eat raw eggs or eggs that are soft-boiled or scrambled but runny. Avoid foods prepared with uncooked or undercooked eggs, such as Caesar salad dressing, chocolate mousse, some frostings, homemade eggnog, and homemade mayonnaise. If you eat homemade ice cream, check to see whether raw eggs are an ingredient. If they are, do not eat it.

■ When cooking eggs, make sure the yolk and white are firm. Follow these cooking times and temperatures:

  ♦ Scrambled eggs: Cook for one minute at medium setting (250°F or 121°C for electric frying pans).

- Sunny-side up eggs: Cook for seven minutes (or four minutes if covered) at medium setting.

- Fried, over-easy eggs: Cook for three minutes at medium setting on one side, then for one minute on the other side.

- Poached eggs: Cook for five minutes in boiling water.

- Hard-boiled eggs: Cook for at least seven minutes in boiling water.

■ Use a pasteurized, frozen egg product—not raw eggs—when a recipe for an uncooked dish calls for eggs.

Milk and dairy products

■ Buy only pasteurized milk and dairy products. Read the labels on cheeses, as not all of them are pasteurized.

■ Check the expiration date. Buy products before the expiration date, and use within the next several days.

■ Don't eat soft-ripened cheeses or cheese that has mold on it. Throw away moldy cheese.

Fruits and vegetables

■ Choose fresh fruits and vegetables with unbroken skins.

■ Wash all fruits and vegetables thoroughly and peel those with skin.

■ Avoid fruits and vegetables that are moldy or have soft spots that show signs of rotting or mold.

■ Refrigerate to reduce spoilage.

Eating Out

■ Be sure your eating utensils, place settings, and beverage glasses are clean. Don't be shy about returning dirty utensils or food that is not hot enough or not cooked thoroughly.

■ In a restaurant, avoid eating the same foods that you avoid eating at home.

■ Avoid salad bars. You can't be sure how well the vegetables or fruits have been washed or handled, or how long they have been sitting out. If you are given a choice between salad and soup, choose the soup.

■ Order meats medium-well to well-done. To check doneness, cut into the center of the meat. If it is pink or bloody, it needs to be cooked more. Fish should be flaky, not rubbery, when cut.

■ Order eggs cooked on both sides, and don't eat runny-looking eggs.

■ If you are not sure about the ingredients and preparation of a dish, ask before ordering.

■ Don't eat raw or lightly steamed seafood.

Traveling Abroad

■ Boil all water before drinking.

■ Drink only beverages made with boiled water, and canned or bottled carbonated drinks. Use only ice cubes that have been made from boiled water.

■ Avoid uncooked vegetables and salads.

■ Peel all fruit.

■ Eat cooked foods while they are still hot.

For more detailed information on food safety, check out the U.S. Department of Agriculture's guidelines on Food Safety for People with HIV/AIDS (see "Additional Resources" below).

For people with HIV and other long-term conditions, it can sometimes be challenging to get all the nutrients that are so important to robust health and still enjoy our meals. In this chapter, we have shown you ways to manage these challenges and to make sure you get the nutrition that your body needs. Along with the information in the previous chapter, you now have a custom "menu" of healthy eating practices and ways to prepare tasty, nutritious meals that are a big part of living healthy and well. As we said before, mealtime *can* be one of the best parts of your day!

Additional Resources

Academy of Nutrition and Dietetics: www.eatright.org

AIDS.gov, "Staying Healthy with HIV/AIDS, Nutrition and Food Safety": www.aids.gov/hiv-aids -basics/staying-healthy-with-hiv-aids/taking-care-of-yourself/nutrition-and-food-safety

AIDS Info: https://aidsinfo.nih.gov/guidelines/html/4/adult-and-adolescent-oi-prevention-and -treatment-guidelines/362/appendix-a—preventing-exposure

American Diabetes Association, CreateYourPlate: www.diabetes.org/food-and-fitness and www.diabetes.org/food-and-fitness/food/planning-meals/create-your-plate

The Body—The Complete HIV/AIDS Resource, "Outsmarting HIV with Healthy Eating": www.thebody.com/content/65773/outsmarting-hiv-with-healthy-eating.html

Canadian AIDS Treatment Information Exchange: "A Practical Guide to Nutrition for People Living with HIV": www.catie.ca/en/practical-guides/nutrition

Food and Agriculture Organization of the United Nations, "Living Well with HIV/AIDS— A Manual on Nutritional Care and Support for People Living with HIV/AIDS": www.fao.org/docrep/005/y4168e/y4168e00.HTM

Healthy Weight Network: www.healthyweight.net

NAM AIDSmap, Nutrition: www.aidsmap.com/Nutrition/page/1060877

National Weight Control Registry: www.nwcr.ws

Shape Up America: www.shapeup.org

U.S. Department of Health and Human Services, "Living with HIV/AIDS—Diet, Nutrition, and Food Safety": http://aids.nlm.nih.gov/topic/1141/living-with-hiv-aids/1144/diet,-nutrition,-and-food

U.S. Food and Drug Administration, "Food Safety for People with HIV/AIDS": www.fda.gov/Food/FoodborneIllnessContaminants/PeopleAtRisk/ucm312669.htm

Weight-Control Information Network (WIN): http://win.niddk.nih.gov/index.htm

Weight Watchers: https://welcome.weightwatchers.com

Suggested Further Reading

To learn more about the topics discussed in this chapter, we suggest that you explore the following resources:

Ferguson, James M., and Cassandra Ferguson. *Habits, Not Diets*, 4th ed. Boulder, Colo.: Bull Publishing, 2003.

Hensrud, Donald D., ed. *Mayo Clinic Healthy Weight for Everybody*. Rochester, Minn.: Mayo Clinic Health Foundation, 2005.

Nash, Joyce D. *Maximize Your Body Potential*, 3rd ed. Boulder, Colo.: Bull Publishing, 2003.

Schoonen, Josephine Connolly. *Losing Weight Permanently with the Bull's-Eye Food Guide*. Boulder, Colo.: Bull Publishing, 2004.

Zentner, Ali. *The Weight-Loss Prescription: A Doctor's Plan for Permanent Weight Reduction and Better Health for Life*. Toronto: Penguin Canada, 2013.

CHAPTER 16

Communicating with Family, Friends, and Everyone Else

"You just don't understand!"

HOW OFTEN HAS THIS STATEMENT SUMMED UP a frustrating discussion for you? Whenever you talk with someone, you want the person to understand. And you are frustrated when you feel you have not been understood. Failure to communicate effectively can lead to anger, helplessness, isolation, and depression. Such feelings can be even worse when you have a stigmatizing health problem like HIV. When communication breaks down, symptoms may worsen. Negative feelings such as frustration, depression, and anger can grow stronger, blood sugar and blood pressure levels may rise, and there is increased strain on your heart. Worry caused by conflict and misunderstanding can make you irritable, interfere with concentration, and sometimes lead to accidents. Clearly, poor communication is bad for your physical, mental, and emotional health.

285

Healthy communication is the lifeblood of relationships, and relationships are a lifeline to healthy coping. Poor communication is the biggest reason for bad relationships between spouses or partners or among family members, friends, and coworkers, or between patients and members of their health care team.

Good communication is necessary when you have a long-term condition. Your health care team, in particular, must understand you. And when you don't understand the advice or recommendations from your doctor, the results can be life threatening. As a self-manager, effective communication skills are essential.

In this chapter we discuss tools to improve communication. Specifically, these are tools to help you express your feelings in a positive way, to minimize conflict, to ask for help, and to say no. We also discuss how to listen, how to recognize body language and different styles of communication, how to get more information from others, and how to tell people that you have HIV.

Keep in mind that communication is a two-way street. As uncomfortable as you may feel about expressing your feelings, asking for help, or sharing that you have HIV, chances are that others are also feeling the same way. It may be up to you to make sure the lines of communication are open. Here are two very important keys to better communication to keep in mind as you read the rest of the chapter:

- Do not make assumptions regarding others because you think "they should know." People are not mind readers. If you want to be sure they know something, tell them.

- You cannot change the way others communicate or react to you. What you can do is change your communication to be sure you are understood.

Expressing Your Feelings

When communication is difficult, take the following steps. First, review the situation. Exactly what is bothering you? What are you feeling? It is important to try to express your feelings clearly and positively. Consider the following example, which shows what can happen when people don't express their feelings effectively:

Miguel and Steve had agreed to go to a football game. When Miguel came to pick Steve up, Steve was not ready. In fact, Steve was not sure that it was a good idea to go because he was feeling tired and having trouble getting up and ready. The following conversation took place.

Steve: *You just don't understand. If you had fatigue like I do, you wouldn't be so quick to criticize. You don't think of anyone but yourself.*

Miguel: *Well, I can see that I should just go by myself.*

In this conversation, neither Miguel nor Steve stopped to think about what was really bothering them or how they felt about it. Each blamed the other for an unfortunate situation, and neither one of them expressed their feelings in a clear and positive way.

The following is the same conversation, but with both people using more thoughtful communications:

Miguel: *When we have made plans and then at the last minute you are not sure you can go, I feel frustrated and angry. I don't know what to do—go on without you, change the plan and just stay here with you, or decide to not make future plans.*

Steve: *When this fatigue hits me like this, I am confused too. I keep hoping I can go so I don't call you because I don't want to disappoint you, and I really want to go. I keep hoping that I will feel better as the day wears on.*

Miguel: *I understand.*

Steve: *Let's go to the game. You can let me off at the gate before parking so I won't have to walk as far. Then I can do the steps slowly and be in our seats when you arrive. I really want to go to the game with you. In the future, I will let you know sooner if I'm not feeling up to it.*

Miguel: *Sounds good to me. I really do like your company and knowing how I can help. It is just that being caught by surprise sometimes makes me angry.*

In this dialogue, Miguel and Steve talked about the situation and how they felt about it. They both expressed their feelings and neither blamed the other.

Unfortunately, most people are often in situations where the other person uses blaming communications. For example, a person may not be listening and when they get caught, they blame the other person. Even in this situation, thoughtful communication and expressing your feelings can be helpful. Consider the following example:

Carolyn: *Why do you always spoil my plans? At least you could have called. I am really tired of trying to do anything with you.*

Ayesha: *I understand. When my anxiety acts up at the last minute, I am confused. I keep hoping I can go and so I don't call you because I don't want to disappoint you. I really want to go. I keep hoping that I will feel less anxious as the day wears on.*

Carolyn: *Well, I hope that in the future you will call. I don't like being caught by surprise.*

Ayesha: *I understand. If it is okay with you, let's go shopping now. If I start feeling too anxious, I'll take a break in the coffee shop with my book while you continue to shop. I do want us to keep making plans. In the future, if I am too anxious, I will let you know sooner.*

In this example, only Ayesha is using thoughtful communication and expressing feelings well. Carolyn continues to blame. The outcome, however, is still positive. Both people got what they wanted.

The following are some suggestions for expressing your feelings and using good communications to create supportive relationships:

■ **Show respect.** Always show respect and regard for people when you are communicating with them. Try not to preach or be excessively demanding. Avoid demeaning or blaming comments such as, "Why do you always spoil my plans?" The use of the word *you* is a clue that your communication might be blaming. A bit of tact and courtesy can go a long way in defusing situations (see "Anger" in Chapter 11, "Understanding the Symptom Cycle," pages 158–160.)

- **Be clear.** Describe a specific situation or your observations using the facts. Avoid words like *always* and *never*. In the previous example, Ayesha clearly describes the situation and the emotions it involves by saying, "When anxiety acts up at the last minute, I am confused. I keep hoping I can go and so I don't call you because I don't want to disappoint you. I really want to go. I keep hoping that I will feel better as the day wears on."

- **Don't make assumptions.** Ask for more detail. Carolyn did not do this. She assumed that Ayesha was rude because there was no phone call. It would have been better if Carolyn asked Ayesha why there was no call earlier. Assumptions are the enemy of good communication. Many arguments arise from one person expecting the other person to be a mind reader. One sign that you are making assumptions is thinking, "This person should know . . ." Don't rely on mind reading. Express your own needs and feelings directly and clearly, and ask questions if you don't understand something.

- **Open up.** Express your feelings openly and honestly. Don't make others guess what you

are feeling—chances are they may be off base. Ayesha did the right thing when talking about wanting to go on the outing, not wanting to disappoint Carolyn, and hoping that the anxiety would get better.

- **Accept the feelings of others.** Try to understand them. This is not always easy. Sometimes you need to think about what was said instead of answering at once. You can always stall a bit by saying, "I think I understand" or "I'm not sure I understand; could you explain some more?"

- **Use humor—sparingly.** Sometimes gently introducing a bit of humor works wonders. But don't use sarcasm or demeaning humor, and know when to be serious.

- **Avoid the role of victim.** You become a victim when you do not express your needs and feelings or when you expect that someone else should act in a certain way. Unless you have done something to hurt another person, you should not apologize. Apologizing all the time is a sign that you view yourself as a victim. You deserve respect and you have a right to express your wants and needs.

- **Listen first.** Good communicators are good listeners who seldom interrupt. Wait a few seconds when someone is finished talking before you respond. They may have more to say.

Using "I" Messages

Many people are uncomfortable expressing feelings, especially when it may seem like they are being critical of someone else. When people

feel very emotional, attempts to express frustration can be full of "you" messages. These suggest blame and can cause the other person to feel under attack. Suddenly, the other person is on the defensive, and barriers go up. The situation just escalates from there, leading to anger, frustration, and bad feelings.

"I" statements are direct, assertive expressions of your views and feelings; whereas "you" sentences are accusative and confrontational. For example, "I try very hard to do the best work I can," not "You always criticize me." Or "I appreciate it when you turn down the television while I talk," not "You never pay attention."

Notice that "I feel that you are not treating me fairly" is actually a disguised "you" statement. A true "I" statement you could make in this situation is, "I feel angry and hurt."

The following are some more examples of how you can convert "you" statements into "I" statements:

"You" message: *"Why are you always late? We never get anywhere on time."*

"I" message: *"I get really upset when I'm late. It's important to me to be on time."*

"You" message: *"There's no way you can understand how lousy I feel."*

"I" message: *"I'm not feeling well. I could really use a little help today."*

"You" message: *"You never are interested in sex anymore. I wish you would just try to show some interest."*

"I" message: *"I really miss having sex with you. It's been a while, hasn't it?"*

Watch out for hidden "you" messages. These are "you" messages with "I feel . . ." stuck in front of them. Here's an example:

"You" message: *"You always walk too fast."*

Hidden "you" message: *"I feel angry when you walk so fast."*

"I" message: *"I have a hard time walking fast."*

The trick to successful "I" messages is to avoid the use of the word *you* and instead report your personal feelings using the word *I*. Of course, like any new skill, crafting "I" messages takes practice. Start by really listening, to yourself and to others. (Grocery stores are a good place to here lots of "you" messages as parents talk to their children.) In your head, take some of the "you" messages and turn them into "I" messages. You'll be surprised at how fast "I" messages become a habit. When using "I" statements seems difficult, adopt this format:

"I notice . . ." (state just the facts)

"I think . . ." (state your opinion)

"I feel . . ." (state what you are feeling)

"I want . . ." (state exactly what you'd like the other person to do)

For example, imagine you have made cookies to bring as a gift to a friend. Somebody comes along in the kitchen, sees them on the counter, and takes several of the cookies. You're upset because, with several of the cookies missing, the gift is ruined. You might say to the cookie eater: "I see that you took the cookies I baked for my friend [fact]. I think you should have asked me about it first [opinion]. I'm really upset and disappointed because I can't give them as a gift now [feeling]. I'd like an apology, and I'd like for you to ask me before you eat anything I bake in the future [want]."

There are some "I" message cautions. First, they are not a cure-all for communication problems. Sometimes the listener has to have time to

Exercise: "I" Messages

Change the following statements into "I" messages. (Watch out for hidden "you" messages.)

1. "You expect me to wait on you hand and foot!"

2. "Doctor, you never have enough time for me. You're always in a hurry."

3. "You hardly ever touch me anymore. You haven't paid any attention to me since my heart attack."

4. "Doctor, you didn't tell me the side effects of all these drugs or why I have to take them."

hear them. This is especially true if the person is used to hearing blaming "you" messages. If using "I" messages does not work at first, continue to use them. Things will change as you gain skill and old patterns of communication are broken.

Second, some people use "I" messages as a means of manipulation. They may often express that they are sad, angry, or frustrated in order to gain sympathy from others. If used in this way, interpersonal problems can escalate. Effective "I" messages must report honest feelings.

Finally, note that "I" messages are not just for tense communication; they are also an excellent way to express positive feelings and compliments. For example, "I really appreciate the extra time you gave me today, doctor."

Good communication skills help make life easier for everyone, especially those with long-term health problems. Table 16.1 summarizes some words that can help or hinder this communication.

Table 16.1 **Ensuring Clear Communication**

Words That Aid Understanding	Words That Hinder Understanding
I	You
Right now, at this time, at this point	Never, always, every time, constantly
Who, which, where, when	Obviously . . .
What do you mean, please explain, tell me more, I don't understand	Why?

Minimizing Conflict

In addition to using "I" messages, there are other ways to reduce conflict and improve communication. The following tips can help you minimize conflict when you communicate with the people in your life:

- **Shift the focus.** If a discussion gets off topic and emotions are running high, shift the focus of the conversation. That is, bring the discussion back to the agreed topic. For example, you might say something like, "We're both getting upset now and drifting away from the topic we agreed to discuss." Or "I feel like we are bringing up things other than what we agreed to talk about, and I'm getting upset. Can we discuss these other things later and just talk about what we originally agreed to discuss?"

- **Buy time.** For example, you might say, "I think I understand your concerns, but I need more time to think about it before I can respond." Or "I hear what you are saying, but I am too frustrated to respond now. I need to find out more about this before I can respond."

- **Make sure you understand each other's viewpoints.** Do this by summarizing what you heard and asking for clarification. You can also switch roles. Try arguing the other person's position as thoroughly and thoughtfully as possible. This will help you understand all sides of an issue, as well as convey that you respect and value the other person's point of view. It will also help you develop tolerance and empathy for others.

- **Look for compromise.** You may not always find the perfect solution to a problem or reach complete agreement. Nevertheless, it may be possible to compromise. Find something on which you can both agree. For example, you can do it your way this time and the other person's way the next time. Agree to accept part of what you want and part of what the other person wants. Or decide what you'll do and what the other person will do in return. These are all forms of compromise that can help you through difficult times.

- **Say you're sorry.** We have all said or done things that have, intentionally or unintentionally, hurt others. Many relationships are hurt—sometimes for years—because people have not learned the powerful social skill of apologizing. Often all it takes is a simple, sincere apology to restore a relationship. Rather than a sign of weakness, an apology shows great strength. To be effective, an apology must do all of the following:

  - *Admit the specific mistake and accept responsibility for it.* You must name the offense; no glossing over with just "I'm sorry for what I did." Be specific. You might say, for example, "I'm very sorry that I spoke behind your back." Explain the particular circumstances that led you to do what you did. Don't offer excuses, make light of your behavior, or sidestep responsibility.

  - *Express your feelings.* A genuine, heartfelt apology involves some suffering. Sadness shows that the relationship matters to you.

- *Acknowledge the impact of wrongdoing.* You might say, "I know that I hurt you and that my behavior cost you a lot. For that I am very sorry."

- *Offer to make amends.* Ask what you can do to make the situation better, or volunteer specific suggestions.

Apologizing sincerely is not fun, but it is an act of courage, generosity, and healing. It brings the possibility of a renewed and stronger relationship, and it can also bring you peace within yourself.

Asking for Help

Getting and giving help is a part of life, but it is an aspect of life that can cause many problems. Even though most of us sometimes need help, few of us like to ask for it. We may not want to admit that we are unable to do things for ourselves. We may not want to be a burden on others. As a result, we may hedge or make a very vague request: "I'm sorry to have to ask this . . ." "I know this is asking a lot . . ." "I hate to ask this, but . . ." Hedging tends to put the other person on the defensive: "Gosh, what is the big deal, anyway?" To avoid this response, be specific. A general request can lead to misunderstanding. The person being asked to help may react negatively if the request is not clear. This leads to a further breakdown in communication and no help. A specific request is more likely to have a positive result.

Consider the following example:

General request: *"I know this is the last thing you want to do, but I need help moving. Will you help me?"*

Reaction: *"Uh . . . well . . . I don't know. Um . . . can I get back to you after I check my schedule?" (probably next year!)*

Specific request: *"I'm moving next week, and I'd like to move my books and kitchen stuff ahead of time. Would you mind helping me load and unload the boxes in my car Saturday morning? I think it can be done in one trip."*

Reaction: *"I'm busy Saturday morning, but I could give you a hand Friday night."*

Sometimes you don't want the help that is offered and the challenge isn't asking for help but kindly and politely refusing it. People with health problems sometimes deal with offers of help that are not needed or desired. In most cases, these offers come from important people in your life. These people care for you and genuinely want to help. A well-worded "I" message allows you to decline the help without embarrassing the other person or seeming ungrateful. You could say, for example, "Thank you for being so thoughtful, but today I think I can handle it myself. I hope I can take you up on your offer another time."

Saying No

Let's look at the other side: you are the one being asked for help. It is generally best not to answer a request right away. You may need more information. The example of helping a person move is a good one. "Help me move" can mean anything from moving furniture up stairs to picking up the pizza for the hungry troops. Using communication skills that get at specifics will avoid problems. It is important to understand any request fully before responding. Asking for more information or having the person restate the request will often bring more clarity: "Before I answer . . ." will not only clarify the request but also prevent the person from assuming that you are going to say yes.

If you decide to say no, it is important to acknowledge the importance of the request. In this way, the person will see that you are rejecting the request rather than the person. Your turndown should not be a putdown. For example: "That sounds like a worthwhile project you're doing, but it's beyond what I can do this week." Again, specifics are the key. Try to be clear about the conditions of your refusal: Will you always turn down this request, or is it just that today or this week or right now is a problem? If you are feeling overwhelmed and put upon, being able to say no can be a useful tool. If you simply cannot help the person but would like to help in some other way, you may wish to make a counteroffer, such as, "I won't be able to drive today, but I will next week." But if a request leaves you feeling negative, trust your feelings. Remember, you always have the legitimate right to decline a request, even if it is a reasonable one.

Accepting Help

We often hear "How can I help?" Our answer is often "I don't know" or "Thank you, but I don't need any help." We may say these things but the entire time we are thinking, "If they really care, they should know how to help . . ." Wishing and hoping other people will be able to anticipate your needs is not a positive way to spend your time. Instead, be prepared to accept help when it is offered by having a specific answer. For example, "It would be great if we could go for a walk together once a week" or "Could you please take out the garbage? I can't lift it." Remember that people cannot read your mind; you need to tell them what help you want and thank them for it. Think about how each person can help. If possible, give people a task that they can easily accomplish. You are giving them a gift. People like being helpful and they feel rejected when they cannot assist someone for whom they care. It is also beneficial to be grateful for the help you receive (see "Practicing Gratitude," in Chapter 12, "Using Your Mind to Manage Symptoms").

Listening

Good listening is the counterpart to being able to express your feelings effectively and is another important skill you can practice to improve communications. Most of us are much better at talking than we are at listening. When others talk to us, we are often preparing a response instead of just listening. There are several steps to being a good listener:

1. **Listen to the words and tone of voice, and observe body language** (see page 296). There may be times when the words being used don't tell the whole story. Is the voice wavering? Is the speaker struggling to find the right words? Do you notice body tension? Does the person seem distracted? Do you hear sarcasm? What is the facial expression? If you pick up on some of these signs, the speaker probably has more on their mind.

2. **Let people know that you heard what they said.** This may be a simple "uh-huh." Many times the only thing the other person wants is acknowledgment or just someone to listen. Sometimes it is helpful simply to talk to a sympathetic listener.

3. **Let the person know you heard both the content and the emotion behind the words.** You can do this by restating the content. For example, "Sounds like you are planning a nice trip." Or you can respond by acknowledging the emotions: "That must be difficult" or "How sad you must feel." When you respond on an emotional level, the results are often startling. These responses tend to open the gates for more expression of feelings and thoughts. Responding to either the content or the emotion can help communication. It discourages the other person from simply repeating what has been said. But don't try to talk people out of their feelings. They are real to them. Just listen and reflect.

4. **Respond by seeking more information** (see below). This is especially important if you are not completely clear about what was said or what is wanted.

Getting More Information

Getting more information is a bit of an art. It can involve both simple and more complicated techniques.

The simplest way to get more information is to ask. "Tell me more" will probably get you more, as will "I don't understand; please explain," "I would like to know more about . . . ," "Would you say that another way?" "How do you mean?"

"I'm not sure I got that," and "Could you expand on that?"

Paraphrasing

Another way to find out additional information is to paraphrase, or repeat what you heard in your own words. This is a good tool if you want to make sure you understand what the other person meant (the actual meaning behind what they said). Paraphrasing can either help or hinder effective communication. This depends on the way you word the paraphrase. It is important to remember to paraphrase in the form of a question, not a statement. For example, imagine someone says:

"I don't know. I'm really not feeling great. This party will be crowded, there'll probably be smokers, and I really don't know the hosts very well."

A provocative paraphrase would be:

"Obviously, you're telling me you don't want to go to the party."

This response might provoke an angry response such as "No, I didn't say that! If you're going to be that way, I'll stay home for sure." Or the response might be no response—a total shutdown because of either anger or despair ("Shane just doesn't understand"). People don't like to be told what they meant.

Here's a better paraphrase, expressed as a question:

"Are you saying that you'd rather stay home than go to the party?"

The response to this paraphrase might be:

"That's not what I meant. I'm just feeling a little nervous about meeting new people. I'd appreciate it if you'd stay near me during the party. I'd feel better about it, and I might have a good time."

As you can see, the second paraphrase helps communication. The paraphraser discovers the real reason the speaker is expressing doubt about the party. In short, you get more information when you paraphrase with questions.

Asking for Specifics

When you are asking for more information, it helps to be specific. If you want specific information, you must ask specific questions. People often speak in generalities. For example:

Doctor: *"How have you been feeling?"*

Patient: *"Not so good."*

The doctor has not gotten much information. "Not so good" isn't very useful. The following example shows how the doctor gets more information:

Doctor: *"Are you still having those sharp pains in your feet?"*

Patient: *"Yes. A lot."*

Doctor: *"How often?"*

Patient: *"A couple of times a day."*

Doctor: *"How long do they last?"*

Patient: *"A long time."*

Doctor: *"About how many minutes would you say?"*

. . . and so on.

Health care providers are trained to get specific information from patients, although they sometimes ask general questions. Most of us are not trained to do this, but we can learn to ask specific questions. Simply asking for specifics often works: "Can you be more specific about . . . ?" "Are you thinking of something special?"

Avoid asking, "Why?" This is far too general a question. "Why?" makes a person think in terms of cause and effect and can put them on the defensive. A person may respond at an entirely different level than you had in mind.

Most of us have had the experience of being with a three-year-old who just keeps asking "Why?" over and over again. This goes on until the child gets the wanted information (or the person being questioned runs from the room, screaming). The poor adult doesn't have the faintest idea what the child has in mind, so they answer "Because . . ." in an increasingly specific order until the child's question is answered. Sometimes, however, the adult's answers are very different from what the child really wants to know, and in these situations children never get the information they were seeking. Rather than using *why*, begin your responses with *who*,

which, *when*, *where*, or *what*. These words promote a specific response.

We should point out that sometimes we do not get the correct information because we do not know what question to ask. For example, you may be seeking legal services from a senior center. You call and ask if there is a lawyer on staff and hang up when the answer is no. If instead you had asked where you might get low-cost legal advice, you might have gotten some referrals. Thinking carefully about what information you want and the best way to ask for it is an important step in communication.

Understanding Body Language and Conversational Styles

Part of listening to what others are saying includes observing how they are saying it. Even when we say nothing, our bodies are talking; sometimes they are even shouting. Research shows that our body language is more than half of what we communicate. If we want to communicate really well, we must be aware of body language, facial expressions, and tone of voice. These should match what we say in words. If we do not do this, we are sending mixed messages and creating misunderstandings. For example, if you want to make a firm statement, look at the other person, and keep your expression friendly. Stand tall and confident, relax your legs and arms, and breathe. You may even lean forward to show your interest. Try not to roll your eyes or bite your lips; this might indicate discomfort or doubt. Don't move away or

slouch, as these communicate disinterest and uncertainty.

When you notice that the body language and words of others do not match, gently point this out. Ask for clarification. For example, you might say, "Dear, I hear you saying that you would like to go with me to the family picnic, but you look tired and you're yawning as you speak. Would you rather stay home and rest while I go alone?"

In addition to reading people's body language, it is helpful to recognize and appreciate that we all express ourselves differently. Our conversational styles vary according to where we were born, how we were raised, our occupations, our cultural backgrounds, and especially our genders.

For example, some people tend to ask questions that are more personal. These show interest and help form relationships. Other people are more likely to offer opinions or suggestions and to state facts. They tend to discuss problems just to find solutions, whereas some other people want to share their feelings and experiences.

No one style is better or worse; they're just different. By acknowledging and accepting these differences, we can reduce some of the misunderstanding, frustration, and resentment we feel in our communications with others.

Telling Others You Have HIV: Disclosure

Telling others you have HIV is probably one of the most important and difficult life decisions you will have to make. Sharing something this private is a daunting experience, but it can also be liberating. You will no longer have to worry about keeping it secret, and the experience can bring you closer to others. The decision you make about whom to tell is a personal choice. (In many states and countries, however, people with HIV do have the legal duty to disclose their status to any past, present, and potential sex partners. This is necessary to help with early detection and treatment, as well as to prevent the spread of infection. In addition, some states require disclosure to doctors and dentists.) While there is no absolute or best way to disclose your HIV status, the communication skills presented in this chapter, as well as the decision-making, action-planning, and problem-solving tools discussed in Chapter 2, "Becoming an HIV Self-Manager," can help you with this process. The following additional suggestions may also be helpful:

■ **Take your time to decide whom to tell— weigh the pros and cons.** Be selective, and remember you do not have to tell everyone you encounter. You might start by telling people in order of their closeness to you. Think about *whom* you really need to tell, *what* (or *how much*) you want to share with

each person, *when and where* you should have this conversation, and *why* you feel the need to tell this person. Answers to these questions will vary depending on whom you decide to tell, and can help you determine if and when you tell each person in your life. For example, you want to inform a spouse or partner if they are at risk and should be tested, but you also want to tell them because you need to ask for their emotional support. Your primary care physician will know your status, but you may also choose to tell your other health care providers so you can get the best treatment and care from them. It is important to know that your employer does not need to know unless your HIV status affects your current ability to perform your job. See "Making Decisions: Weighing the Pros and Cons" in Chapter 2, "Becoming an HIV Self-Manager," for some tips on making important choices.

■ **Prepare and think ahead about what you are going to say.** Do some research so you feel confident enough to explain HIV to someone who may not know much about it. Also, be clear in your mind about what you want this person to know about you. For example, what you choose to tell a relative or friend is different from what you tell an employer. Keep it simple; you do not need to share your life story. You may want to bring printed information from a reputable website, pamphlets from your doctor's office, or a hotline number for them to get more information (see "Additional Resources" at the end of this chapter).

- **Choose your time and place.** Share this information in person, not on the phone or via e-mail. Find a safe and calm place where both of you can focus on the conversation. If people have lots of questions, answer what you can, but also provide them with a few pamphlets about HIV or a hotline number.

- **Expect and accept that not everyone's reaction to your news will be positive or helpful.** Some people may be shocked or overwhelmed and will not know what to say. Others may be angry and say or do hurtful things. (If you anticipate that someone may react with physical violence, plan ahead about how you will handle it. For example, take someone with you, or leave and call 911 for help immediately.) You cannot control how others feel or how they respond. All you can do is give each

person time to process the information. But, whether peoples' reactions are negative or positive, remember their first reactions will probably not be their last. People's feelings often change with time.

- **Trust your instincts.** If you are not ready to tell close friends, family members, or others about your HIV status yet, it is okay. But be sure to take steps to protect yourself and others (practice safer sex, don't share needles, etc.) to prevent new infections or reinfections. In many places there are laws about disclosing your HIV status to sexual partners and health care providers. Ask a social worker or case manager at your HIV clinic about pertinent laws. Also, try not to isolate yourself by keeping your status a secret from everyone you encounter. Rather, look for support through organized groups for people with HIV, or call an HIV hotline. Hopefully, with their support and by sharing their disclosure experiences, they can help you find the words and courage to tell others over time. Some useful resources related to disclosure are listed in the "Additional Resources" section that follows.

Suggested Further Reading

To learn more about the topics discussed in this chapter, we suggest that you explore the following resources:

Beck, Aaron T. *Love Is Never Enough: How Couples Can Overcome Misunderstandings, Resolve Conflicts, and Solve Relationship Problems Through Cognitive Therapy*. New York: HarperCollins, 1989.

Davis, Martha, Kim Paleg, and Patrick Fanning. *The Messages Workbook: Powerful Strategies for Effective Communication at Work and Home*. Oakland, Calif.: New Harbinger, 2004.

Additional Resources

AIDS.gov: https://aids.gov/hiv-aids-basics

AIDSMap: www.aidsmap.com/Disclosing-HIV-status-at-work/page/1497956

AIDSmeds: www.aidsmeds.com/articles/disclosure_7568.shtml

American with Disabilities Act: 1-800-669-4000 for employment information and 1-800-514-0301 for questions about workplace discrimination

The Body—The Complete HIV/AIDS Resource: www.thebody.com/content/art32375.html

Gay Men's Health Crisis (GMHC): www.gmhc.org or 1-800-243-7692.

Lambda Legal: www.lambdalegal.org

National AIDS Hotline: 1-800-232-4636 (English and Spanish)

Positive Women's Network: www.pwn.bc.ca/hiv-community/disclosing-your-hiv-status

Donoghue, Paul J., and Mary E. Siegel. *Are You Really Listening? Keys to Successful Communication.* Notre Dame, IN: Sorin Books, 2005.

Donoghue, Paul J., and Mary E. Siegel. *We Really Need to Talk: Steps to Better Communication.* Notre Dame, IN: Sorin Books, 2010.

Gottman, John M., and Joan DeClaire. *The Relationship Cure: A 5-Step Guide to Strengthening Your Marriage, Family, and Friendships.* New York: Three Rivers, 2001.

Gottman, John M., and Nan Silver. *The Seven Principles for Making Marriage Work: A Practical Guide from the Country's Foremost Relationship Expert.* New York: Harmony Books, 2015.

Hendrix, Harville. *Getting the Love You Want: A Guide for Couples* (20th anniversary edition). New York: Henry Holt, 2008.

McKay, Matthew, Martha Davis, and Patrick Fanning. *Messages: The Communication Skills Book.* Oakland, Calif.: New Harbinger, 2009.

Nichols, Michael P. *The Lost Art of Listening: How Learning to Listen Can Improve Relationships*, 2nd ed. New York: Guilford Press, 2009.

Robinson, Jonathan. *Communication Miracles for Couples: Easy and Effective Tools to Create More Love and Less Conflict.* San Francisco: Conari Press, 2012.

Tannen, Deborah. *You Just Don't Understand: Women and Men in Conversation.* New York: HarperCollins, 2001.

CHAPTER 17

Planning for the Future: Fears and Reality

PEOPLE LIVING WITH HIV often worry about what will happen to them if their disease becomes truly disabling. If HIV is not their most serious or their only health problem, other conditions can cause worry and concerns about the future. People fear that at some time in the future they may have problems managing their lives and their illnesses.

One way people can deal with fears of the future is to take control and plan for it. You may never need to put your plans into effect, but there is reassurance in knowing that you will be in control if the events you fear happen. In this chapter, we examine the most common concerns people with chronic illnesses have and offer some suggestions that may be useful. These suggestions are not necessarily related to HIV, but to any chronic health problem. Please note that the services described in this chapter apply to the United States. Check with an HIV organization in your own country for information on similar services.

What If I Can't Take Care of Myself Anymore?

Regardless of our state of health, most of us fear becoming helpless and dependent. But this fear is even greater among people with potentially disabling health problems. And it usually has physical as well as financial, social, and emotional components.

Physical Concerns of Day-to-Day Living

As your health changes, you may need to consider changing your living situation. This may involve getting help from friends or family, hiring someone to help you in your home, or moving to a place where more help is provided. How you make this decision depends on your needs and how they can best be met. Keep in mind that when we say needs, we are talking about physical, social, and emotional needs. All must be considered.

Start by evaluating what you can do for yourself and which activities of daily living (ADLs) require some kind of help. ADLs are everyday things such as getting out of bed, bathing, dressing, preparing and eating meals, cleaning house, shopping, and paying bills. Most people can do all of these things, even though they may have to do them slowly, with some modification, or with some help from gadgets or assistive devices.

Some people, though, may eventually find one or more of these tasks no longer possible without help from somebody else. For example, you may still be able to fix meals but no longer be able to do the shopping. Or, if you have problems with fainting or sudden bouts of unconsciousness, you might need to have somebody around at all times. You may also find that some

things that you enjoyed in the past, such as gardening, are no longer pleasurable.

Problem Solving about Your Living Situation

Using the problem-solving steps discussed in Chapter 2, "Becoming an HIV Self-Manager," analyze and make a list of what your potential problems might be. Once you have this list, solve the problems one at a time, first writing down every solution you can think of. For example:

Can't go shopping

- Get a friend to shop for me.
- Find a volunteer shopping service.
- Shop at a store that delivers.
- Use the Internet to order just about anything, from groceries to clothing to electronics.
- Get home-delivered meals.

Can't be by myself

- Hire an around-the-clock attendant.
- Move in with a friend or relative.
- Get an emergency response system such as Lifeline, Alert1, or LifeAlert.
- Move to a board-and-care home.
- Move to a retirement community.

Sometimes a social worker, occupational therapist, or visiting nurse can help you identify problems as well as resources and solutions. When you have listed your problems and the possible solutions to those problems, select the solution that seems the most workable, acceptable, and within your financial means. Review "Steps in Problem Solving" (page 21); this is step 3—pick an idea to try.

Your selection will depend on your finances, the family or other resources you have, and how well the potential solutions will solve your problem. Sometimes one solution will be the answer for several problems. For instance, if you can't shop, can't be alone, and household chores are becoming increasingly difficult, you might consider moving into a retirement community that will solve all of these problems. In this case, you'd look for a home that offers meals, regular house cleaning, and transportation for errands and medical appointments.

Even if you are not of retirement age, many facilities accept younger people, depending on the facility's particular policies. Some facilities take residents at age 50 or younger if another member of the household is the minimum age. If you are a young person, the local center for people with disabilities or "independent living center" should be able to direct you to an out-of-home care facility appropriate for you. When looking at your options, consider the levels of care that are offered. These usually include independent living, where you have your own apartment or small house; assisted living, where you get some help with dressing, taking medications, and other tasks; and skilled nursing, which includes help with all ADLs and some medical care.

It may help to discuss your wishes, abilities, and limitations with a trusted friend, relative, or social worker. Sometimes another person can spot things we ourselves overlook or would like to ignore. A good self-manager often makes use of other resources, which is step 6 in the problem-solving steps in Chapter 2, "Becoming an HIV Self-Manager."

Exploring Care Options

Make changes in your life slowly, one step at a time. You don't need to change your whole life to solve one problem. Remember that you can always change your mind. If possible, try not to burn your bridges behind you. If you think that moving out of your own place to another living arrangement (relatives, care home, or elsewhere) is the thing to do, don't give up your present home until you are settled in your new home and are sure you want to stay there.

If you think you need help, hiring someone to help you at your present home is easier to try out and reverse than moving into a new place. If you can't be alone and you live with a family member who is away from home during the day, consider an adult or senior day care center. In fact, adult day care centers can be ideal places to make new friends and participate in activities geared to your abilities.

A social worker at your HIV clinic or service organization, local senior center, or center for people with disabilities can be very helpful in providing information about resources in your community. This person can also give you ideas about how to deal with your care needs. There are several kinds of professionals who can be of great help. Social workers are good for helping you decide how to solve financial and housing problems and locating appropriate community resources. Some social workers are also trained in counseling emotional and relationship problems that may be associated with your health problem.

An occupational therapist (OT) can assess your daily living needs and suggest assistive devices or rearrangements in and around your home to make life easier. OTs can also help you figure out how to keep doing pleasurable activities that are limited because of disability. Physical therapists (PTs) can also be helpful in designing safe and easier ways for you to move about inside and outside your home.

No matter with whom you work, it is very important that you are honest with this person. If you have concerns about your ability to care for yourself, say so. Be specific about the nature and scope of your problems. Solutions are almost always available, but people can help you find a solution only if you share your concerns.

Finding In-Home Care

If you find that you cannot manage alone, the first option usually is to hire somebody to help. Many people just initially need a home aide or someone with a similar title and job description. These are people who do not provide medically related services that require special licensing but do help with bathing, dressing, meal preparation, and household chores.

Home Health Care Agencies

There are a number of ways to find somebody to help you in your own home. The easiest, but most expensive, is to hire someone through a home care agency, usually listed under "home care" or "home nursing" online or in the phone book. These agencies are usually (but not always) private, for-profit businesses that supply caregiver staff to individuals at home. Fees vary by region and with the skill and license of the caregiver, but they are usually about double what you would expect to pay for someone you hire directly without the help of an agency (which has to cover taxes, insurance, bonding, and profit for the agency). The advantage, if you can afford it, is that the agency assumes all payroll responsibilities, including Social Security and federal and state taxes, as well as responsibility for the skill and integrity of the attendant, and can replace an ill or no-show attendant right away. The agency pays the staff directly. As the client, you pay the agency and have no involvement with paying the attendant.

Other types of agencies act as referral services. They maintain lists of prescreened caregivers and you select the one you wish to hire from their lists. The agency will charge a "placement fee," usually equal to one month's pay of the person hired. The agency assumes no liability for the skill or honesty of these people, and it will be necessary to check references and to interview carefully, just as you would for someone from any other source. You can find agencies in resource directories under the listing for "home nursing agencies" or "home nursing registries." Some agencies provide both their own staff and registries of other staff for you to select from.

Registered nurses (RNs) hired this way are expensive, but it is rare that home care for a chronically ill person requires a registered nurse. Licensed vocational nurses (LVNs) cost less but are still expensive. LVNs are also usually not needed unless nursing services (such as dressing changes, injections, or ventilator management) are required. Certified nursing assistants (CNAs) have some basic training in nursing, are much less expensive, and can provide satisfactory care for all but the most critically ill person at home. In some cases, Medicare or Medicaid may cover some of the expense.

Most agencies supply home aides as well as the licensed staff we just listed. Unless you are very ill and must stay in bed or require some procedure that must be done by someone with a certain category of medical license, a home aide will most likely be the most appropriate choice for your needs.

Other Resources for Home Health Care

Other resources that may provide help at home include senior centers and centers serving the disabled. They often have lists of people who have called them to say they are seeking work as a home attendant or who have posted a notice on a bulletin board there. These job seekers are not screened and must be interviewed carefully and have their references checked before they start on the job.

Many experienced home care attendants use the local newspaper's classified "employment wanted" section to find new jobs. They may also advertise online at websites such as Monster.com, Craigslist, or other job search sites. Home attendant jobs tend to be temporary because clients usually progress to a need for more or sometimes less care than the attendant provides, so the attendant must then look for a new job. Again, you can find a competent helper through the newspaper or on the Internet, but take to heart our advice to interview carefully when following this route.

Probably the best source of help is word of mouth—a recommendation from someone who has employed a person or knows of a person who has worked for a friend or relative. Putting the word out through your family and social network may give you some good leads.

Home sharing may be an option if you have space and could offer a home to someone in exchange for help. This works best if the help you need consists mainly of household and garden chores. Some people may be willing to provide personal care, such as assistance with dressing, bathing, and meal preparation. Some communities have agencies or government bureaus that help match up home sharers and home seekers.

It is important to know that every county in the United States has an Area Agency on Aging. You can find yours in the phone book or online. These are excellent agencies to call when you are looking for assistance with finding the right type of home care for your needs.

Finding Out-of-Home Care

If you are considering moving out of your home, you have several options to find the lifestyle and level of care you need.

Retirement communities

The person who needs very little personal care but recognizes the need to live in a more protected setting, with security, emergency response services, and so on, and who is older (usually over 50), may wish to consider a retirement community. These may be owned units, rental units, or so-called life care facilities. The life care facility requires a substantial advance payment (called an endowment, an accommodation fee, or something similar), plus a monthly charge that covers living space, services, and in some cases personal or nursing care when or if the need for that arises.

Some facilities are subsidized by the federal government for lower-income clients. The criteria for what constitutes "low income" are determined by the rules governing the federal subsidy that finances the organization. Don't assume that you will not qualify for these subsidies because of income. Qualification depends on the community in which you live and other factors. It can't hurt to ask.

There are almost always waiting lists for retirement communities, even before they are built and ready for occupancy. If you think such a place would be right for you, add your name to the waiting list right away, or at least a couple of years before you think you want to move. You can always change your mind or decline if you are not ready when a space is available for you. To locate a facility in your area, call your senior center or go to the library or the Internet and consult the directory of LeadingAge (formerly the American Association of Homes and Services for the Aging). Your reference librarian should be able to help you find this publication. If you have friends living in nearby retirement communities, ask to be invited for a visit and a meal. In this way you can get an inside view of the facilities. Some communities have guest accommodations where you can arrange to stay for a night or two before you commit to a lease or contract.

Residential Care Homes

Residential care homes, also known as board-and-care homes, are licensed by a state or county social services agency. They provide nonmedical care and supervision for individuals who cannot live alone. The smaller homes have about six residents, who live in a family-like setting in a neighborhood residence. The large ones have more residents, sometimes hundreds, who live in a boardinghouse or hotel-like setting. They take meals in a central dining room and have individual or shared rooms, with activities conducted in large common rooms.

In either type of facility, the services for the residents are the same: all meals, assistance with bathing and dressing as needed, laundry, housekeeping, transportation to medical appointments, supervision, and assistance with taking medications. The larger facilities usually have professional activities directors. Residents of the larger facilities usually need to be more independent because they do not receive as much personal attention as in the smaller homes.

These homes are licensed in most states for either "elderly" (over 62) or "adult" (under 62). The adult category is further divided into facilities for the mentally ill, the developmentally delayed, and the physically disabled.

It is important when considering a residential care home to evaluate the type of residents already living there to make sure you will fit in with them. For example, some of these facilities may cater to individuals who are mentally confused. If you are mentally clear, you would not find much companionship there. Similarly, if everybody is hard of hearing, you might have trouble finding somebody to talk to.

Although all homes are required by law to provide wholesome meals, you should make sure the cuisine is to your liking and can meet your dietary needs. If you need a salt-free or diabetic diet, for instance, be sure the operator is willing to prepare your special meals.

The monthly fees for residential care homes vary, depending on whether they are basic or luxurious. The most basic facilities cost about the same as the government Supplemental Security Income (SSI) benefit and will accept SSI beneficiaries, billing the government directly. The more luxurious the home is with respect to furnishings, neighborhood, services, and so on, the higher the cost. However, even the nicest residential care homes typically cost less than full-time, 24-hour, 7-days-a-week at-home care.

Skilled Nursing Facilities

Sometimes called a "nursing home" or "convalescent hospital," the skilled nursing facility provides the most comprehensive care for people who are severely ill or disabled. Typically, a person who has had a stroke or a hip or knee replacement will be transferred from the acute care hospital to a skilled nursing facility for a period of rehabilitation before going home. Recent studies have shown that almost half of all people over 65 will spend some time in a nursing home, many of them only for a short time. No care situation seems to inspire more fear than the prospect of having to go to a nursing home. Horror stories in the news media help foster anxiety about the awful fate that will befall anyone who has the misfortune to have to go there. But it must be remembered that nursing homes serve a critical need. When one really needs a nursing home, usually no other care situation will do.

Public scrutiny is valuable in helping ensure that standards of care and humane and competent treatment are provided. In fact, each nursing home is required by law to post in a prominent place the name and phone number of the "ombudsman," a person assigned by the state licensing agency to assist patients and their families with problems related to their nursing

home care. Fortunately, many facilities provide excellent care in safe, welcoming environments.

Skilled nursing facilities provide medical care for people who can no longer function without such care. This means that they may take medications that are administered by injection or intravenously or need to be monitored by professional nursing staff. A nursing home patient is usually very physically limited and needs help getting in and out of bed, eating, bathing, or dealing with bladder or bowel control. Skilled nursing facilities can also manage the care of feeding tubes, respirators, and other high-tech equipment.

For people who are partially or temporarily disabled, skilled nursing facilities also may provide physical, occupational, and speech therapy, wound care, and other services. Not all nursing homes provide all types of care. Some specialize in rehabilitation and therapies, and others specialize in long-term custodial care. Some are able to provide high-tech nursing services, and others do not.

In selecting a nursing home, seek out the help of the hospital discharge planner, a social worker, or a similar professional from a home care agency or center for seniors or the disabled. They should be able to point you to organizations that monitor and often rate local nursing homes. You can also look under "social service organizations" in the Yellow Pages or online for agencies that can help you with this, or contact the Area Agency on Aging in your county. If possible, have family or friends visit several facilities and make recommendations. They know you well and may be able to tell right away which nursing facility will best fit your needs.

Will I Have Enough Money to Pay for My Care?

After the fear of physical dependence, the next fear on many peoples' lists is not having enough money to pay for their needs. Being sick often requires expensive care and treatment. If you are too ill or disabled to work, the loss of income, and especially the loss of your health insurance coverage, may present an overwhelming financial problem. You can, however, avoid some of the risks by planning ahead and knowing your resources.

Health insurance and Medicare may meet only a part of the ultimate cost of your care. There are many needs that Medicare does not meet at all, and most private "Medigap" insurance policies cover only the 20 percent that Medicare does not cover. For example, do not count on Medicare to pay for skilled nursing facilities. It usually has very limited or no coverage.

Supplemental insurance policies offer the kind of coverage that provides for care needs that Medicare and Medigap insurance do not cover. Due to the Affordable Care Act, you cannot be turned down for insurance because of preexisting conditions. If you are considering long-term care insurance, be sure that the policy covers care at a realistic rate for your community.

If you are too sick to work—either permanently or for some extended period—you may be entitled to draw Social Security on the basis of your disability. If you have dependent children, they also receive benefits. If you have been disabled for a specified period (as of this writing, it is two years), you may be entitled to Medicare coverage for your medical treatment needs. Disability payments are based only on disability, not on need.

If you have minimal savings and little or no income, there are federal and state programs for medical treatment and long-term skilled or custodial care. The eligibility rules and what is covered differs from state to state. Consult your local social services department to see if you are entitled to benefits. If Social Security benefits are unavailable or insufficient, the Supplemental Security Income (SSI) program is available to individuals who meet the eligibility criteria for Medicaid.

The social services department in a hospital where you have obtained treatment can advise you about your own situation and the probability of your being eligible for these programs. The local agency serving the disabled usually has advisers who can refer you to programs and resources for which you may be eligible. Senior centers often have counselors knowledgeable about health care insurance.

If you own a home, you may be able to get a reverse mortgage, whereby the bank pays you a monthly amount based on the value of your home. A reverse mortgage is a loan that lets older people tap the equity they have built up in their homes. Usually you must be at least 62 to qualify. The nice thing is that no matter how long you live, you can never be thrown out of your home because no principal or interest payments are due until the borrower dies or moves out of the house. Reverse mortgages are not for everyone, and they are complex, so be sure to look closely at the details of any financial transaction you enter into, and get friends and family advice if you need it. If possible, it's always a good idea to have the contract reviewed by an attorney.

I Need Help but Don't Want Help—Now What?

Let's talk about the emotional aspects of needing help. We all value our independence. Nearly everyone emerges from childhood reaching for and cherishing every possible sign of independence—the driver's license, the first job, the first credit card, the first time we go out and don't have to tell anybody where we are going or when we will be back, and so on. In these and many other ways, we demonstrate to ourselves as well as to others that we are "grown up"—in charge of our lives and able to take care of ourselves without any help from parents.

If a time comes when we must face the realization that we can no longer manage completely on our own, it may seem like a return to childhood and having to let somebody else be in charge of our lives. This can be very painful and embarrassing.

Some people in this situation become extremely depressed and can no longer find any joy in life. Others fight off the recognition of their need for help, placing themselves in possible danger and making life difficult and frustrating for those who would like to be helpful. Still others give up completely and expect others to take total responsibility for their lives, demanding attention and services from their children or other family members. If you are having one or more of these reactions, you can help yourself feel better and develop a more positive response.

The concept of "changing the things I can change, accepting the things I cannot change, and being able to know the difference" is fundamental to being able to stay in charge of your life. You must be able to evaluate your situation accurately and honestly. You must identify the activities that require the help of somebody else (going shopping and cleaning house, for instance) and those that you can still do on your own (getting dressed, paying bills, writing letters). Another way to look at this is that you are getting help from others for the things you least like to do. This gives you the time and energy to do the things you want to do.

This means making decisions, and as long as you are making the decisions, you are in charge. It is important to make decisions and take action while you are still able to do so, before circumstances intervene and decisions get made for you. That means being realistic and honest with yourself. Decision-making tools can be found in Chapter 2, "Becoming an HIV Self-Manager," on pages 22–23 and 31.

Some people find it comforting and helpful to talk with a sympathetic listener, either a professional counselor or a sensible close friend or family member. An objective listener can often point out alternatives and options you may not have known about or had overlooked. The person can provide additional information or contribute another point of view or interpretation of a situation. Listening to the opinions of others can be an important part of the self-management process.

Be very careful, however, in evaluating advice from somebody who has something to sell you. There are many people whose solution to your problem just happens to be whatever it is they are selling—health or burial insurance policies, annuities, special and expensive furniture, "sunshine cruises," special magazines, or foods with magical curative properties.

In talking with family members or friends who offer to be helpful, be as open and reasonable as you can be. At the same time, try to make them understand that you reserve for yourself the right to decide how much and what kind of help you will accept. They will probably be more cooperative and understanding if you can say, "Yes, I do need some help with _____, but I still want to do _____ myself." More tips on asking for help can be found in Chapter 16, "Communicating with Family, Friends, and Everyone Else."

No matter who you speak with, lay the ground rules early on. Insist on being actively involved. Ask to be presented with choices so that *you* can decide what is best for you. If you try to objectively weigh the suggestions made to you and not dismiss every option out of hand, people will consider you able to make reasonable decisions and will continue to give you the opportunity to do so.

Be appreciative. Recognize the goodwill and efforts of people who want to help. Even though you may be embarrassed, maintain your dignity by accepting with grace the help that is offered if you need it. If you are truly convinced you are being offered help you don't need, decline it with tact and appreciation. For example, you can say, "I appreciate your offer to have Thanksgiving at your house, but I'd like to continue having it here. I could really use some help, though—maybe with the cleanup after dinner."

If you are unable to come to terms with your increasing dependence on others, consult a professional counselor. This should be someone who has experience with the emotional and social issues of people with disabling health

problems. Your local HIV agency can refer you to the right kind of counselor. The local or national organization dedicated to serving people with your specific health condition (Project Inform, the Well Project, AIDS.gov, American Lung Association, American Heart Association, American Diabetes Association, etc.) can also direct you to support groups and classes to help you in dealing with your condition. Locate the agency you need through the resource directories under the listing "social service organizations," or see "Additional Resources" at the end of this chapter. AIDS.gov, for example, has an interactive map that can help you find local resources in the United States.

Similar to the fear and embarrassment of becoming physically dependent is the fear of being abandoned by family members who would be expected to provide needed help. Many people are haunted by tales of being "dumped" in a nursing home by family who never come to visit. They worry that this may happen to them.

We need to be sure that we do reach out to family and friends and ask for the help we need when we recognize that we can't go on alone. It sometimes happens that fearing rejection, people fail to ask for help. Some people try to hide their need because they are worried that their need will cause loved ones to withdraw. Families often complain "If we'd only known . . ." when it is revealed that a loved one had unmet needs.

If you really cannot turn to close family or friends because they are unable or unwilling to become involved in your care, there are agencies dedicated to providing for such situations. Through your local social services department's "adult protective services" program or Family

Service Association, you should be able to locate a "case manager" who will be able to organize the resources in your community to provide the help you need. The social services department in your local hospital can also put you in touch with the right agency.

Making tough decisions and preparing for possible health care needs in advance is hard work, but it can relieve a great deal of worry about the future. There are other times in life when emotions are very high. We'll talk about some of those times next.

Grieving: A Normal Reaction to Bad News

When people experience any kind of a loss—small ones (such as losing one's car keys) or big ones (such as losing a life partner or facing a disabling or terminal illness)—we go through an emotional process of grieving and coming to terms with the loss. A person with a chronic, disabling health problem experiences a variety of losses. These include loss of confidence, loss of self-esteem, loss of independence, loss of a known and cherished lifestyle, and perhaps the most painful of all, loss of a positive self-image if the condition has an effect on appearance. Psychiatrist Elisabeth Kübler-Ross, who has written extensively about this process, describes the stages of grief:

- **Shock,** when a person feels both a mental and a physical reaction to the initial recognition of the loss.

- **Denial,** when the person thinks, "No, it can't be true," and proceeds to act for a time as if it were not true.

- **Anger,** when the person fumes "Why me?" and searches for someone or something to

blame (if the doctor had diagnosed it earlier, the job caused me too much stress, etc.).

- **Bargaining,** when the person promises, "I'll never smoke again," or "I'll follow my treatment regimen absolutely to the letter," or "I'll go to church every Sunday, if only I can get over this."

- **Depression,** when awareness sets in, and the person confronts the truth about the situation and experiences deep feelings of sadness and hopelessness.

- **Acceptance,** when the person recognizes that they must deal with what has happened and make up their minds to do what they have to do.

People do not pass through these stages in a straight line or one step after another. You are more apt to flip-flop between them. Don't be discouraged if you find yourself angry or depressed again when you thought you had reached acceptance.

I'm Afraid of Death

Fear of death is something most of us begin to experience only when something happens to bring us face-to-face with the possibility of our own death. Losing someone close, having an accident that might have been fatal, or learning we have a health condition that may shorten our lives usually causes us to consider the inevitability of our own eventual passing. Many people, even then, try to avoid facing the future because they are afraid to think about it.

Our attitudes about death are shaped by our own central attitudes about life. This is the product of our culture, our family's influences, perhaps our religion, and certainly our life experiences.

If you are ready to think about your own future—about the near or distant prospect that your life will most certainly end at some time—then the ideas that follow will be useful to you. If you are not ready to think about it just yet, put this aside and come back to it later.

The most useful way to come to terms with your eventual death is to take positive steps to prepare for it. This means to get your house in order by attending to all the necessary details, large and small. If you continue to avoid dealing with these details, you will create problems for yourself and for those involved with your situation.

There are several components to getting your affairs in order, including the following:

- **Decide and then convey to others your wishes** about how and where you want to be during your last days and hours. Do you want to be in a hospital or at home? When do you want procedures to prolong your life stopped? At what point do you want to let nature take its course when it is determined that death is inevitable? Who should be with you—only the few people who are nearest and dearest, or all the people you care about and want to see one last time?

- **Make a will.** Even if your estate is a small one, you may have definite preferences about who should inherit what. If you have a large estate, the tax implications of a proper will may be significant. A will ensures that your assets and belongings go where you would like them to go. Without a will, some distant or "long lost" relative may end up with your estate.

- **Plan your funeral.** Write down your wishes or actually make arrangements for your funeral and burial. Your grieving loved ones will be very relieved not to have to decide what you would want and how much to spend. Prepaid funeral plans are available, and you can purchase your burial space in the location and of the type you prefer.

- **Draw up a durable power of attorney** for health care and also one for managing your financial affairs. (These are discussed later in this chapter.) You should also discuss your wishes with your personal physician, even if they don't seem interested. (Your physician may also have trouble facing the prospect of losing you.) Have some kind of document or notation included in your medical records that indicates your wishes in case you can't communicate them when the time comes.

Be sure that the persons you want to handle things after your death are aware of your wishes, your plans and arrangements, and the location of necessary documents. You will need to talk to them, or at least prepare a detailed letter of instructions and give it to someone who can be counted on to deliver it to the proper person at the appropriate time. This should be a person close enough to you to know when that time is at hand. You may not want your partner or spouse to have to take on these responsibilities, for example, but your partner or spouse may be the best person to keep your letter and know when to give it to your designated agent.

You can purchase at any well-stocked stationery store a kit in which you place a copy of your will, your durable powers of attorney, important papers, and information about your financial and personal affairs. Another useful source to help organize this information is "My Life in a Box," which is noted in the reading and resources lists at the end of this chapter. It contains forms that you fill out about bank and charge accounts, insurance policies, the location of important documents, the location of your safe deposit box and its key, and so on. This is a handy, concise way of getting everything together that anyone might need to know about. Some people keep these documents on computers. If this is the case, be sure others will be able to find your passwords and accounts when the time comes.

Finish your dealings with the world around you. Mend your relationships. Pay your debts, both financial and personal. Say what needs to be said to those who need to hear it. Do what needs to be done. Forgive yourself. Forgive others.

Talk about your feelings about your death. Most family and close friends are reluctant to initiate such a conversation but will appreciate it if you bring it up. You may find that there is much to say to and to hear from your loved ones. If you find that they are unwilling to listen to you talk about your death and the feelings that you are experiencing, find someone who will be comfortable and empathetic in listening to you. Your family and friends may be able to listen to you later. Remember, those who love you will go through the stages of grieving themselves when they have to think about the prospect of losing you.

A large component in the fear of death is fear of the unknown: "What will it be like?" "Will it be painful?" "What will happen to me after I die?" Most people who die of a disease are ready to die when the time comes. Painkillers and the disease process itself weaken body and mind, and the awareness of self diminishes without the realization that this is happening. Most people just "slip away," with the transition between the state of living and that of no longer living hardly identifiable. Reports from people who have been brought back to life after being in a state of clinical death indicate they experienced a sense of peacefulness and clarity and were not frightened.

A dying person may sometimes feel lonely and abandoned. Regrettably, many people cannot deal with their own emotions when they are around people they know to be dying and so deliberately avoid their company, or visitors may engage in superficial chitchat, broken by long, awkward silences. This is often puzzling and hurtful to those who are dying, who need companionship and solace from the people they counted on.

You can help by telling your family and friends what you want and need from them—attention, entertainment, comfort, practical help, and so on. Again, a person who has something positive to do is more able to cope with difficult emotions. If you can engage your family and loved ones in specific activities, they can feel needed and can relate to you around the activity. This will give you something to talk about, to occupy time, or at least provide a definition of the situation for them and for you.

Palliative Care and Hospice Care

In most parts of the United States, as well as in many other parts of the world, both palliative care and hospice care are available. In everyone's life there comes a time when regular curative medical care is no longer helpful and we need to prepare for death. This preparation means that medical and other care is aimed at making the patient as comfortable as possible and providing a good quality of life for their remaining days. Recent research has shown that at least for some diseases, people who receive hospice care actually live longer than those who receive more aggressive treatment.

Palliative care is a medical specialty that improves the quality of life of patients and their families facing a serious illness through the prevention and relief of symptoms. It can be helpful for anyone with a serious condition or who is facing a life-limiting illness, such as cancer. Palliative care services are provided during any stage of disease, including at the onset of diagnosis and throughout treatment.

Palliative care is different than hospice care. The goal of hospice care is to provide the terminally ill patient (someone who is expected to die within months) with the highest quality of life possible. Hospice professionals help both the patient and the family prepare for death with dignity and also help the surviving family members. Today, most hospices are "in-home" programs. This means that patients stay in their own homes and the services come to them. In some places there are also residential hospices where people can go for their last days.

One of the problems with hospice care is that often people wait until the last few days before death to ask for it. They somehow see asking for hospice care as "giving up." By refusing hospice care, they often put an unnecessary burden on themselves, friends, and family. On the other hand, some families say they can cope without help. This may be true, but the patient's life and dying may be much better if hospice takes care of all the medical needs and frees up family and friends to give love and support.

Most hospices only accept people who are expected to die within six months. This does not mean that you will be thrown out if you live longer. It is important that you recognize that if you, a family member, or a friend is in the end stage of illness, you should find and make use of your local hospice. It is a wonderful final gift.

Making Your Wishes Legal: Advance Directives

There are legal documents you can prepare that will make the difficult decisions ahead easier for your family, friends, and health care professionals. Collectively, these documents are referred to as advance health care directives. Everyone, including people who do not have a chronic illness, should think ahead about what might happen in case of accidents or other events. But many people do not have advance directives. Some of these documents don't require an attorney, but seeking legal advice is worthwhile. Many people fear that going to a lawyer will be very expensive. That is not always the case. Many lawyers offer a free initial meeting to discuss your needs and the price of each service. The cost of having a lawyer prepare the documents that we discuss in this section is relatively inexpensive. This is a task that is easy to put off. Resist this temptation and do it now.

Please note that the material in this section is not complete. To learn more about the details of these processes, you should seek legal counsel. In addition, the laws of each state are different. The topics that we discuss below are just the basics to prepare you for a deeper discussion.

Anyone, young or old, could find themselves in a position to need an advance directive. Even if you have don't have HIV, accidents and sudden illness happen. Everyone should have one of these documents, including all those you care about.

Durable Power of Attorney (DPA)

A general durable power of attorney, sometimes shortened to DPA, is a document in which one person (you) assigns another person (usually a family member or friend) as their "attorney in fact." This is the legal authority to act on your behalf when you cannot. The authority can be limited to something specific such as selling the house or using a specific bank account, or it can be general. DPAs can be changed any time you wish, and you should review them on a regular basis to make sure they continue to state your wishes. There is a separate power of attorney for health care, which we will discuss shortly.

A general power of attorney gives the designated person the power to make all legal decisions, including handling all the money. There are two types of general powers of attorney: a *durable* power of attorney and a *simple* power of attorney. A simple power of attorney is valid only as long as the person signing the document is able to understand its meaning. A durable power of attorney, on the other hand, continues to be valid even if the person signing no longer can think or act for themselves or understands the document.

There are also two types of durable powers of attorney. Both types are valid if the person cannot act on their own behalf. The difference between these DPAs is when they take effect.

1. One is legal when it is signed and stays legal if the person becomes completely incapacitated.

2. The second type is legal only when the person is incapacitated.

A DPA can help you avoid the need for a conservator. Conservatorship involves a court hearing where one person, the "conservatee," is found to be unable to handle their own affairs, and another person, the "conservator" (caregiver or some other person), is appointed to handle these affairs. This is expensive and usually means going to court many times.

A DPA is not usually used for medical care decisions. For this there is another document called the advance health care directive, which we will talk about next.

Advance Health Care Directive

An advance health care directive helps you keep control over medical care when you are not able or competent to express your wishes. There are two types of this directive: living will, and power of attorney for health care. Both directives express your wishes about the health care you do or do not want when you are unable to express those wishes yourself.

Living Wills

A living will is not the same document as a last will and testament. A living will only applies to end of life medical care, and it does not appoint anyone to act on your behalf. It is a document that you prepare for your doctor that states what types of medical care you do and do not wish when you have reached the end of life. You should supply a copy and discuss your living will with your doctor and family, and make sure hospitals have a copy if you are admitted to one. You do not need a living will if you have a power of attorney for health care.

Power of Attorney for Health Care

The power of attorney for health care, sometimes known as a health care proxy, is not the same as the plain power of attorney that we dis-

cussed earlier. The power of attorney for health care *only* applies to health care decisions. It gives a person (called an agent or proxy) the right to make health care decisions for you. For example, you may become the agent for a friend or family member, and a family member or friend could become your agent.

Note that it is especially important to have an advance health care directive if you wish to choose your nonlegal partner or someone who is not a blood relative as your agent. Otherwise, it's possible that your medical decisions will end up being made by a family member who may be unaware of or disagree with your wishes. In the material that follows, we discuss some things to think about as you prepare a power of attorney for health care.

Choosing a Health Care Agent

Begin by deciding whom you want as your agent. The person can be a friend or family member, but it cannot be the physician who is providing your care. The following are some things to think about as you choose your agent:

- First, the person should be available in the geographic area where you live. If the agent is not available to make decisions for you, they are not much help. Just to be on the safe side, you can also name a backup agent who will act on your behalf if your first-choice agent is not available.

- Second, you must be sure that this person shares your values or at least is willing to carry out your wishes.

- Third, the person must be someone who you feel would be able to carry out your wishes. Sometimes a partner or child is not

Your Health Care Agent

Look for these characteristics in a health care agent:

- Someone who is available if called upon to act on your behalf
- Someone who understands your wishes and is willing to carry them out
- Someone who is emotionally prepared and able to carry out your wishes
- Someone who will not be emotionally burdened by carrying out your wishes

the best agent because this person is too close to you emotionally. For example, if you do not wish to be resuscitated while in a severe coma, your agent has to be able to tell the doctor not to resuscitate. This decision could be difficult or impossible for a family member or partner to make. Be sure the person you choose as your agent is up to such a task.

- Finally, you want your agent to be someone who will not find this job too much of an emotional burden. The person has to be comfortable with the role, and willing and able to carry out your wishes.

Finding the right agent is a very important task. You may want to talk to several people before making your choice; these may be the most important interviews you ever conduct. We talk more about discussing your wishes with family, friends, and your doctor later in this chapter.

Your Wishes Concerning Medical Treatment

The other major decision you need to make has to do with the kind of medical care you would like, and under what circumstances. In other words, what are your directions to your agent?

Some power of attorney for health care forms give you several statements to choose from, or leave a space in which you can write your own statement. The following are some sample statements:

- I do *not* want my life to be prolonged and I do *not* want life-sustaining treatment to be provided or continued if:

  (1) I am in an irreversible coma or persistent vegetative state;

  (2) I am terminally ill and the application of life-sustaining procedures would serve only to artificially delay the moment of my death; or

  (3) under any other circumstances where the burdens of treatment outweigh the expected benefits. I want my agent to consider the relief of suffering and the quality and extent or possible extension of my life in making decisions concerning life-sustaining treatment.

- I want my life to be prolonged and I want life-sustaining treatment to be provided *unless I am in a coma or vegetative state* that my doctor reasonably believes to be irreversible. Once my doctor has reasonably concluded that I will remain unconscious for the rest of my life, I do *not* want life-sustaining treatment to be provided or continued.

■ I want my life to be prolonged to the greatest extent possible without regard to my condition, my chances for recovery, or the cost of the procedures.

Some of these forms simply make a "general statement of authority granted," in which you give your agent full power to make decisions. You do not write out the details of these decisions; you simply trust your agent to follow your wishes. Because these wishes are not explicitly written, it is very important that you discuss them in detail with your agent.

Forms for advance health care directives are easy to find. You can get them from your health care provider, hospital, senior or community center, or on the Internet. You do not need a lawyer to complete an advance health care directive; you just need to have it witnessed. Get the appropriate forms for your state by asking your doctor or lawyer or by contacting CaringInfo, a program of the National Hospice and Palliative Care Organization (see "Additional Resources" at the end of this chapter).

Other Statements of Desires, Special Provisions, or Limitations

All power of attorney for health care forms have a space in which you can write out specific wishes that either limit or add to the authority you have given your agent. You are not required to give specific details but may wish to. Knowing what details to write is a little complicated because you do not know the exact circumstances in which the agent will have to act. However, you

can get some idea by asking your doctor about what they think are the things most likely to happen to someone with your condition. Then you can direct your agent how to act in those situations. Your directions can cover outcomes, specific circumstances, or both. If you discuss outcomes, the statement should focus on which types of outcomes would be acceptable and which would not—for example, "Resuscitate if I can continue to fully function mentally."

Two of the more common circumstances encountered by people with HIV are HIV- or AIDS-associated dementia and poor lung function. There are decisions you may want to make about each of these circumstances:

■ HIV-associated dementia is a disease that can leave you with little or no mental function. In spite of this, it is generally not life threatening, at least not for a long time. It can be prevented or delayed by consistently taking your HIV medications. However, people with HIV-associated dementia may be vulnerable to other ailments that can become life threatening, such as pneumonia, meningitis, and wasting. You need to decide how much treatment you would want if you were to have HIV dementia complex. For example, would you want antibiotics if you got pneumonia? Would you want to be resuscitated if you died in your sleep? Would you like a feeding tube if you become unable to feed yourself? Remember, it is your choice how to answer each of these questions. You may not want to be resuscitated, but you may want a feeding tube. You may want to use all means to sustain life, or you may not want any special means to sustain life.

■ You may have very poor lung function that will not improve. Should you be unable to breathe on your own, would you want to be placed in an intensive care unit on mechanical ventilation (a breathing machine)? Remember, this is a situation that will not improve. To say that you never want ventilation is very different from saying that you don't want it if it is used to sustain life when no improvement is likely. Obviously, mechanical ventilation can be lifesaving in crises such as a severe asthma attack, when it is used for a short time while the body regains normal function. Here the issue is not whether to use mechanical ventilation *ever*, but rather when—under what circumstances—you wish it to be used.

These examples give you some idea of the directions to give in your durable power of attorney for health care. Again, to better understand how to write such directions and how to personalize them to your own condition, talk with your physician about the most common problems and decisions for people like you.

In summary, there are several decisions you need to make when directing your agent how to act on your behalf:

■ Generally, *how much treatment do you want?* This can range from the very aggressive—that is, doing many things to sustain life—to the very conservative, doing almost nothing to sustain life, except to keep you clean and comfortable.

■ Given the types of life-threatening things likely to happen to people with your condition, *what sorts of treatment do you want and under what conditions?*

■ If you become *mentally incapacitated*, what sorts of treatment do you want for *other illnesses*, such as pneumonia?

Many people get this far. That is, they have thought through their wishes about dying and have even written them down in a power of attorney for health care. This is an excellent beginning, but it's not the end of the job. A good self-manager has to do more than just write a memo. They have to see that the memo gets delivered. If you really want your wishes carried out, you must share them fully with your agent, your family, and your doctor. This is often not an easy task. In the following pages, we discuss ways to make these conversations easier.

Talking with Your Family, Friends, and Your Agent

Before you can discuss your wishes with family, friends, and agent, all interested parties need to have copies of your power of attorney for health care. Once you have completed the documents, have them witnessed and signed. In some states, they may also need to be notarized. Make several copies. Besides one for yourself, you need copies for your agent, family members, and your doctor and hospital. You may also want to give one to your lawyer.

Once everyone has their copy of your advance health care directive, you are ready to talk about your wishes. Nobody likes to discuss their own death, or that of a loved one. Therefore when you bring up this subject, do not be surprised if the response is, "Oh, don't think about that," or "That's a long time off," or "Don't be so morbid, you're not that sick." This is usually enough to end the conversation, but don't let it end there.

Your job as a self-manager is to keep the conversation open. Here are some suggestions to begin your discussion of this subject:

- Once you have prepared your durable power of attorney for health care and given copies to the appropriate friends or family members, *ask them to read it and then set a specific time to discuss it.* If they give you one of those responses mentioned above, tell them that you understand this is a difficult topic, but insist that it is important to you to discuss it with them. This is a good time to practice the "I" messages discussed in Chapter 16, "Communicating with Family, Friends, and Everyone Else." Practice a simple image like this one: "I understand that death is a difficult thing to talk about. However, it is very important to me that we have this discussion."

- Get blank copies of the form for those who are close to you and suggest that you each *fill one out and share them with each other.* Present this task as an important aspect of being a mature adult or family member. Making this a group project involving everyone may make it easier to discuss. And it will help to clarify everyone's values about the topics of death and dying.

- If the first two suggestions seem too difficult or are for some reason impossible to carry out, *write a letter* or *prepare a recording* to send to the people closest to you or members of your family. In the letter or recording, state why you feel your death is an important topic to discuss and tell them that you want them to know your wishes.

Then state your wishes, providing reasons for your choices. At the same time you share the letter or recording, send each person a copy of your directive. Ask that they each respond to the material you have sent in some way or set aside some time to talk in person or on the phone.

Talking with Your Doctor

From our research, we have learned that, in general, people have a much more difficult time talking to their doctors about their wishes surrounding death than to their families. In fact, only a very small percentage of people who have health care directives ever share them with their physicians. There are several reasons why it is important that such a discussion take place. First, you need to *be sure that your doctor has values that are compatible with your wishes.* If you and your doctor do not have the same values, it may be difficult for the doctor to carry out your wishes. Second, *your doctor needs to know what you want.* This allows your physician to take appropriate actions, such as writing orders to resuscitate or not to use mechanical resuscitation should this be needed. Third, *your doctor needs to know who your agent is and how to contact this person.* If an important decision has to be made and your wishes are to be followed, the doctor must talk with your agent. It is important to give your doctor a copy of your durable power of attorney for health care so that it can become a permanent part of your medical record.

As surprising as it may seem, many physicians also find it difficult to discuss death and how death may occur with their patients. After all, they are in the business of helping to keep people alive and well. They don't like to think about their patients dying. On the other hand, most doctors want their patients to have durable powers of attorney for health care because this relieves the pressure they feel about end-of-life issues and their worry.

If you wish, *plan a time with your doctor when you can discuss your wishes*. This should not be a side conversation at the end of a regular visit. Rather, start a visit by saying, "I want a few minutes to discuss my wishes about what should happen in the event of a serious problem or my impending death." When you put it this way, most doctors will make time to talk with you. If the doctor says that they do not have enough time, ask when you can make another appointment to talk about it. This is a situation in which you may need to be a little assertive. Sometimes a doctor, like your family members or friends, may say, "Oh, you don't have to worry about that, let me do it," or "We'll worry about that when the time comes." Similarly, you have to take the initiative, using an "I" message to communicate that this is important to you and that you do not want to put off the discussion.

Sometimes doctors do not want to worry you. They think they are doing you a favor by not describing all the unpleasant things that may happen to you, or the potential treatments, in the case of serious problems. You can help your doctors by letting them know that having control and making some decisions about your future will ease your mind. Tell your doctor that not knowing or not being clear on what will happen is more worrisome than being faced with the facts, unpleasant as they may be, and dealing with them.

Even if you are aware of all the information we have just discussed, it can still be difficult sometimes to talk with your doctor. Therefore, it may be helpful to *bring your agent with you* when you have this discussion. The agent can facilitate the discussion and, at the same time, meet your doctor. This way, everyone has a chance to clarify any misunderstandings about your wishes. It opens the lines of communication so that if your agent and physician have to act to carry out your wishes, they can do so with few problems.

Making your wishes known about how you want to be treated in case of a serious or life-threatening illness is one of the most important tasks of self-management. The best way to do this is to prepare an advance directive and share it with your family, close friends, and physician.

Once you have taken care of your advance directives, you have done all the important things. You can rest easy. The hard work is over. However, remember that you can still change your mind at any time. Your agent may no longer be available, or your wishes may change. Be sure to keep your durable power of attorney for health care updated. Like any legal document, you can revoke or change it at any time.

Storing Your Advance Health Care Directives

It is important to have copies of your health care directive where they can easily be found. If the paramedics are called to your home, they will want to know your wishes, as well as your medical particulars (medications, medical conditions, etc.). One idea is to put the information in your freezer or refrigerator with a sign on the refrigerator door that says "emergency information inside." You can also get "My Life in a Box," which stores all the important information you would need in case of an emergency, including natural disasters. *Never* put your advance health care directive in your safe deposit box. If the bank is closed, no one can get to it in an emergency!

Additional Resources

AARP, Advance Directives: www.aarp.org/relationships/caregiving/info-03-2012/free-printable-advance-directives.html

Aging with Dignity, Five Wishes: www.agingwithdignity.org

AIDS.gov: https://aids.gov

Benefits Check Up: www.benefitscheckup.org

Center for HIV Law and Policy: www.hivlawandpolicy.org

The Conversation Project: www.theconversationproject.org

Greater Than AIDS: www.greaterthan.org/about

Growth House—Improving Care for the Dying: www.growthhouse.org

Integrating Palliative Care Into HIV Services: A Practical Toolkit for Implementers: www.fhi360.org/sites/default/files/media/documents/Integrating%20Palliative%20Care%20into%20HIV%20Services%20Toolkit.pdf

Lambda Legal, Long-Term Care and People Living with HIV: www.lambdalegal.org/sites/default/files/publications/downloads/fs_long-term-care-and-people-living-with-hiv_1.pdf

LeadingAge: www.leadingage.org

My Life in a Box: A Life Organizer: www.mylifeinabox.com

National Council on Aging: www.ncoa.org

National Hospice and Palliative Care Organization: www.caringinfo.org or 1-800-658-8898

National Resource Center on Psychiatric Advance Directives: www.nrc-pad.org

Suggested Further Reading

To learn more about the topics discussed in this chapter, we suggest that you explore the following resources:

Doukas, David John, and William Reichel. *Planning for Uncertainty: Living Wills and Other Advance Directives for You and Your Family*, 2nd ed. Baltimore: Johns Hopkins University Press, 2007.

Gawunde, Atul. *Being Mortal: Medicine and What Matters in the End*. New York: Henry Holt, 2014.

Kübler-Ross, Elisabeth. *On Death and Dying: What the Dying Have to Teach Doctors, Nurses, Clergy, and Their Own Families*. New York: Scribner, 2014.

Long, Laurie Ecklund. *My Life in a Box—A Life Organizer: How to Build an Emergency Tool Box*, 4th ed. Fresno, Calif.: AGL, 2010.

Merlin, Jessica S., Rodney O. Tucker, Michael S. Saag, and Peter A. Selwyn. "The Role of Palliative Care in the Current HIV Treatment Era in Developed Countries." *Topics in Antiviral Medicine*, vol. 21, no. 1 (February-March 2013): 20–26, www.iasusa.org/sites/default/files/tam/21-1-20.pdf.

Schwalbe, Will. *The End of Your Life Book Club*. New York: Vintage, 2013.

Speerstra, Karen, and Herbert Anderson. *The Divine Art of Dying*. Studio City, Calif.: Divine Arts, 2014.

CHAPTER 18

Finding Resources

A MAJOR PART OF BECOMING A SELF-MANAGER is knowing when you need help and how to find it. When you seek help, you are not a victim of your condition; you are a good self-manager. Start by evaluating your condition—figure out what you can do and what you want to do. You may find that there is a difference between what you can do and what you want to do (or have done). If so, it may be time to get help so that you have more time and energy to do the things that are most important to you.

When most people begin to look for help, they start by asking family or friends. Sometimes this can be difficult. You may be afraid that others will see you as weak or needy. Sometimes your pride may get in the way. The truth is that most people want to be helpful but do not know how. Your job is to tell them what you need. Finding the right words to ask for help is discussed in Chapter 16, "Communicating with Family, Friends, and Everyone Else."

Unfortunately, some people either do not have family or close friends or cannot bring themselves to ask. Sometimes family or friends cannot offer all the help that is needed. Thankfully, you have another wonderful resource at your disposal: your community.

Finding Clues and Networking

Finding resources can be a little like hunting for treasure. As in a treasure hunt, creative thinking is the key to success. Finding what you need may be as simple as looking up phone numbers and making a couple of calls or using the Internet. Other times, finding help may take some detective work. The community resource detective must find clues and follow them. Sometimes this involves starting over when a clue leads to a dead end.

The first step is defining the problem and deciding what you want. For example, suppose you love to cook but are finding it difficult to prepare meals because standing for a long time is too tiring or painful. After some thought, you decide that you really want to continue cooking for yourself rather than have someone else prepare meals for you. You realize that you could cook comfortably if you were able to sit while cooking. The goal of your treasure hunt is figuring out how to do this.

You look at kitchen stools and do not think this solution will work to prevent your discomfort, so you decide that you need to redesign the kitchen. Now the hunt is on. Where can you find an architect or contractor who has experience in kitchen alterations for people with physical limitations? You need a starting point for your treasure hunt. The newspaper and Yelp (the online directory) have pages of ads and listings for architects and contractors. Some advertisers say they specialize in kitchens. None of the ads mention designing to accommodate physical limitations. So you call and ask.

After calling a few contractors, you come to realize that none are experienced in kitchens for the physically limited. Next you return to the Internet and broaden your search beyond just Yelp. You find a company that seems to be just what you need, but it is located more than 200 miles away.

Now what? You have a couple of choices. You can contact all the general renovation businesses listed for your area until you find what you need. This could be time consuming. And that won't be the end of your hunt because even if you find someone suitable, you would still have to check references.

Who else might have the information you need? Maybe someone who works with people with physical disabilities would know. This opens a long list of possibilities: occupational and physical therapists, medical supply stores, the local Center for Independent Living, and voluntary organizations such as AIDS Action. You decide to start by asking your friend Hank, who is a physical therapist.

He does not have the answer but says, "Gosh, Jack So-and-So just had his kitchen remodeled to accommodate a wheelchair." This is an excellent tip. Jack will almost certainly be able to give you the name of the person who apparently does the kind of work you are seeking. Jack can also probably give you some ideas about the cost and hassle before you go any further.

Unfortunately, though, this lead turns out to be not much help because the contractor is booked too far in advance to be of use to you. Now what?

There are people in every community who are natural resources. These "natural connectors" seem to know everyone and everything about their community. They tend to be folks who have lived a long time in the community and have been closely involved in it. They are also natural problem solvers. The natural connector is the one who other people turn to for advice. This person always seems to be helpful. The connector could be a friend, a business associate, another person with HIV, the mail carrier, your physician, your pet's veterinarian, the checker at the corner grocery, the pharmacist, a bus or taxi driver, the school secretary, a real estate agent, the chamber of commerce receptionist, or the librarian.

Think of this person as an information resource. Sometimes the natural connector will taste the thrill of the hunt and, like a modern-day Sherlock Holmes, announce that "the game is afoot!" and promptly join you in your search.

Say the person who fills this role in your community is Michelle, the mail carrier. One day, you are home when the mail is delivered and you tell Michelle about your search. She tells you about a contractor whose wife uses a wheelchair. Michelle knows this because the contractor just did a great job on a kitchen on her postal route. You call the contractor and find everything you need. From the conversation, you learn that some very simple adjustments can be made to your existing kitchen to keep you cooking, which is great news!

Let's review the take-away lessons from this example. The most important steps in finding the resources you need are these:

1. Identify the problem.

2. Identify what you want or need to solve the problem.

3. Look at resources such as the newspaper and the Internet.

4. Ask friends, family, people at your clinic, others living with HIV, and neighbors for ideas.

5. Contact organizations that might deal with similar issues.

6. Identify and ask "natural connectors" in your community.

One last note: the best sleuth follows several clues at the same time. This will save you lots of time and shorten the hunt. Once you get good at thinking about community resources creatively, you may even become a natural connector in your own right, and then you will have to find time in your schedule to help others who seek your advice!

Getting Started: Resources for Resources

When you need to find goods or services, there are certain go-to resources you may think to call on first. One resource often leads to another. The community resource "detective's kit" should include a variety of useful tools.

The phone book and Internet search engines are the most frequently used tools. These are particularly helpful if you are looking for someone to hire. For most searches, this is where to start. In the material that follows, we describe some additional places to look for resources.

Organizations and Referral Services

Almost all communities have one or more information and referral service. Sometimes these are related to a geographic area such as a city or county. Other times they are specific to an age group, such as the Area Agency on Aging, or are specific to a condition such as HIV. There are several types of agencies that operate these services. Search under "United Way Information and Referral," "Senior Information and Referral" (or "Area Agency on Aging" or "Council on Aging"), and "information and referral." If you are using a phone book, be sure to check your county or city government listings. Once you have an information and referral telephone number, your searches will become much easier. These services maintain huge files of referral addresses and telephone numbers for just about any help you might need. Even if they don't have the answer, they will almost always be able to refer you to another agency that might.

HIV service organizations are excellent resources. The national organizations maintain telephone hotlines that offer information about all kinds of resources in your community. In addition, local HIV organizations often publish resource guides and provide information about local services.

As people with HIV grow older and find that they have other chronic conditions as well, agencies such as the American Heart Association, American Diabetes Association, and the American Cancer Society become useful resources. Organizations like these exist in most countries. Funded by contributions from individuals and corporate sponsors, these agencies provide up-to-date information about specific health problems, as well as support services for people with the illness. They also fund research intended to help people live better with their illness and to someday lead to a cure. For a small fee, you can become a member of one of these organizations. This entitles you to receive regular bulletins by mail or e-mail. You do not, however, have to be a member to qualify for their services; the organizations exist to serve you. Many of these organizations have wonderful websites, allowing a person living in, say, rural North Dakota to access help from AIDS organizations in Victoria, Australia.

Other organizations in your community offer information and referral services along with direct services. These include the local chapter of AARP (formerly known as the American Association of Retired Persons), senior centers, community centers, and religious social service agencies. These organizations provide information, classes, recreational opportunities, nutrition programs, legal and tax help, and social programs. There is probably such a community or senior center close to you. Your city government office or local librarian knows where to find such resources, and the calendar section of your newspaper usually publishes information about programs these organizations offer.

Most religious groups offer information and social services to persons who need it, either directly through the place of worship or through organizations such as the Council of Churches, Catholic Charities or the local diocese, Jewish Family Service, or Muslim Social Services. To get help from religious organizations, start with the local place of worship, which can help you directly or refer you to someone who can help you. You usually need not be a member of the congregation or even of the religion to receive help.

Another option is to call your local hospital, clinic, or health insurance plan and ask for the social service department. Doctors are also aware of the physical and mental health services available in the health care organizations they are affiliated with.

Libraries

Your public library is a particularly good resource if you are looking for information about HIV or some other chronic condition. Even if you think you are an excellent library detective, it's a good idea to ask the reference librarian to make sure you haven't overlooked something. These people see volumes of material cross their desks constantly and are knowledgeable about the

community (they're probably among the ranks of the local natural connectors). Even if you cannot get to the library, you can call or e-mail. Libraries are no longer just collections of books.

In addition to city or county libraries, there are other, more specialized health libraries. Ask your information and referral service if there is a health library in your community. Such libraries specialize in health-related resources and usually have a computerized database search service available along with the usual print, audiotape, and videotape materials. Nonprofit organizations and hospitals usually maintain health libraries,which sometimes charge a small fee for use.

Universities and colleges also have libraries available to the public. By law, the regional "government documents" sections of these libraries must be open to the public at no charge. Government publications exist on just about any subject, and the health-related publications are particularly extensive. These publications represent "your tax dollars at work." You can find everything from information on organic gardening to detailed nutritional recipes. The librarians are usually very helpful.

If you are fortunate enough to have a medical school in your community, you may be able to use its medical library. This is a place to go for information rather than to look for help with tasks. Naturally, you can expect to find a great deal of information about disease and treatment at a medical library. Use medical libraries with care, though. Unless you have special knowledge about medicine, the detailed information you find in a medical library can be confusing and even frightening.

Books

Books can be useful—indeed, you are reading a book now! Many books about diseases and other health topics contain reading and resource lists, either at the ends of chapters or at the back of the book. These lists can be very helpful. Because research in the field of HIV is rapidly changing, it is important to check the publication date of the book (usually located in front, on the copyright page). Try to find HIV books published in the last five years in order to ensure that you have the most recent, relevant information.

Newspapers and Magazines

Your local newspaper, especially if you live in a smaller community, can be an excellent resource. Be sure to look in the calendar of events. Even if you are not interested in a particular featured event, calling the contact telephone number or visiting the website may help you find what you are looking for if the event is about the same topic. (Don't overlook weekly "alternative" newspapers in your community, which often contain extensive calendars of events.) Look for news stories that might also be of interest, especially the pages around the calendar section. For example, if you are looking for an exercise program for people with your health problem, look in the sports and fitness section.

Sometimes you can find clues in the classified section. Look under "announcements," "health," or any other heading that seems promising. Review the index of classified headings, which is usually printed at the front of the section near the rate information, to see which headings your newspaper uses.

There are a variety of general health magazines that can be useful, as well as some publications focusing on specific conditions, including HIV. POZ is a magazine for people living with HIV; you can order it online or you may be able to read a copy in your doctor's office.

The Internet

Today most people have access to the Internet. Even if you are not an Internet user yourself, you most likely know a number of people who are. If you do not have a computer, you can use one in your local library or ask a friend for help. Most people can also access the Internet with their smartphones or other electronic devices.

The Internet is the fastest-growing source of information today. Information is being added every second of every day. The Internet offers information about health and anything else you can imagine. It also provides several ways to interact with people all over the world. For example, someone who is receiving treatment for both HIV and hepatitis C might find it difficult to find others living locally with both diseases. The Internet can put the person in touch with a whole group of such people; it doesn't matter whether they are across the street or on the other side of the world.

The good thing about the Internet is that anyone can maintain a website, a Facebook or other social network page, a blog, or a discussion group. That is also the bad thing about the Internet. There are virtually no controls over who is posting information or whether the information is accurate or even safe. This means that although there is a lot of information out there that is very useful, you will also probably encounter incorrect or even dangerous information. You should never assume that information found on the Internet is entirely trustworthy. Approach information obtained online with skepticism and caution. Ask yourself: Is the author or sponsor of the site clearly identified? Is the author or source reputable? Is the information contrary to what other reliable sources are saying about the subject? Does common sense support the information? What is the purpose of the site? Is someone trying to sell you something or win you over to a particular point of view?

One way to start analyzing the purpose of a website is to look at the URL (the site's "address" on the Internet, located in a bar at the top of the page and usually starting with http:// or www). The URL will usually look something like this:

http://patienteducation.stanford.edu

At the end of the main part of a U.S.–based website's URL, you will most commonly see .edu, .org, .gov, or .com. This will give you a clue about the nature of the organization that owns the site. A college or university site ends with .edu, nonprofit organizations use .org, a governmental agency site ends in .gov, and commercial websites end in .com.

As a general rule of thumb, .edu, .org, and .gov are fairly trustworthy sites, although a nonprofit organization can be formed to promote just about anything. A site that has a URL that ends with .com is trying to sell you a product or service or is selling advertising space on its site to others trying to sell you something. This doesn't mean that a commercial website can't be a good one. On the contrary, there are many outstanding commercial sites dedicated to providing high-quality, trustworthy information. They are often able to cover the costs of providing this service only by selling advertising or by accepting grants from commercial firms. For example, The Body (www.thebody.com) is an excellent resource for people with HIV. We list the URLs for some of our favorite reliable websites at the end of this chapter.

Social Networking Sites

Social networking sites and blogs are exploding on the Internet. Sites such as Facebook, Twitter, Instagram, and Blogspot are currently very popular, but things move quickly online so everything may change by the time this book is published. These sites enable the average person to communicate easily with others who want to listen (or read). Some sites, such as Facebook, require that users determine who is allowed to read what they post on their page. Others, such as Blogspot, are more like personal journals that are open to anyone.

Many such sites have been started by people living with particular health conditions such as HIV, and the authors are eager to share their experiences. Some have discussion forums associated with them. The information and support offered can be valuable, but be cautious: some sites may propose unproven and dangerous ideas.

Discussion Groups on the Internet

Yahoo, Google, and other websites offer discussion groups for just about anything you can imagine. Anyone can start a discussion group about any subject. Groups are run by the people who start them. For any one health problem, you can typically find dozens of discussion groups. You can join them and the discussions if you wish, or just "lurk" (read without interacting). For people with HIV and hepatitis, for example, a discussion group may allow them to connect to people who share their experiences, or even their specific hepatitis C "genotype" (genotype is the exact strain of hepatitis C the person has). This may be some people's only opportunity to talk with others who share their specific conditions. For people with HIV, it may be difficult to talk with others face-to-face about health problems. To find discussion groups, go to the Google or Yahoo (or other) home page and search for a link to "groups."

Keep in mind that the Internet changes by the second. Our guidelines reflect conditions at the time this book was written. Things may have changed by the time you read this.

Becoming an effective resource detective is one of the jobs of a good self-manager. We hope that this chapter has given you some ideas about the process of finding resources in your community. Knowing how to search for resources will serve you better than being handed a list of resource agencies. If you find resources that you think we should add to future editions, kindly send them to us at self-management@stanford.edu. Thank you!

Additional Resources

AIDS Community Research Initiative of America (ACRIA): www.ageisnotacondom.org

AIDS Educator: www.aidseducator.org

AIDS hotlines (by state, including Spanish and deaf services): www.aids.org/topics/aids-factsheets/aids-hotlines

AIDS Info: www.aidsinfo.nih.gov

AIDS InfoNet: www.aidsinfonet.org

AIDS.gov: www.aids.gov

AIDS.org—Information, Education, Action: www.aids.org

AIDSmap: www.aidsmap.com

AIDSmeds: www.aidsmeds.com

Association of Cancer Online Resources (ACOR): www.acor.org

AVERTing HIV and AIDS: www.avert.org

The Body—The Complete HIV/AIDS Resource: www.thebody.com

CarePages: www.carepages.com

CaringBridge: www.caringbridge.org

Center for Advancing Health: www.cfah.org

Centers for Disease Control and Prevention (CDC): www.cdc.gov

Gay Men's Health Crisis (GMHC): www.gmhc.org or 1-800-243-7692

Global Network of People Living with HIV: www.gnpplus.net

Health Resources and Services Administration, HIV/AIDS Programs: www.hab.hrsa.gov

HealthCentral: www.healthcentral.com

HIV and Hepatitis: www.hivandhepatitis.com

HIVInSite: www.hivinsite.ucsf.edu

Mayo Clinic: www.mayoclinic.org

MedlinePlus, Evaluating Health Information: www.nlm.nih.gov/medlineplus/evaluatinghealthinformation.html

Memorial Sloan-Kettering Cancer Center: www.mskcc.org

More ▶

National Association of People with HIV Australia: www.napwha.org.au

National Cancer Institute: www.cancer.gov

National Institutes of Health (NIH): www.nih.gov

National Prevention Information Network (NPIN): https://npin.cdc.gov

Planned Parenthood: www.plannedparenthood.org/learn/stds-hiv-safer-sex/hiv-aids

Positively Aware—The HIV Treatment Journal of TPAN: www.positivelyaware.com

POZ—Health, Life, and HIV: www.poz.com

PrEP Watch: www.prepwatch.org

Project Inform: www.projectinform.org

Psych Central: www.psychcentral.com

QuackWatch: Your Guide to Quackery, Health Fraud, and Intelligent Decisions: www.quackwatch.org

U.S. Department of Health and Human Services (HHS): www.healthfinder.gov

U.S. Department of Veterans Affairs: www.hiv.va.gov/patient

U.S. National Library of Medicine: www.nlm.nih.gov

WebMD: www.webmd.com

The Well Project: www.thewellproject.org

World Health Organization (WHO): www.who.int/hiv/en

Index

Note: Page numbers followed by *b*, *f*, or *t* indicate a box, figure, or table, respectively